THE TAI CHI CLASS

by Richard Morley

CONTENTS

Acknowledgements 5

Introduction.. 6

Chapter One : The History of the Tai Chi Form 8

Chapter Two : Characteristics of the Style.................................... 9

Chapter Three : Tai Chi Chuan Body Principles 10

Chapter Four : Glossary of Tai Chi Terminology 12

Chapter Five : Tai Chi hand shapes 16

Chapter Six : Tai Chi Stances for the legs 18

Bow Stance 18

Cat Stance 19

Parallel Bow Stance.. 20

Single Legged Stances 21

Stepping Sideways 22

Chapter Seven : Tai Chi Movement Exercises 24

Exercise One 23

Exercise Two 27

Exercise Three 29

Exercise Four 31

Exercise Five 33

Exercise Six 35

Exercise Seven 37

Exercise Eight 39

Exercise Nine 41

Exercise Ten 43

Exercise Eleven 45

Exercise Twelve 47

Exercise Thirteen 49

Chapter Eight : Meditation 51

How to Meditate.. 52

Chapter Nine : Standing Post 53

Chapter Ten : The form movements decoded 54

Wu Ji 54

Commencement 55

Heaven and Earth 56

Ward Off Left 57

Ward Off Right 58

Rollback 60

Press 62

Single Whip 64

Lift Hands/Play Guitar 66

Pluck 67

Elbow/Shoulder Stroke 68

White Crane Spreads its Wings 69

Brush Knee and Push 70

Parry and Punch 71

Apparent Close Up 72

Seal the Knot 73

Fist Under Elbow 74

Repulse Monkeys 75

Diagonal Flying 77

Wave Hands Like Clouds 79

Snake Creeps Down 81

Golden Phoenix Stands on Left and Right Legs 83

Separate and Kick with Right Foot and Left Foot 85

Turn and Kick with Heel 87

Punch to Groin 89

Fair Lady Works at Shuttles 91

Step Up to Seven Stars 93

Step back and Ride the Tiger 95

Turn and Sweep Lotus with Leg 96

Bend Bow to Shoot the Tiger 97

Chapter Eleven : The 37 Step Tai Chi Form Movements 98

Chapter Twelve : The 37 Step Tai Chi Form with instructions 100

Commencement 101

1) Heaven and Earth 102

2) Ward Off Left 104

3) Grasp the Sparrows Tail. 105

4) Single Whip 110

5) Lift Hands 116

6) Pluck, elbow, shoulder stroke 117

7) White Crane Spreads its Wings 118

8) Brush Knee and Push 119

9) Play Guitar 120

10) Brush Knee Push 121

11) Parry and Punch 122

12) Seal the Knot 127

13) Carry Tiger Return to Mountain 128

14) Diagonal Single Whip 134

15) Fist Under Elbow. 139

16) Repulse Monkeys 140

17) Diagonal Flying 148

18) Wave Hands Like Clouds 151

19) Snake Creeps Down 158

20) Golden Phoenix Stands on the Left and Right Legs 164

21) Separate and Kick with Right and Left Foot 167

22) Turn and kick with Heel 175

23) Brush Knee and Push Right and Left 180

24) Brush Knee, Punch to Groin 181

25) Grasp the Sparrows Tail. 183

26) Single Whip 191

27) Fair Lady Works Shuttles x 4 196

28) Ward Off Left. 207

29) Grasp Sparrows Tail. Ward Off Right. 210

30) Single Whip 218

31) Snake Creeps Down 223

32) Step Up to Seven Stars 226

33) Retreat to Ride a Tiger 228

34) Turn and Sweep Lotus with Leg 230

35) Bend Bow to Shoot the Tiger 234

36) Deflect Parry and Punch 235

37) Seal the Knot 240

ACKNOWLEDGEMENTS

I want to say massive thank you to my Amazing Family, Shannon and Gabriel, you are Awesome.

Thank you to my Mum Susan for being my Mum.

Thanks to Dr Nibs, for his invaluable help in putting this Book together.

Thank you to my brother Fallon, who I shared so much Joy with.

Massive thanks to my Teachers, Colin and Gaynel Hamilton, without your kindness and sharing of Tai Chi Chuan with me, I would have nothing.

Thank you to my friend Mark Corcoran for sharing Yang Jian Hou's, Tai Chi Chuan with me.

Thanks to everyone else, you know who you are.

INTRODUCTION

I wrote this Book because I want you to enjoy a happier, healthier life through Tai Chi. I know from my own personal experience that Tai Chi really works; in fact, I regained my ruined health through training in this amazing art.

Before I began to practise Tai Chi, I suffered for almost fifteen years from Fibromyalgia, (its symptoms are fatigue, extreme pain, sleeplessness and more), and it ruined my life.

The Medical profession could do nothing for me but pump me full of drugs, which didn't work.

I searched desperately for help, I tried anything and everything in my quest to get well, Hypnosis, Vitamins, Reiki, Massage etc, but nothing worked.

A friend convinced me to try a class, with a Teacher of authentic Tai Chi and it worked like Magic, I went from depressed with deteriorating health, to healthy and feeling great in a very short time.

Since then, I have travelled the world and studied with famous Teachers and Masters of Tai Chi. I eventually went on to become an international level competition Judge, Teacher and gold medal winning Martial artist.

I have been fortunate enough to help thousands of other people to have better lives through my sharing of the art of Tai Chi with them.

Now modern scientific research has proven what I, my students and millions of people already know, that Tai Chi practice gives you robust health and well-being throughout your life.

In fact, Medical studies have proven that Tai Chi...

- Boosts your Immune system
- Helps you to beat Stress
- Reduces the effects of Depression
- Slows down Aging
- Reduces the effects of some illnesses

- Improves your posture
- Builds better Balance
- Improves your Circulation
- Reduces falls in older people
- Improves your Mental focus
- Increases your Bone density
- Lowers high Blood pressure
- Helps your concentration

During my deep research into Tai Chi, I read over 100 Books on the subject and found that while many of them purport to explain a Tai Chi form, the author generally goes into little detail, the explanation is unclear and the pictures are poor quality.

In writing this Book, I have tried to give you a clearer explanation of a Tai Chi form from start to finish, with many full colour pictures to help you in this process. I have also included everything else that you will need to succeed as a new student in my Tai Chi class.

Most people take up Tai Chi when they are ill, or are advanced in years, my advice to you is not to wait before learning Tai Chi, the best time to start is right now.

Follow the instructions in the Book, practise Tai Chi everyday and you too will enjoy the myriad benefits of this Wonderful art.

Rich

WWW.RichMorleyTaiChi.Com

Chapter One: The History of the Tai Chi Form

The style of Tai Chi that you are studying in this book is the simplified Thirty-Seven step Tai Chi form of Professor Cheng man Ch'ing.

(A Tai Chi form is the series of soft flowing movements that most people recognize as Tai Chi).

It is a shortened version of the traditional, Yang family, Tai Chi Chuan (Tai Chi Chuan, is Tai Chi's full title) long form that Professor Cheng Man Ch'ing learned from his teacher, Grandmaster Yang Chen Fu.

In 1938 when he was the director of the Henan Martial Arts academy Professor Cheng shortened the traditional long form and removed some of the more difficult movements. He did this because he wanted to help more people to enjoy the great health and wellbeing that Tai Chi gives to its practitioners.

Professor Cheng Man Ch'ing moved from China to Taiwan where he was one of the foremost teachers of Tai Chi Chuan for many years.

Eventually, Professor Cheng moved to New York City in the late nineteen sixties, where he taught Tai Chi at the United Nations and at his own school, which he called Shr Jung. He was one of the first Chinese Teachers to popularize Tai Chi in America, breaking with convention and teaching westerners for the first time.

His simplified version of Yang style Tai Chi is one of the most popular in the world today.

Chapter Two: Characteristics of the Style

Professor Cheng's version of Yang style Tai Chi Chuan emphasizes softness and relaxation, even more so than other styles of Tai Chi.

The movements of the form are medium sized and less complicated than other authentic styles of Tai Chi, therefore it is easier to learn and takes less time to practice.

Professor Cheng's version of Yang style Tai Chi Chuan emphasizes softness and relaxation the movements of the form are small or medium sized and less complicated than other authentic styles of Tai Chi.

For example the traditional Yang Long Form that Professor Cheng learned from his teacher, Grandmaster Master Yang Chen Fu, was a large frame form. It's movements are more complicated and the postures more open and expanded.

Even more so than other styles of Tai Chi, therefore it is easier to learn and takes less time to practice.

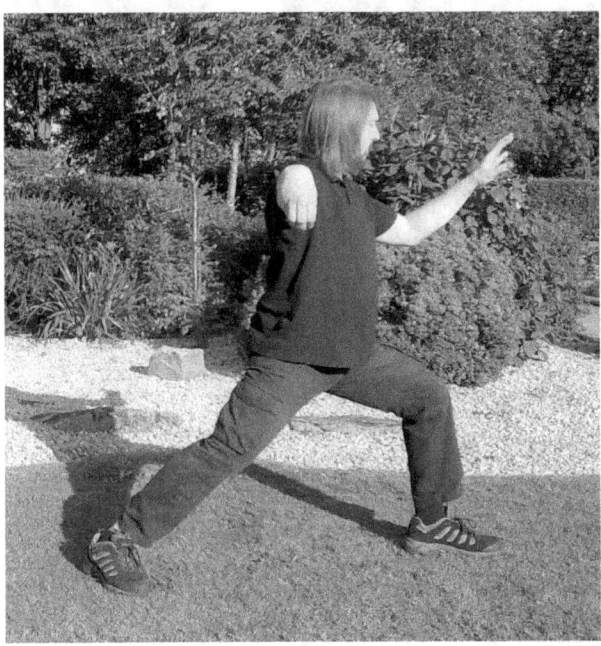 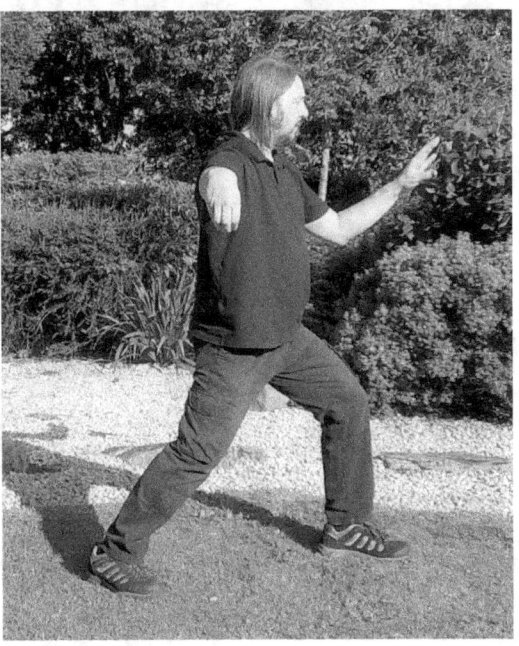

Traditional Yang Long Form, Single Whip   Cheng Man Ch'ing style, Small Frame, Single Whip

Chapter Three: Tai Chi Chuan Body Principles

To get the best results from your Tai Chi practice you need Tai Chi's body principles. You should focus on one body principle at a time when you practice, until they all become second nature to you.

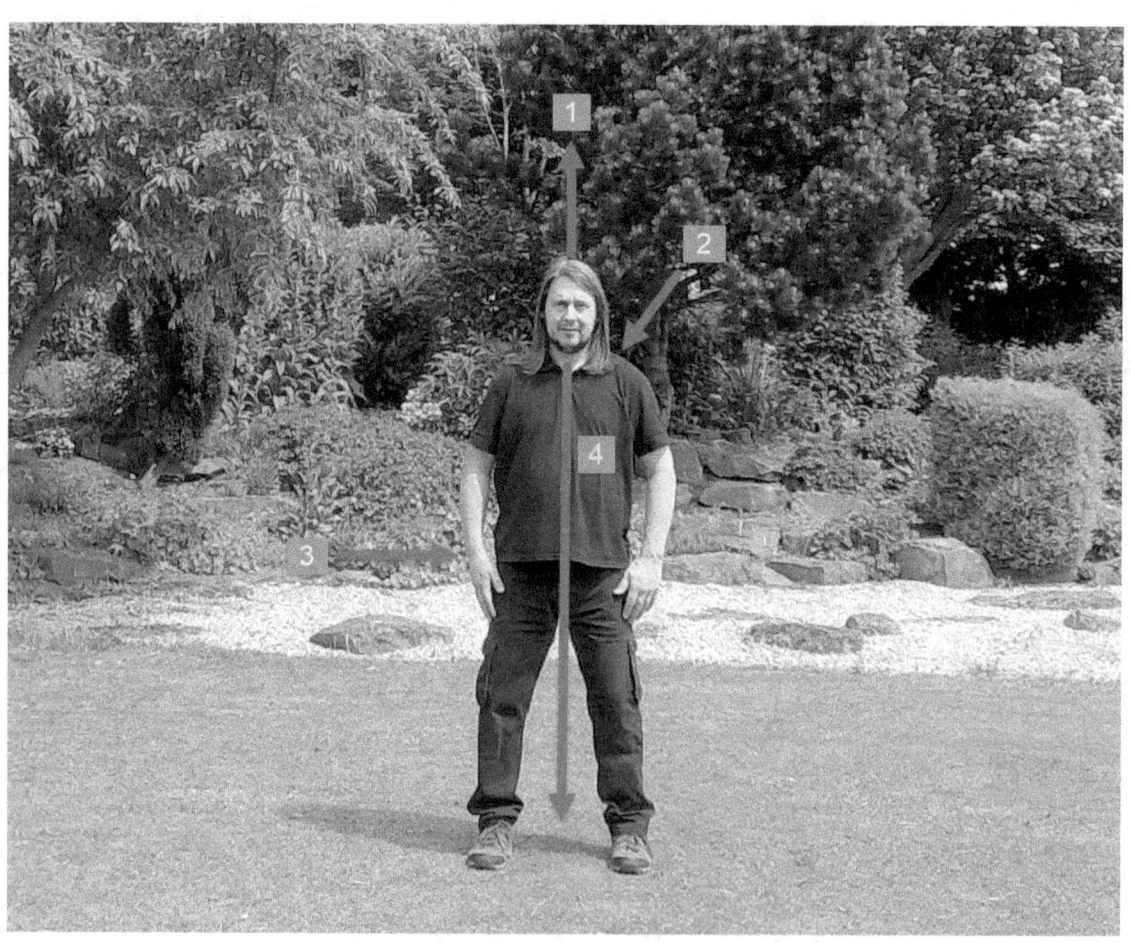

1) Suspend the Crown Point at the top of your head. You should feel as if your head is held up by a rope that is attached to the top most part of your head.

2) Relax your shoulders and let them sink down.

3) Sit down, as if you are sitting on a tall barstool. When you do this, your hips roll forward slightly, flattening out and opening the lower back. This helps you to have a better connection between the upper and lower body.

4) Relax your chest and belly.

Do not stick out your chest and do not let it collapse inward. Keep the chest neutral and relax your chest muscles. Relax the muscles of your lower abdomen so that the Chi can sink to your Dantien.

CHAPTER FOUR: GLOSSARY OF TAI CHI TERMINOLOGY

An: An is the downward energy of Tai Chi. It is one of the eight energies of Tai Chi Chuan and is part of the Grasp the Sparrows Tail sequence.

Bai Hui: The Crown Point is the topmost point of your head.

Bow Stance: The **Bow** stance in Yang Style Tai Chi is a shoulder\hip width posture. The front foot faces forward; the rear foot turns outward at forty-five degrees.

Bubbling Well Point: There is a bubbling well point in each foot. It is located roughly in the center of your foot, slightly behind the big and little ball of the foot. This is the point in the foot where energy enters and rises up through the legs.

Cat Stance: A Cat stance is a rear-weighted stance, with ninety percent of the weight in the back foot and ten percent in the front foot. The back foot is turned out at forty-five degrees, the front foot faces straight forward and the heels are in line. The front foot has the toes or heel lifted up, depending on the form movement.

Chi: Your Chi is the Life Force energy that powers you, in your body, you have pre natal Chi and post natal Chi. Pre-natal Chi comes from your parents and the universe. Post-natal Chi is gained from the air and from the food that you eat.

When you practice Tai Chi Chuan, it rebuilds your store of Pre-natal Chi, which otherwise will deplete throughout your life. Compare the vitality of a child to that of an older person.

Chi Hai: The Chi Hai is called, the "Sea of Chi", it is an important energy point, which is situated two inches below your naval.

Dantien: The lower abdominal area. This is the place where you gather and store your internal energy. Think of it as a reservoir that you fill up with energy.

Dong Jin: The term Dong Jin means being able to understand the information that you get from Ting Jin (Listening Energy) it means being able to understand energy. You gain such sensitivity that you can understand the opponent's movements and direction of force

Fa Jin: Fa Jin is the attacking energy of Tai Chi Chuan.

Fair Maidens Hand: This is the hand shape used in Cheng Man Ch'ing style Tai Chi. Your fingers are spread apart, curved, and relaxed. The palm shape is like a very shallow bowl. This hand shape helps you to relax the hand.

The Five Steps: Gaze left (Stepping to the left), Look right (Stepping to the right), Forward (Stepping forward), Backward (Stepping backward), Central equilibrium (Standing still).

Grasp Sparrows Tail: The series of postures that comprise Grasp the Sparrows Tail are, Ward Off, Roll Back, Press, and Push. These are the most important form movements in Yang Style Tai Chi.

Hu K'uo: The Tigers Mouth, this is the area between your index finger and thumb.

Hua Jin: Hua is used in Tai Chi Chuan to neutralize an opponent's force.

Ji: Ji means to press or squeeze, it is one of the eight energies of Tai Chi Chuan.

Jou: Elbow stroke: One of the eight energies of Tai Chi Chuan.

Kao: Shoulder stroke. One of the eight energies of Tai Chi Chuan

Kua: The Kua are the inguinal creases that run up the inside of your groin at the front from the base right up to the hip crest.

Li: Li is natural muscular power. (Brute strength)

Lieh: Split. Split is one of the eight energies of Tai Chi Chuan.

Lu: Lu is Rollback. This is one of the eight energies of Tai Chi Chuan.

Ming men: The Ming men is the "Gate of life point", it is situated between the kidneys on the spine.

Peng: Peng is pronounced "Pung" Peng is one of the eight energies of Tai Chi Chuan, it is the primary Tai Chi energy.

Pushing: Pushing Hands exercises are two person-training exercises to develop sensitivity and body skills.

Seated Wrist: The wrist sits down slightly.

Shen Fa: Body skills, skilful body movements.

Tai Chi Chuan: Supreme Ultimate Boxing, Tai Chi is the martial art that follows the principles of the Universe.

Ting Jin: The Listening energy of Tai Chi Chuan. Through sensitivity, you can feel the changes inside the opponent's body, you "hear" the direction and duration of his force.

Tsai: Pluck. This is one of the eight energies of Tai Chi Chuan.

Yi: Yi is your mental intention to do something. For example, you can think about closing your hand all day long and nothing will happen, until you have the intention for the hand to close, only then will it close.

Yin: Yin is the soft energy of Tai Chi Chuan. (Corresponding to the feminine)

Yang: Yang is the hard energy of Tai chi Chuan. (Corresponding to the masculine)

CHAPTER FIVE: TAI CHI HAND SHAPES

Three hand shapes are used in the Cheng man Ch'ing style of Tai Chi Chuan.

The Fair Maidens Hand: The fingers are spread slightly apart, gently curved, and relaxed. The palm shape is like a very shallow bowl.

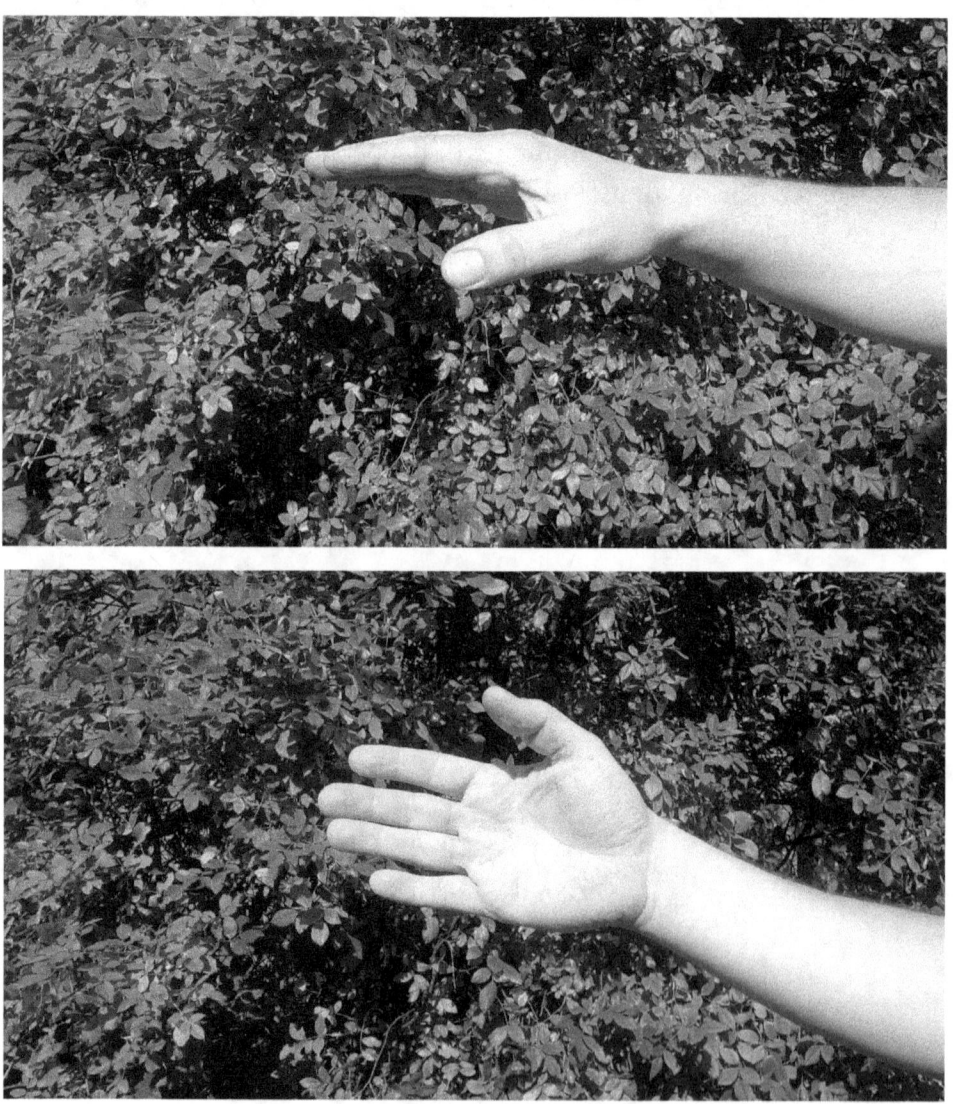

The Relaxed Fist: Make a soft fist, with a tiny space (This is called a Chi cavity) at its centre.

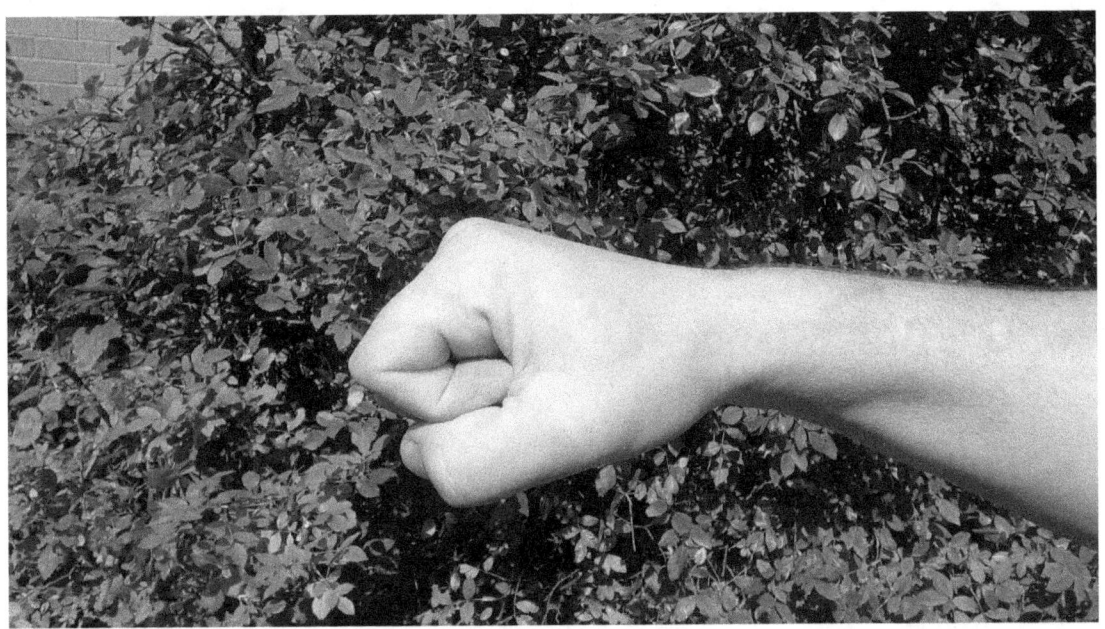

The Beak: Bend your wrist downward, point your thumb towards the floor and put the tips of your fingers around it to form a Beak shape.

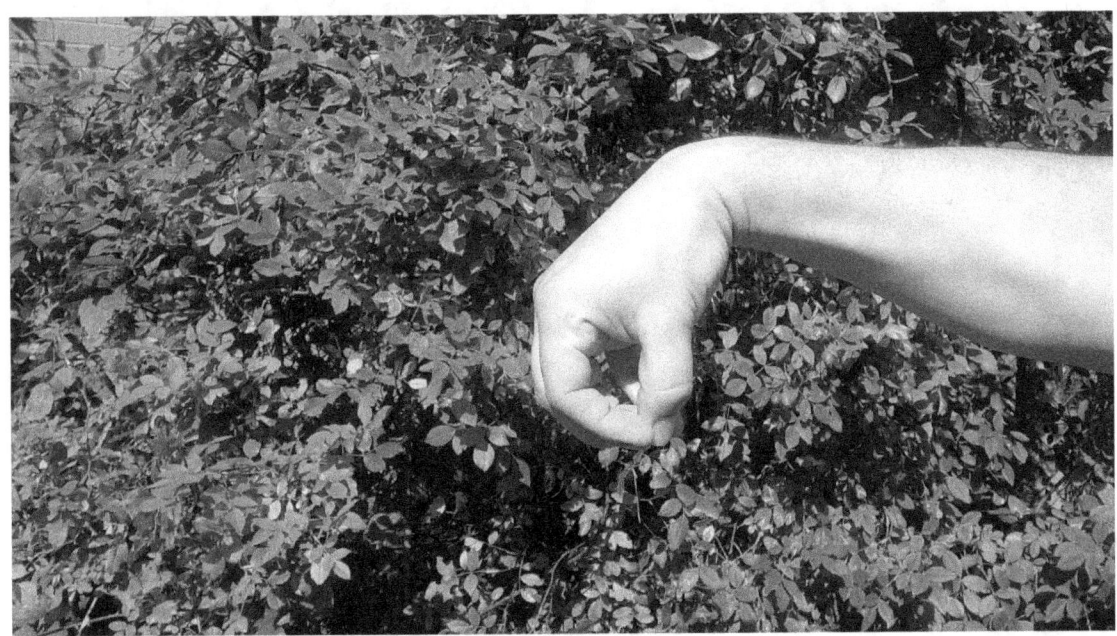

Chapter Six: Tai Chi Stances

There are five stances for your legs in Professor Cheng's style of Tai Chi,

- ## The Bow Stance

- ## The Cat Stance

- ## The Parallel Bow Stance

- ## The Single Legged Stance

- ## Stepping Sideways

Bow Stance

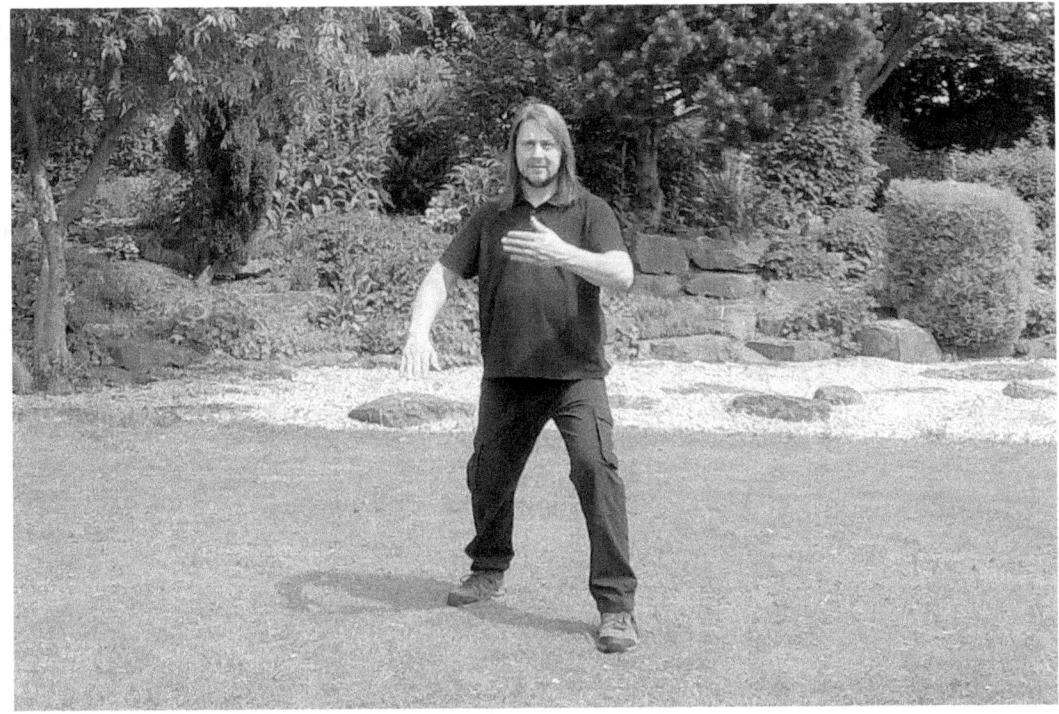

In a Bow stance, either the left or the right foot can be facing straight forward while the back foot turns outwards at a forty-five degree angle

There is a shoulder width space between your feet.

In a forward Bow stance, seventy percent of your weight is on the front leg. When stepping into a forward Bow stance, place the heel down first and roll the rest of the foot gradually down.

Cat Stance

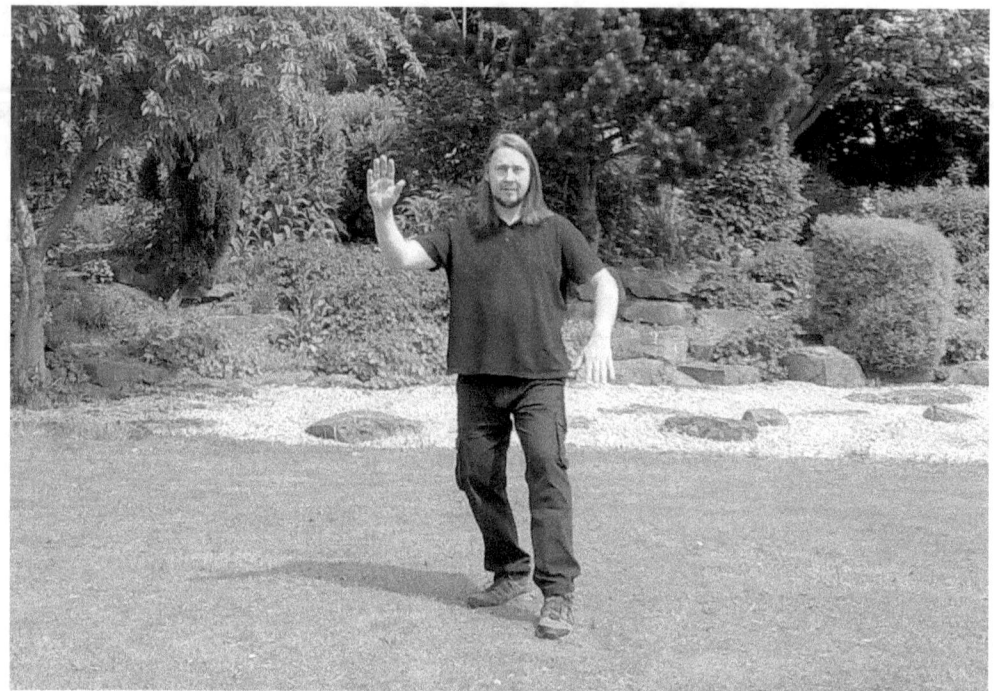

A Cat stance is a ninety to ten percent back weighted stance.

The right or left leg can be the supporting leg. (This depends on the Tai Chi form movement that you are performing)

The rear foot should be at forty-five degrees

The forward foot is square to the front; the heels are in line, or with a little width between them.

In a Cat stance the toes or heel of the front foot is raised, this depends on the posture.

e.g. White Crane Spreads its Wings is a heel raised, Cat stance. Whereas Play Guitar is a toes raised Cat stance.

Parallel Bow Stance

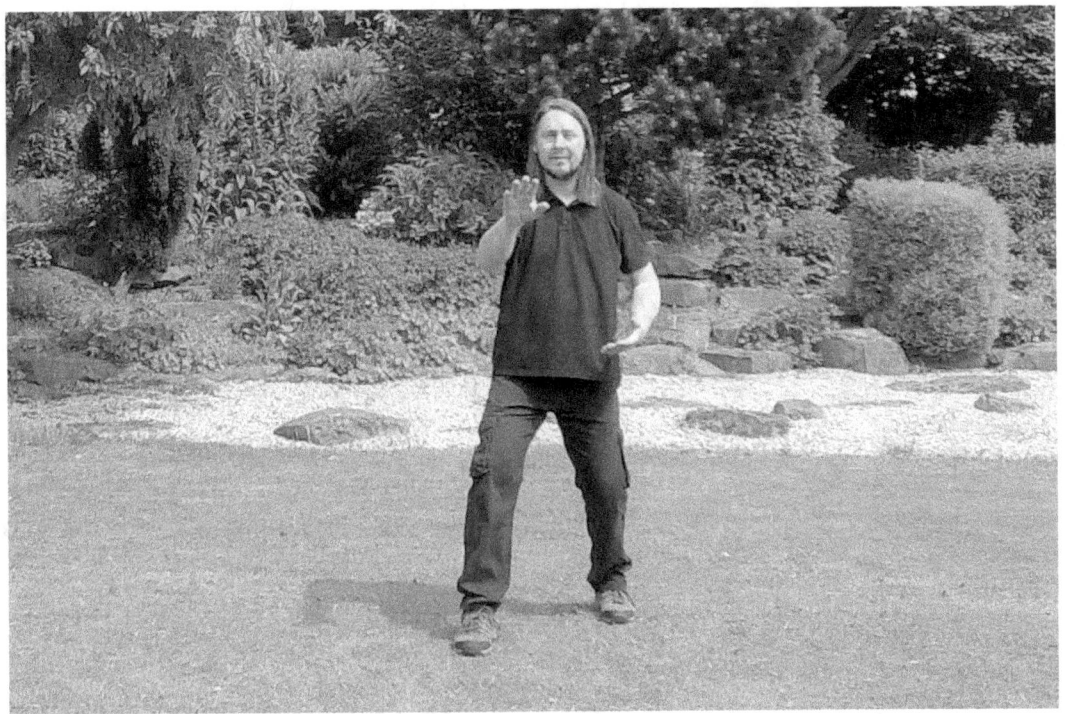

This is a shoulder width Bow stance with both of your feet facing forwards.

In this stance, you step backwards and place the toes down first, gradually rolling the rest of your foot down, and shifting your weight onto it.

The ending point of this posture is a seventy per cent back weighted stance.

This is way of stepping is only used when performing Repulse Monkeys in this style of Tai Chi Chuan.

Single Legged Stances

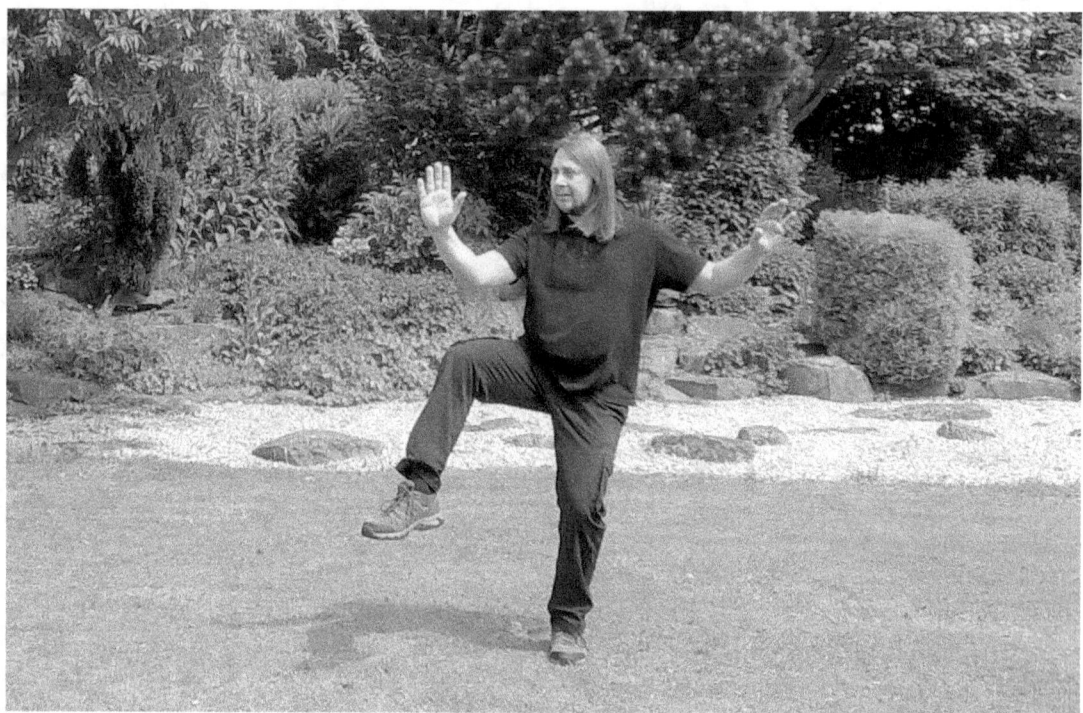

In the single legged stances, you stand with your weight fully on one leg. The foot of the supporting leg should be at forty-five degrees from square. You use this stance for Golden Phoenix Stands on One Leg or Separate and Kick with Heel.

Stepping Sideways

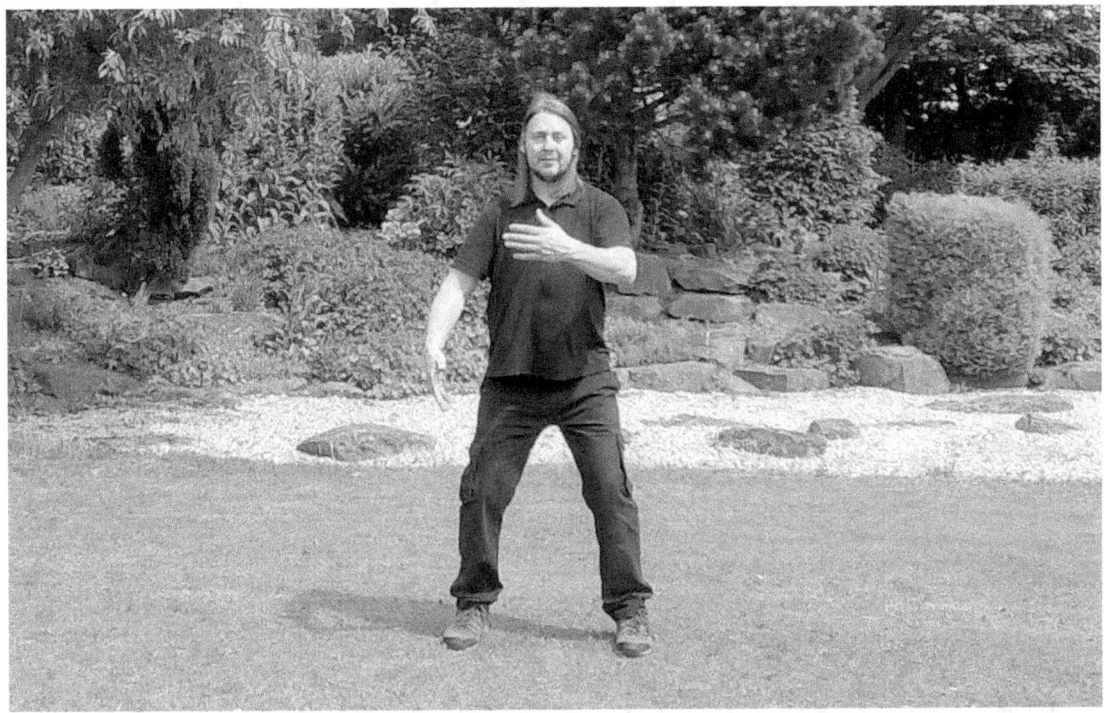

This is a parallel feet posture. The distance between your feet changes from full shoulder width, to half shoulder width as you step. You must roll the heel down first. Your weight shifts fully from one leg to the other as you turn your body from side to side.

You use this step when performing the movement called Waving Hands like Clouds.

CHAPTER SEVEN: TAI CHI MOVEMENT EXERCISES

Movement in Tai Chi Chuan is different to your normal daily way of moving, practise of these simple exercises will help you to develop correct Tai Chi movement.

Exercise One

 Stand in a shoulder width stance, with both feet facing straight forward. (Keep your nose, the centre of your chest and belly button aligned throughout this exercise).

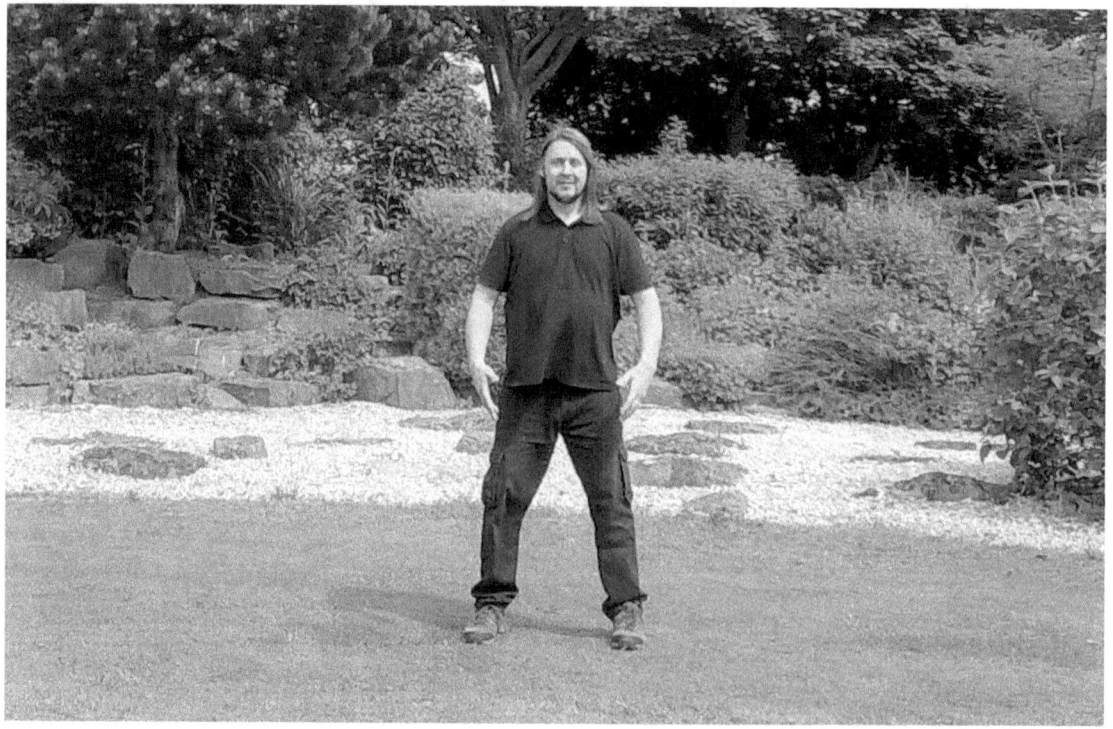

Turn your body to the left, hold the position for a count of five, and return to the forward position.

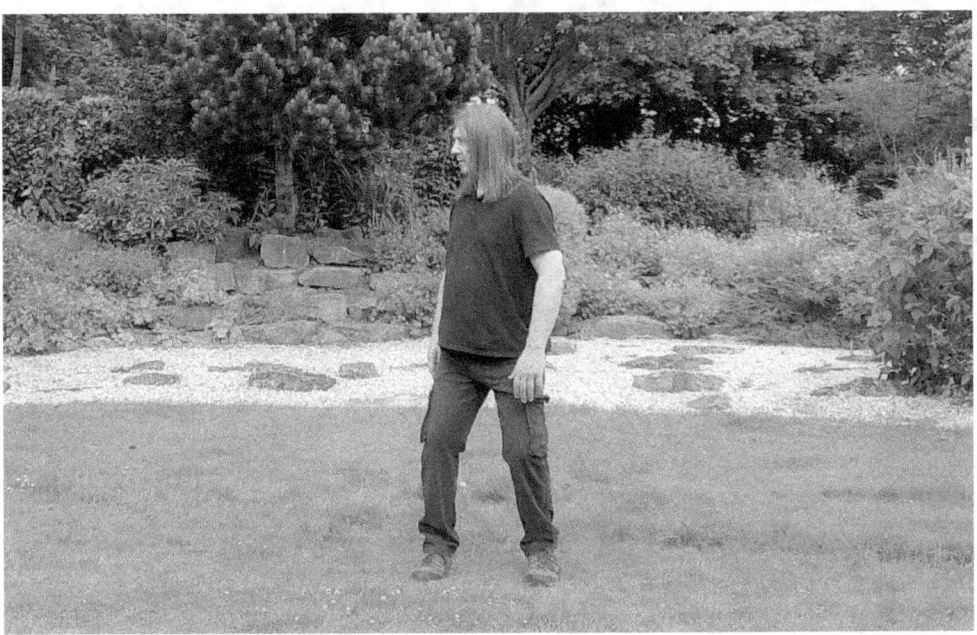

Next, turn to your right, hold the position for five seconds, and return to the forward position.

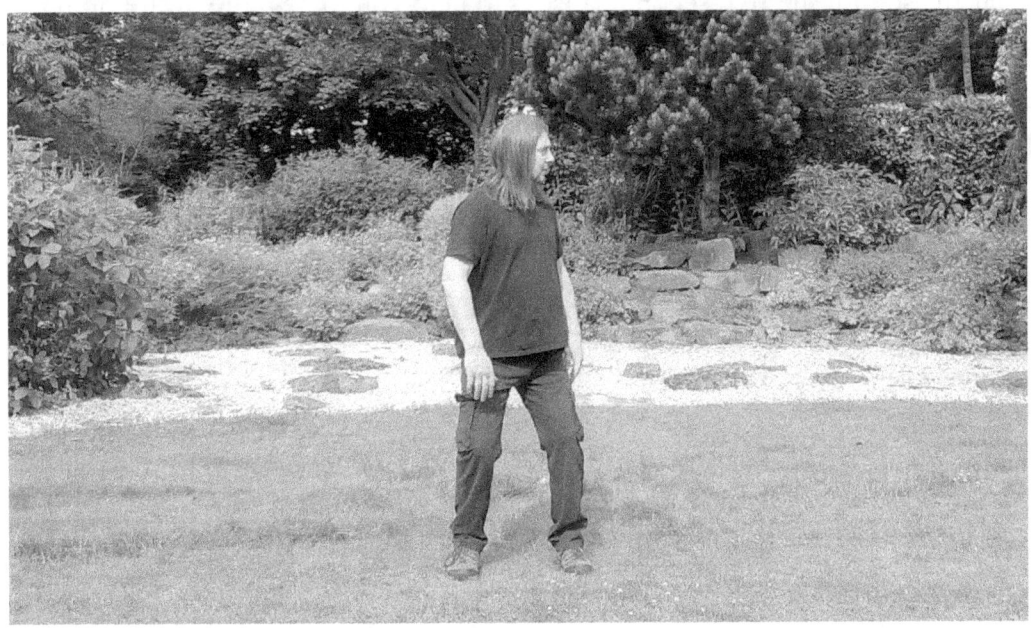

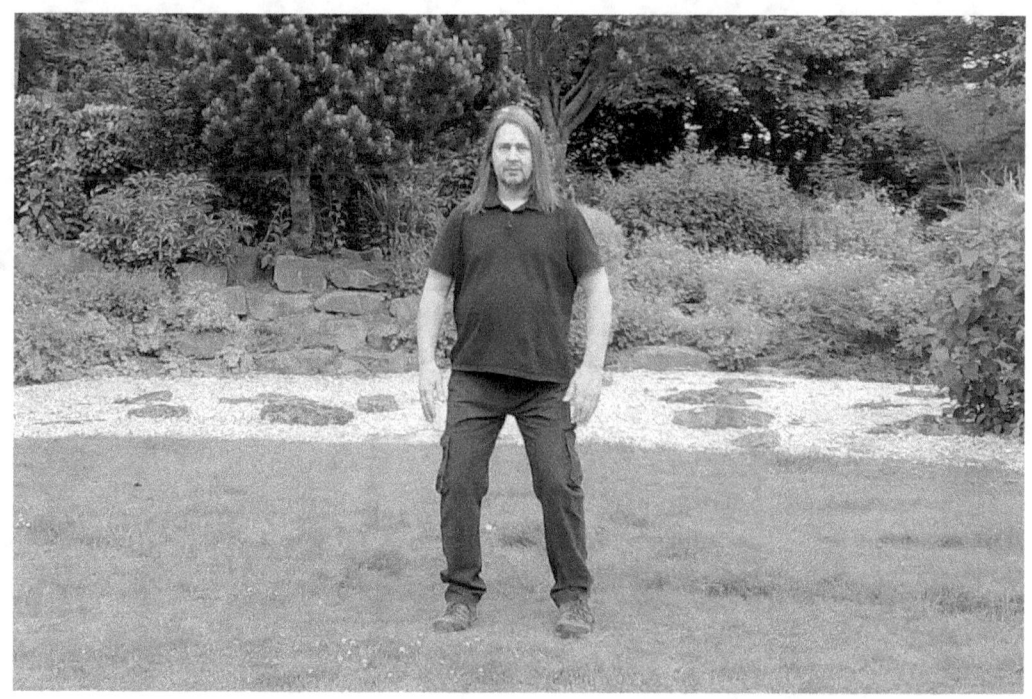

Note: The reason for the five-second pause is to help you to be more aware of the required alignments and to get the correct feeling into your muscle memory.

Repeat 20 times

Exercise Two

In this exercise, repeat the same movements as exercise one, but this time you turn from side to side with no pauses.

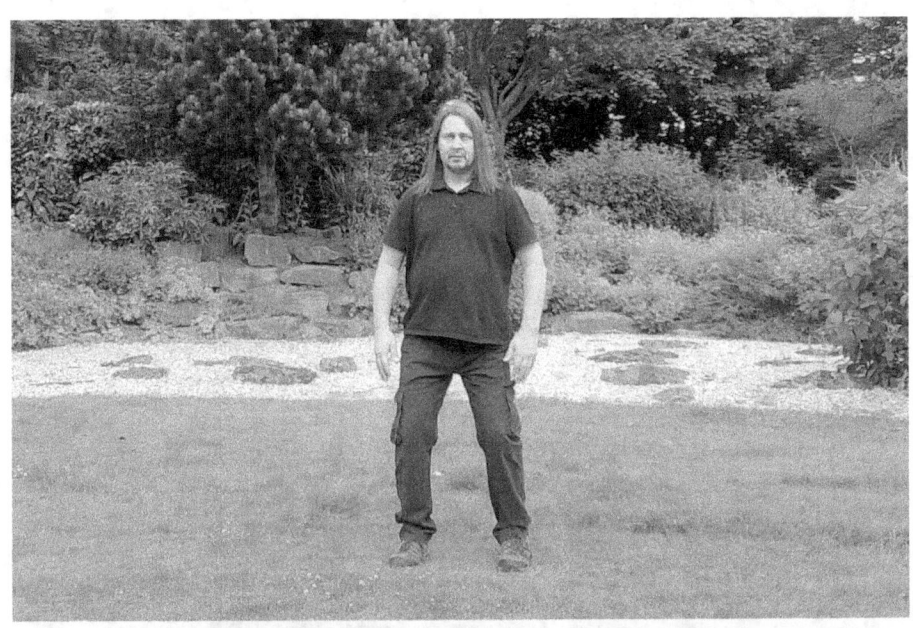

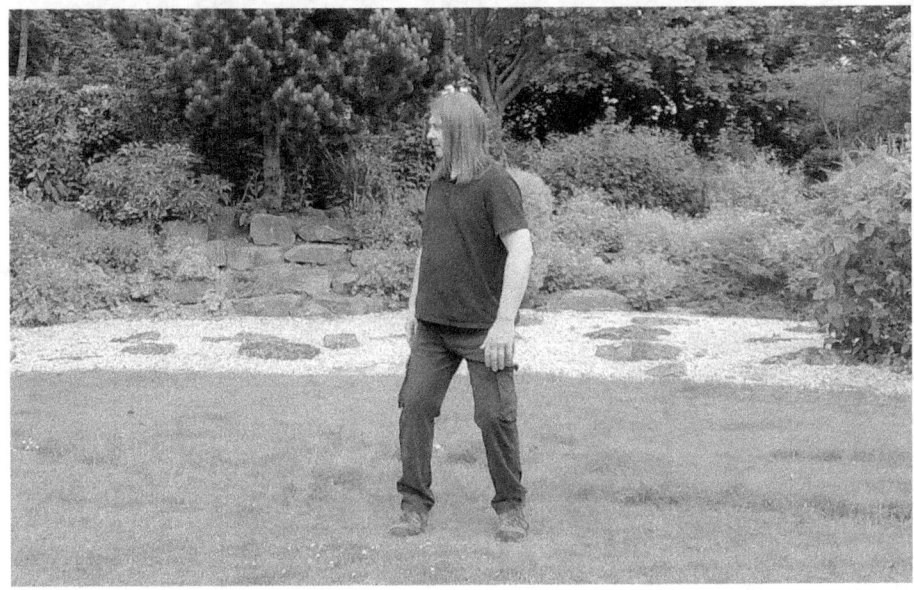

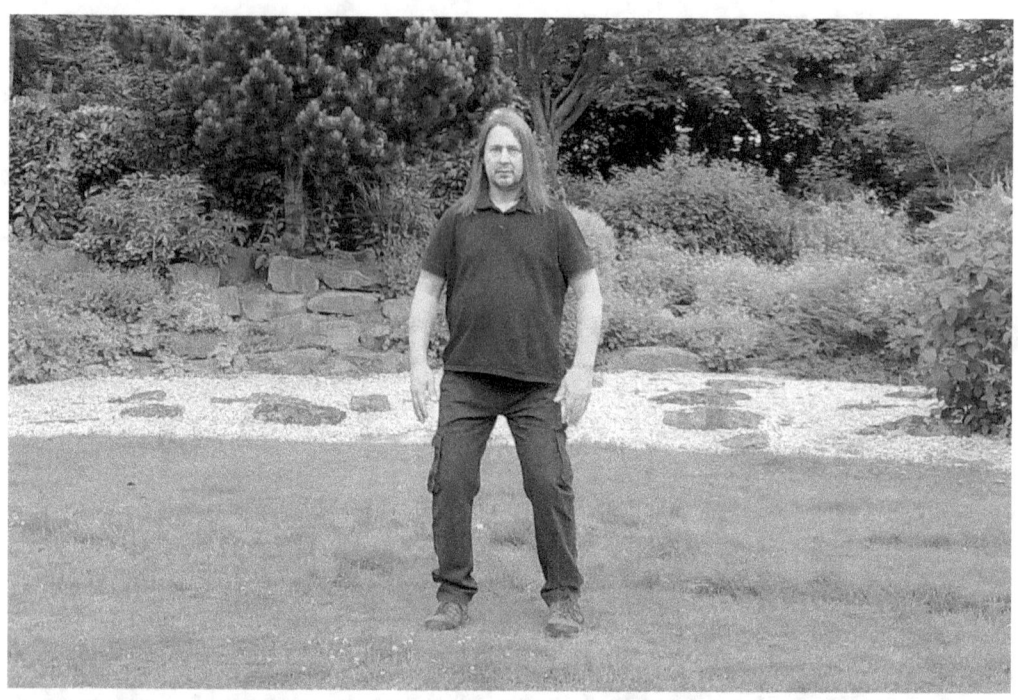

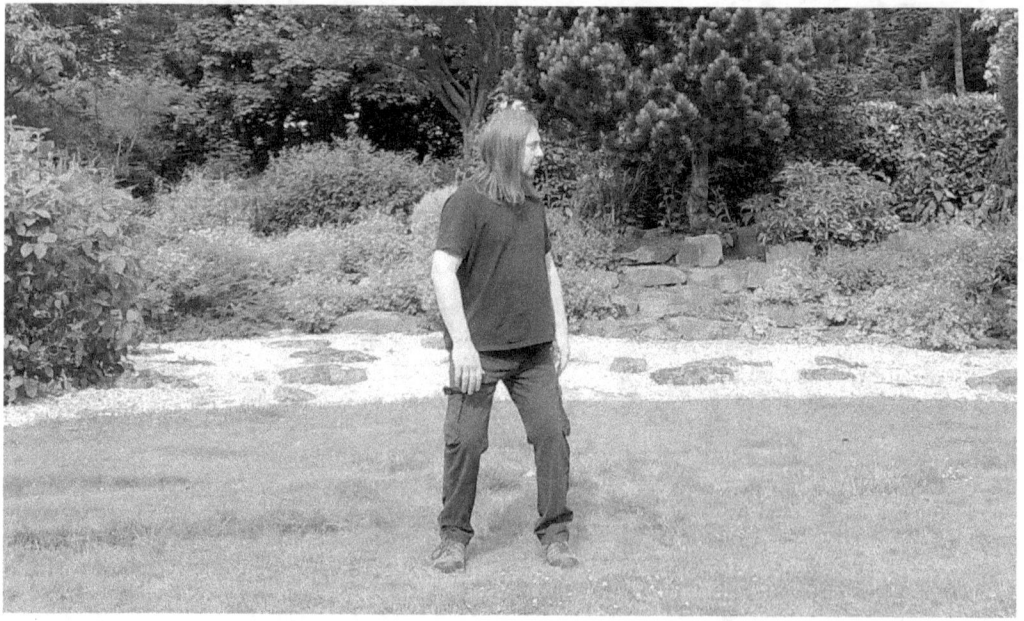

So that you can keep your alignments steady, do not turn too far. Your range of movement will be small to begin with but will increase with time and practice.

Repeat 20 times

Exercise Three

Stand in a shoulder width parallel posture; put your arms out in front of your upper chest, your palms face down.

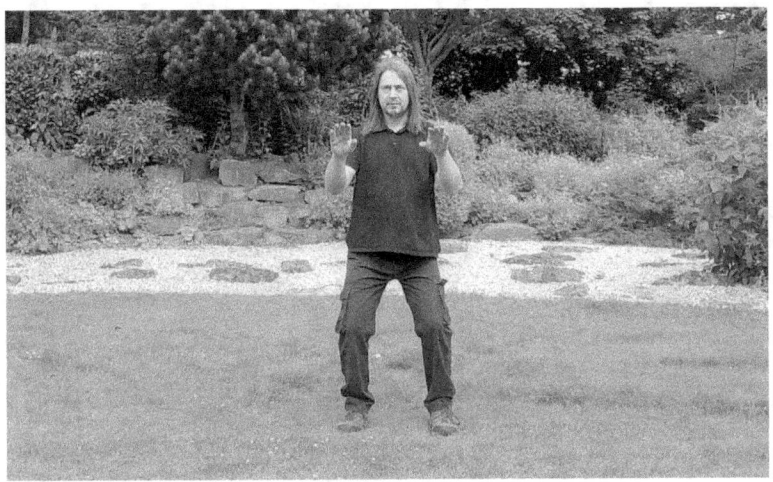

Sink your shoulders and elbows down and make sure that your hands do not rise up above the height of your shoulders. In this exercise, let the arms move with the body as if they are a whole unit.

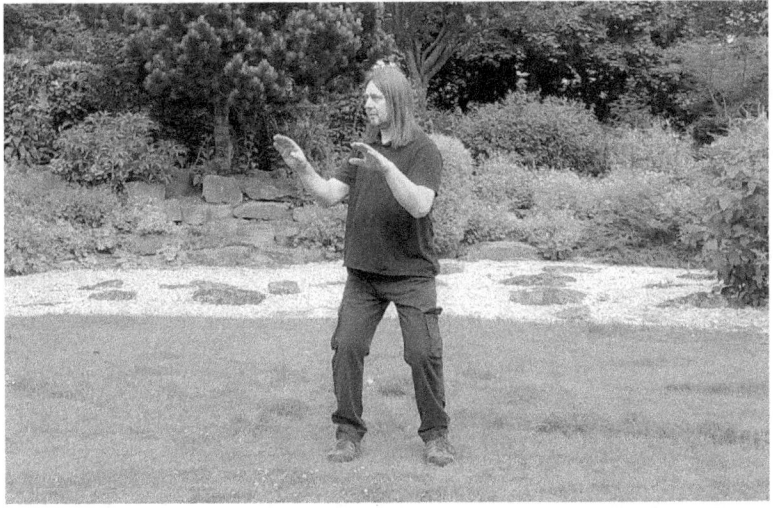

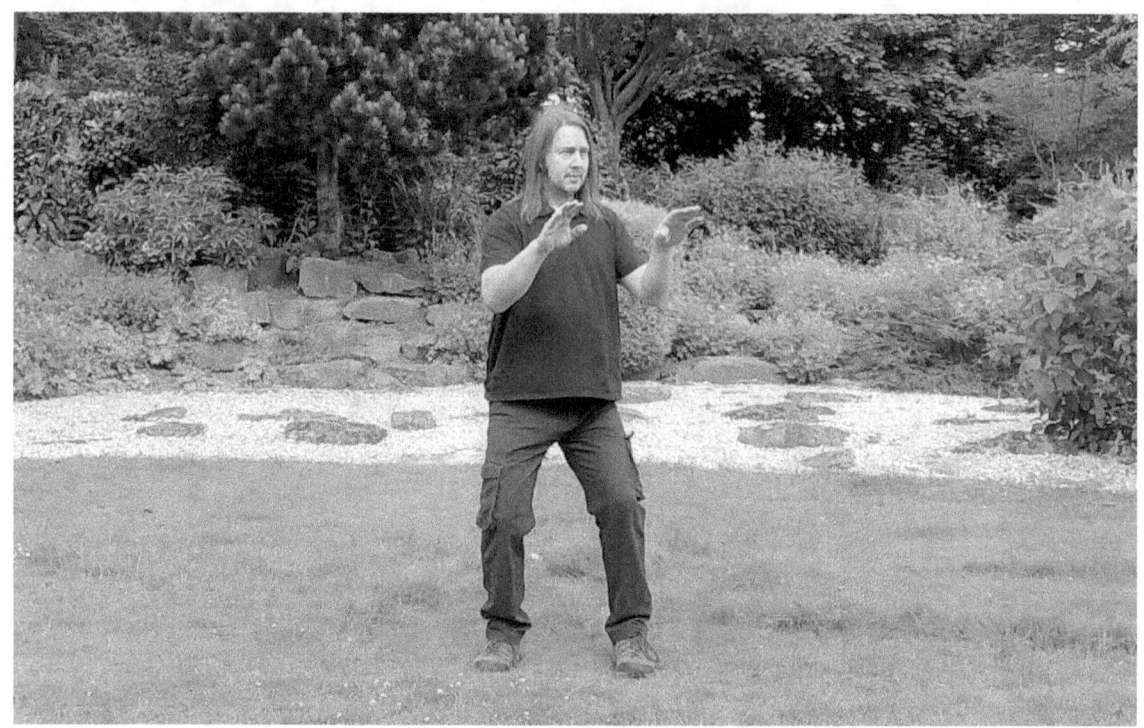

Turn to the left and pause for five seconds, return to the centre and then turn to your right side, hold for five seconds. Continue the exercise from the right to the centre and to the left.

Repeat 20 times.

Exercise Four

Repeat the previous exercise, this time let your arms trail behind the body's movement. You should feel a pulling in the shoulders before the arms move.

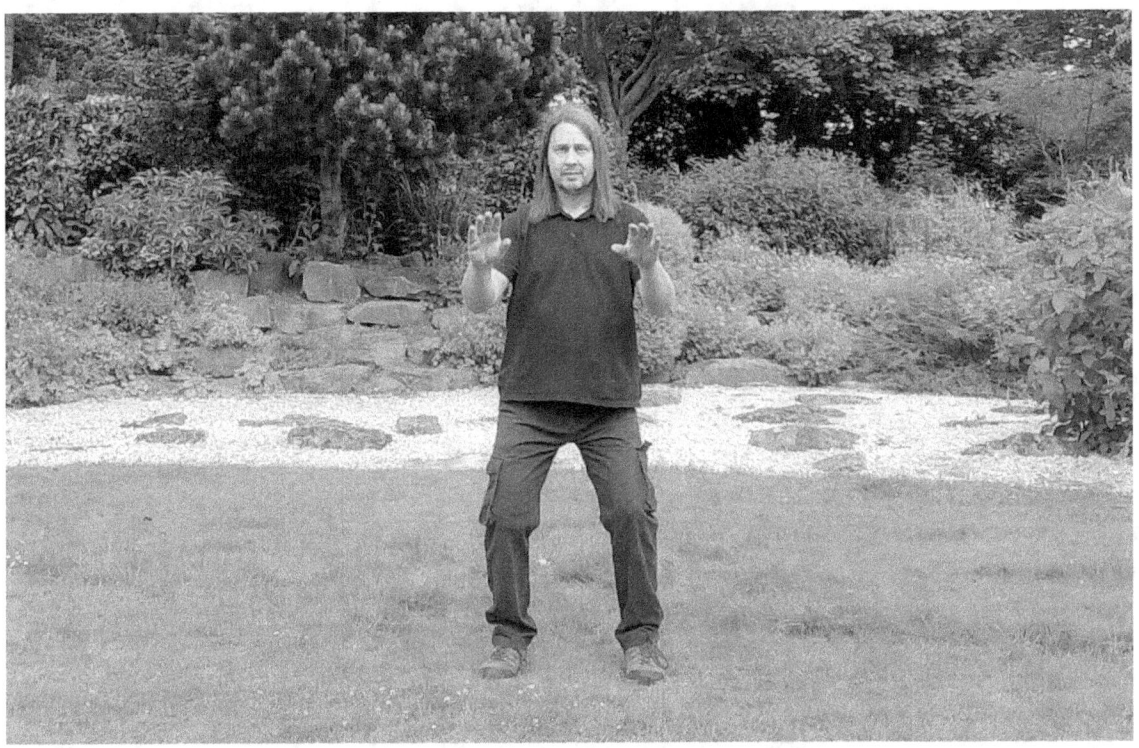

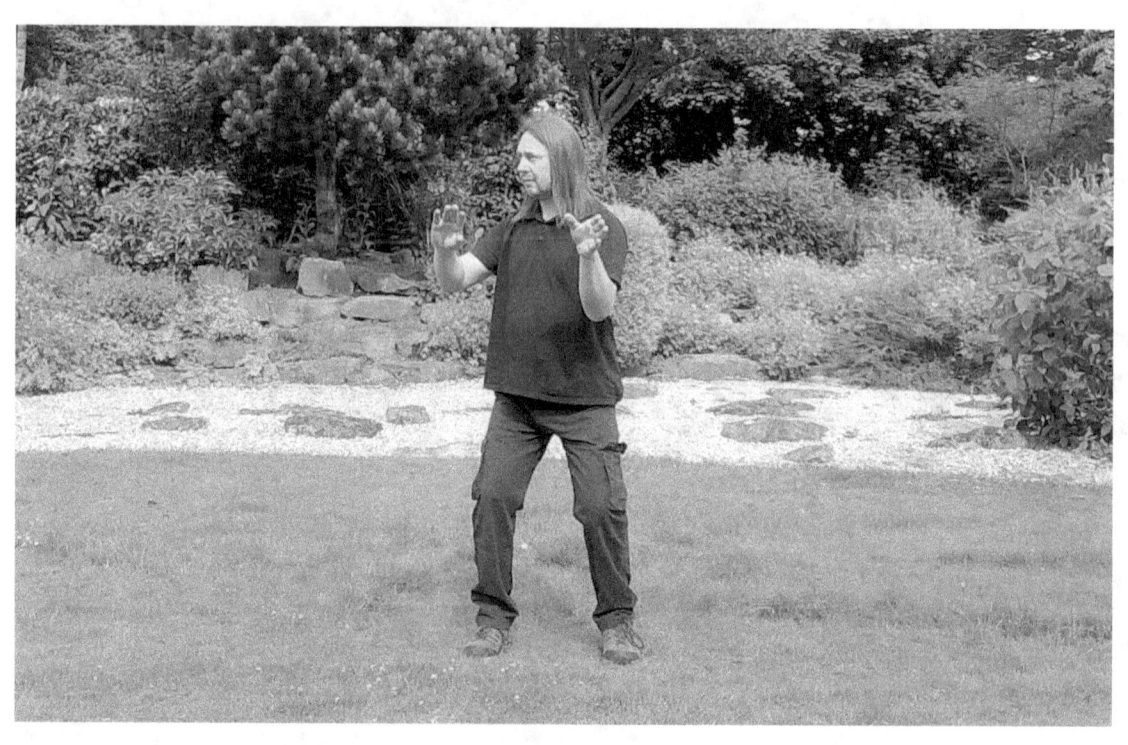

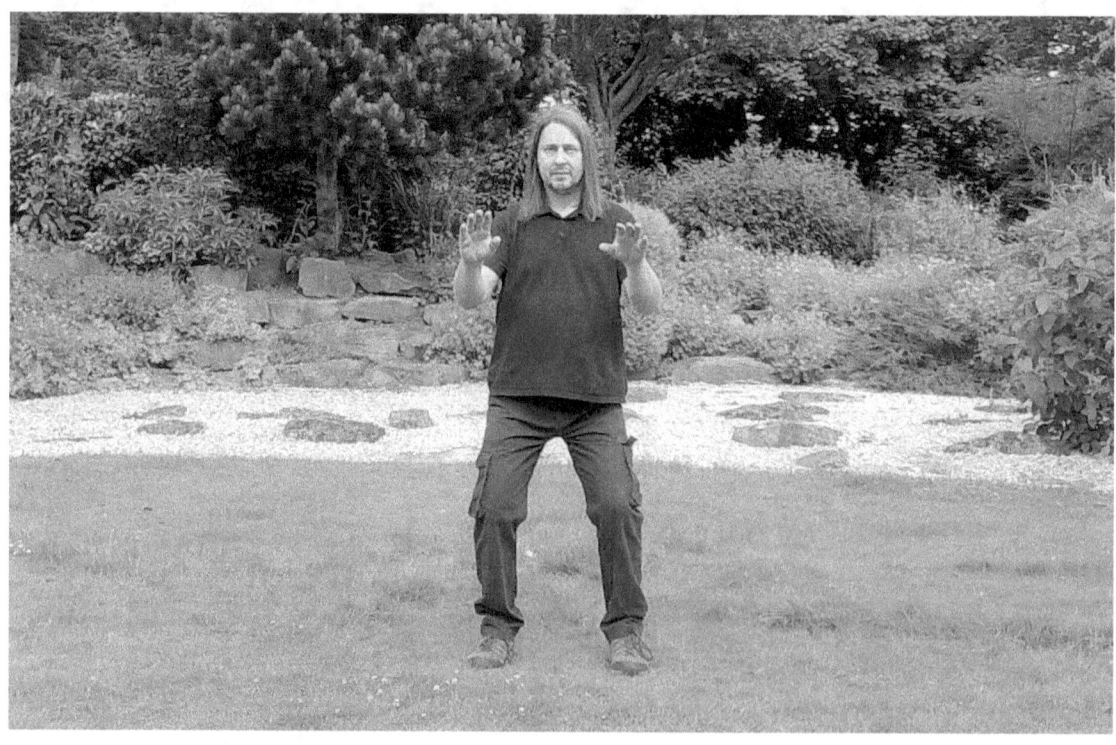

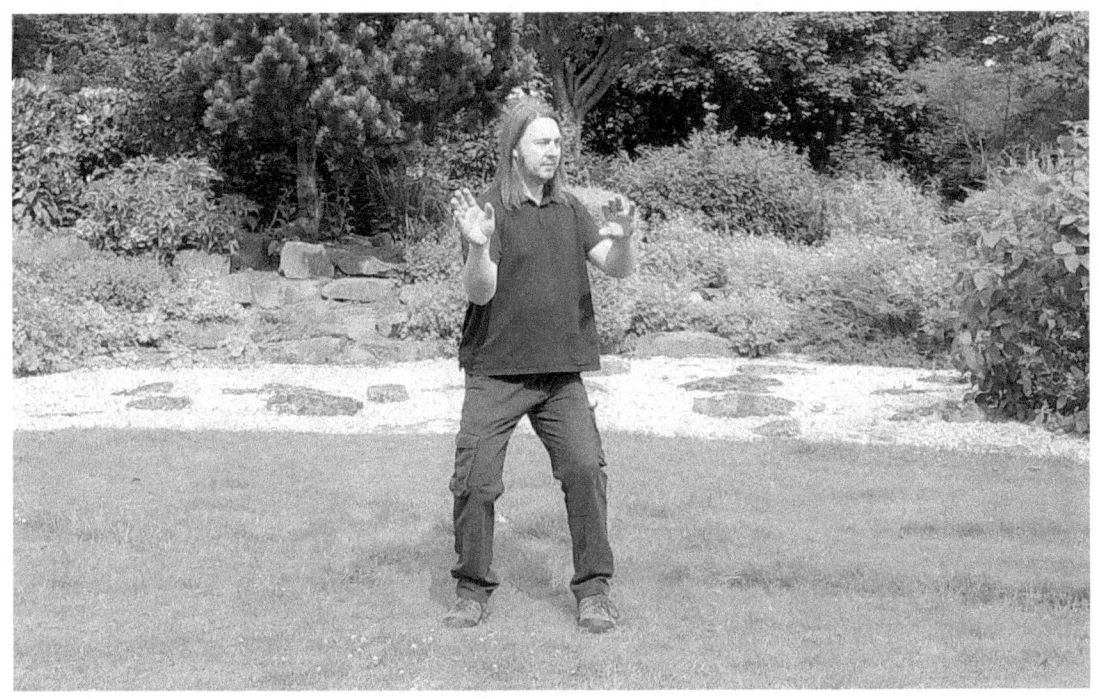

Repeat 20 times

Exercise Five

If you were doing this exercise while standing in water, there would be some resistance, and your arms would trail through the water with some lag between the initial motivating movement and the arms following. Imagine that feeling and turn side to side with the arms trailing in this manner.

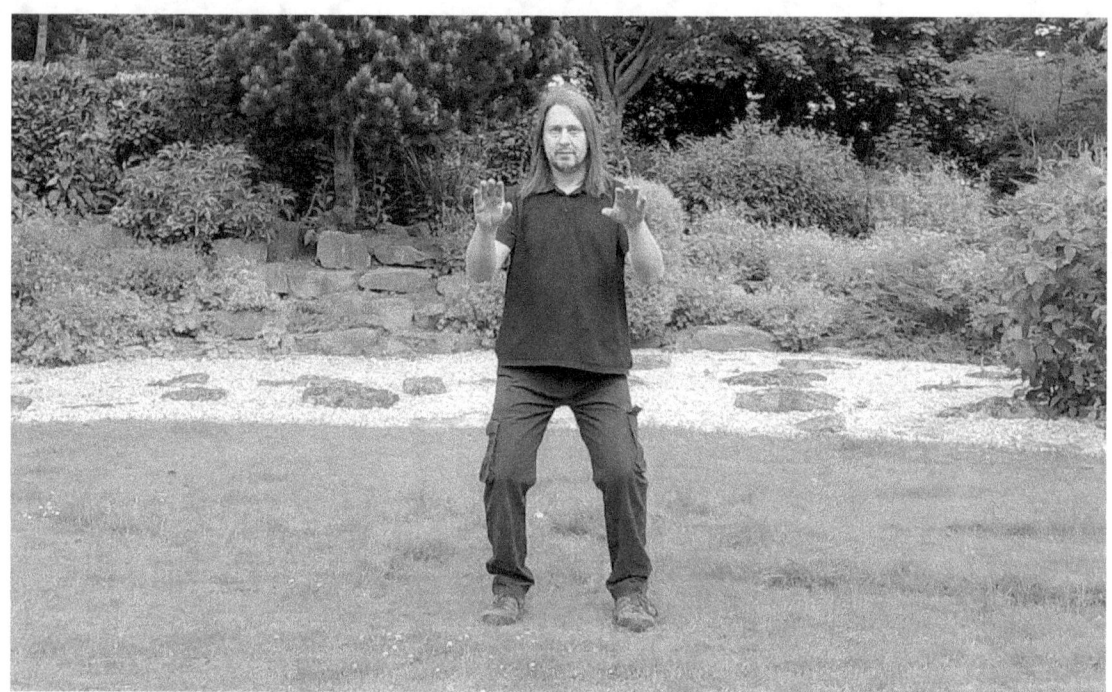

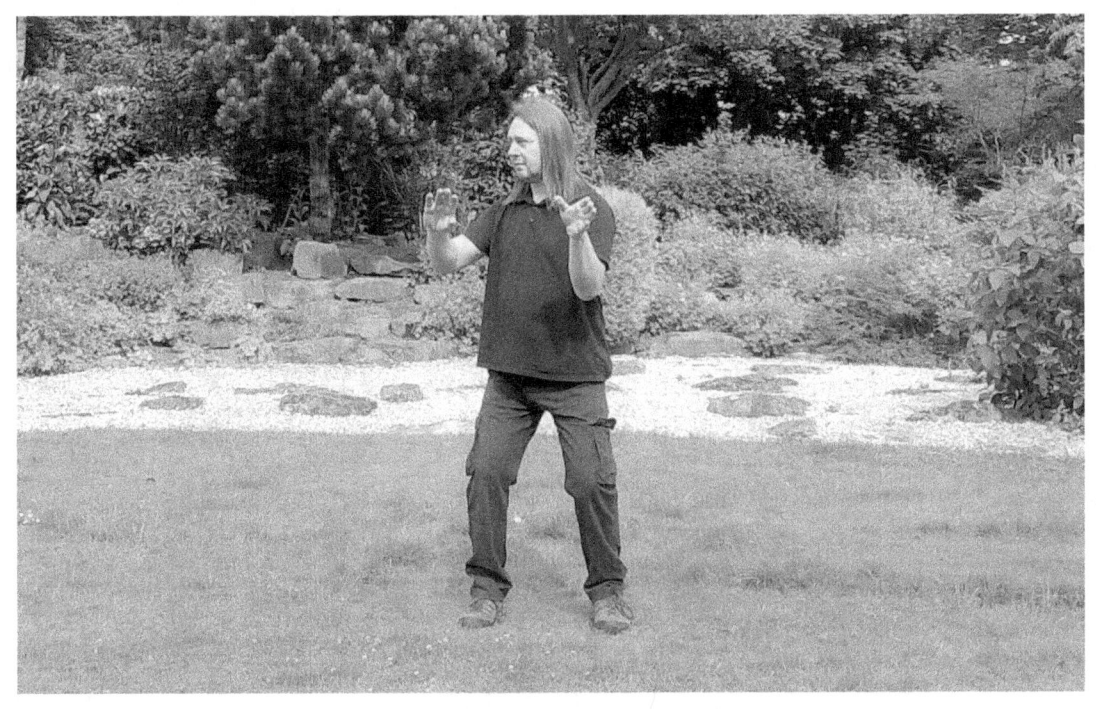

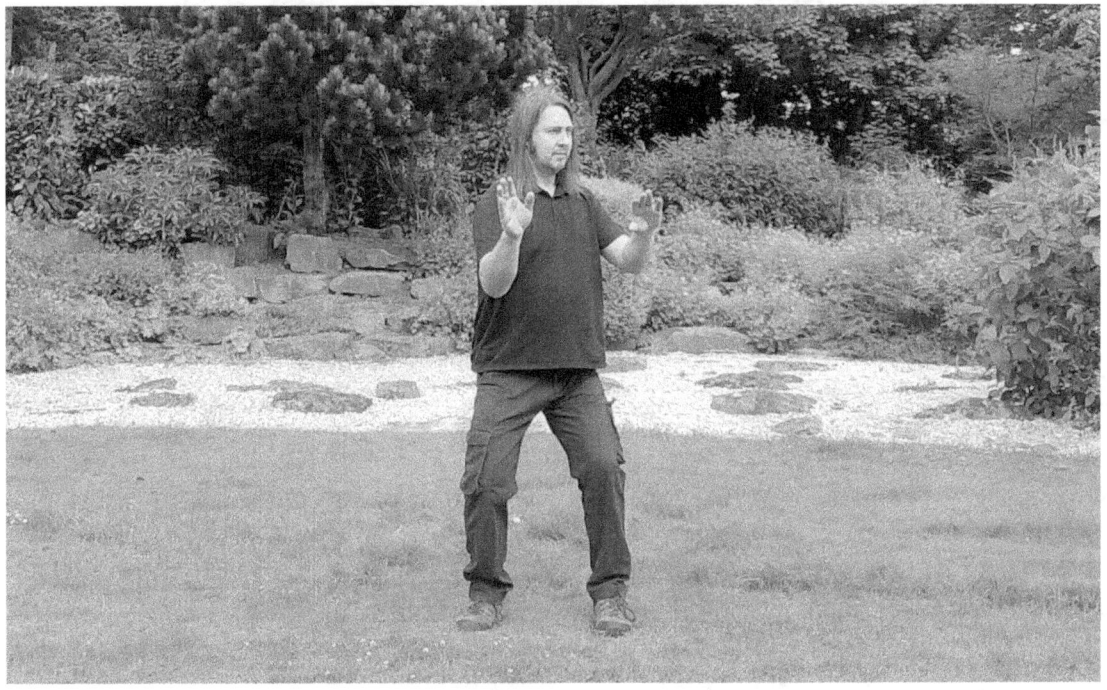

Repeat 20 times

Exercise Six

This Exercise is will help you to understand turning around the centreline of the body.

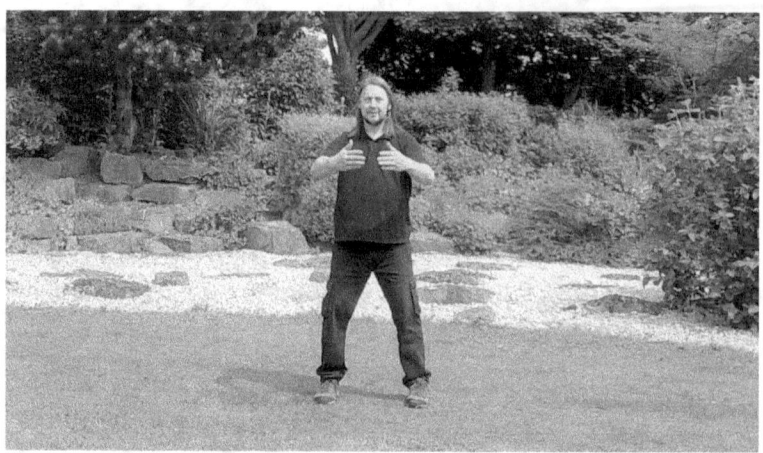

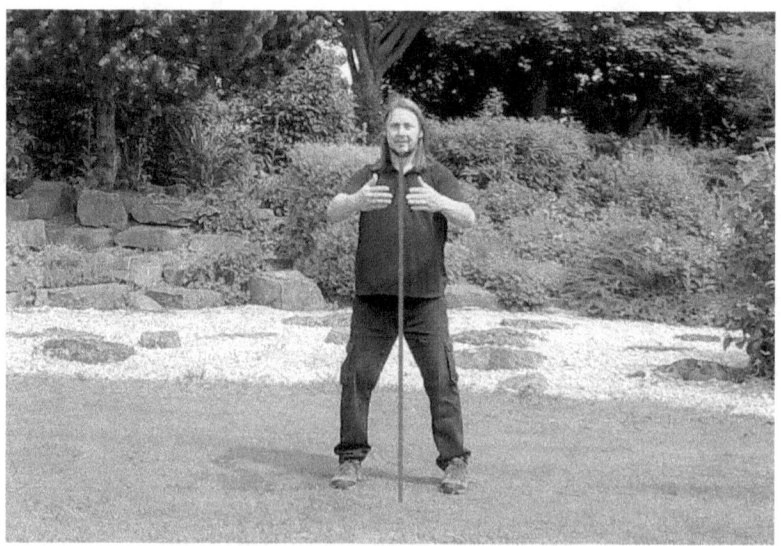

In a parallel stance, make a hold the ball shape in front of your upper chest. Turn from left to right and right to left, keep centred with no shifting from side to side. Feel how your body can rotate smoothly around the centreline.

Repeat 20 times

Exercise Seven

Take a forward Bow stance, your front foot is straight, and the rear foot is angled between 45-35 degrees, your body is square to the front. Put seventy percent of your body weight in the front foot leg.

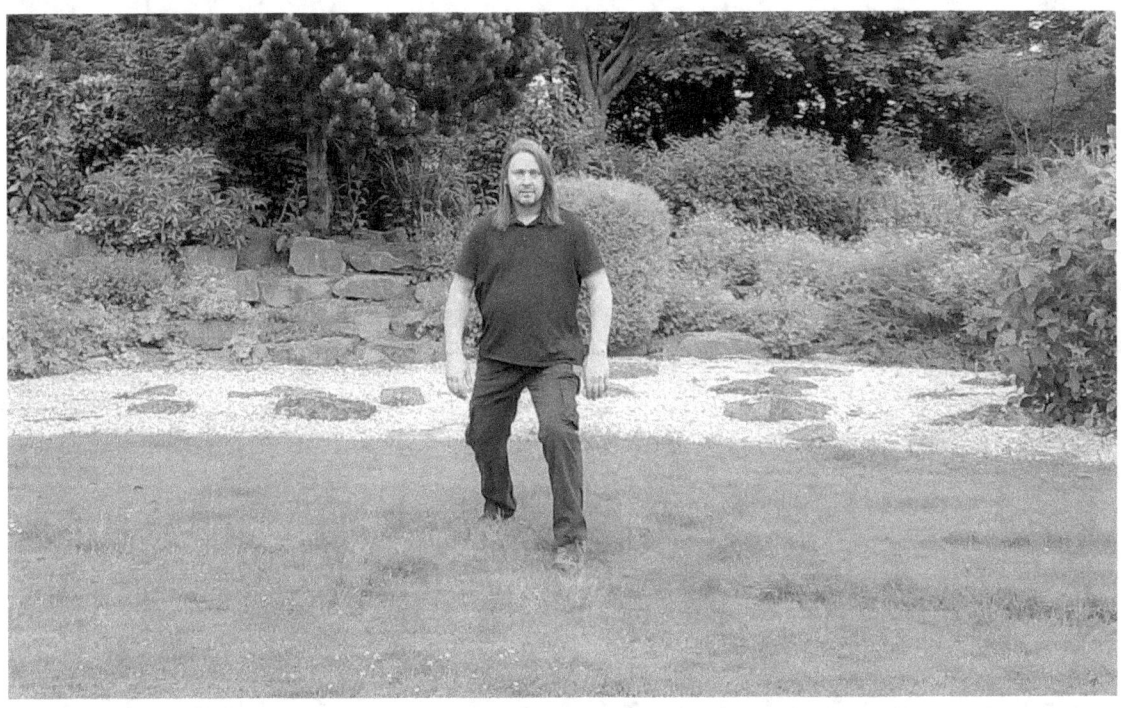

Slowly shift your centre backwards along an imaginary line that goes straight between your feet. (In the Cheng man Ch'ing style of Tai Chi when you are in a Bow stance you move straight forwards and backwards, minimizing side-to-side movement.)

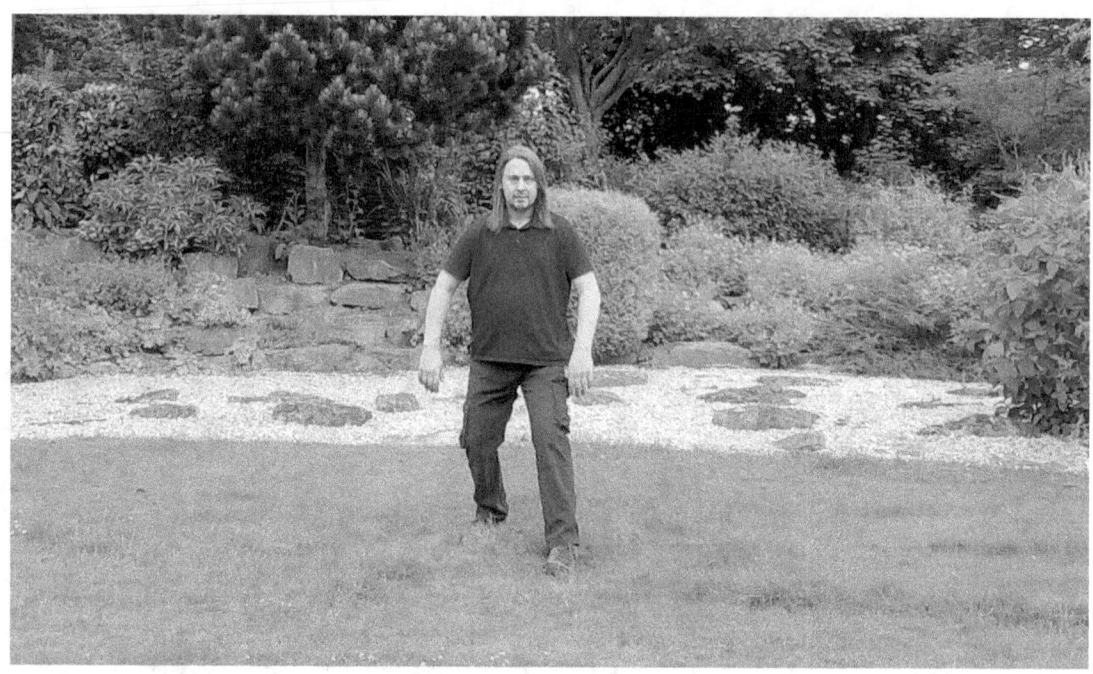

Once you have seventy percent of your weight in the rear foot, return to the front foot. Move slowly back and forth. When you have practiced on the left side, change over into a right forward Bow stance and repeat the exercise.

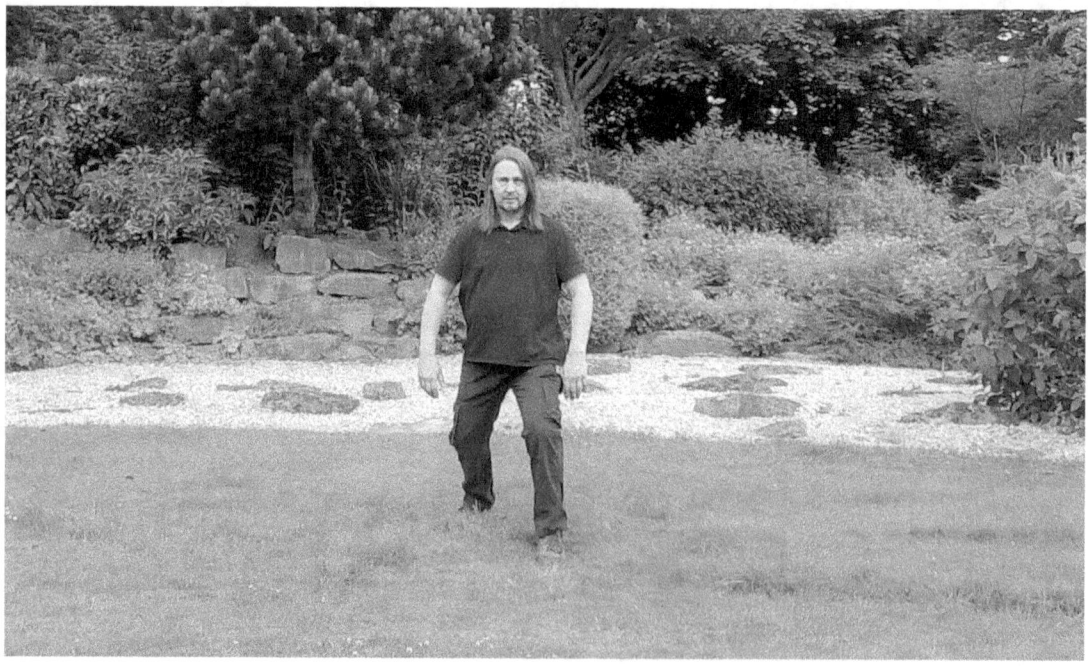

Repeat 20 times

Exercise Eight

Stand in a left forward Bow stance; imagine that both legs are hollow and your front leg is filling with liquid and that your rear leg is emptying. Shift backward and forward feeling the full and the empty in your legs. Practise this exercise on both sides.

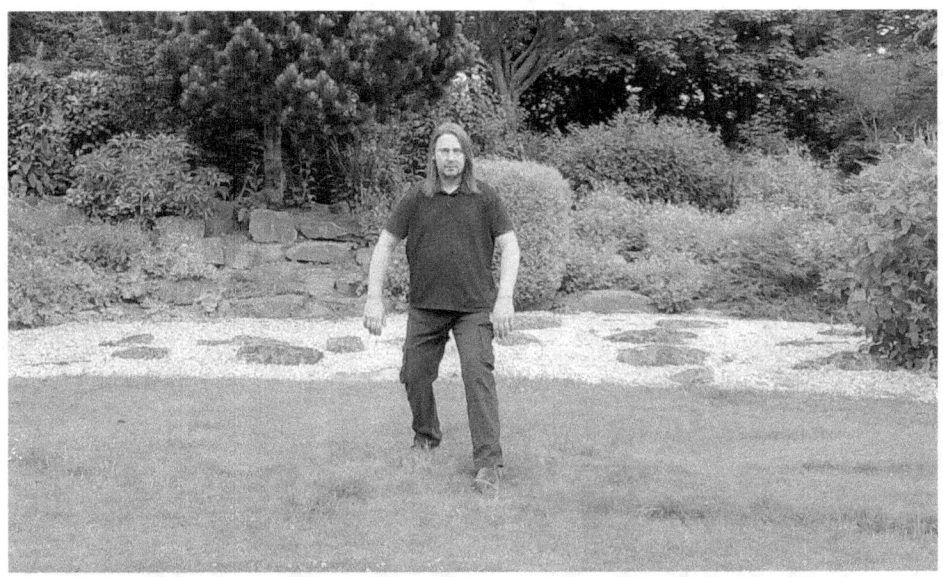

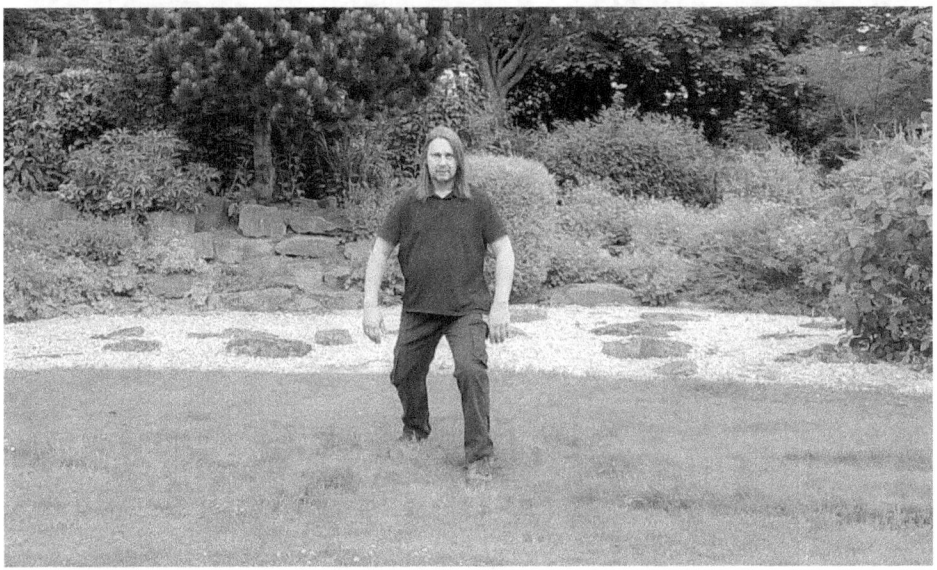

Repeat 20 times

Exercise Nine

Stand in a right Bow stance and move slowly into your left leg. As you move forward and back pay close attention your head keeping it upright, (suspended from the Crown Point) and that your shoulders and hips remain level and do not wobble as you move.

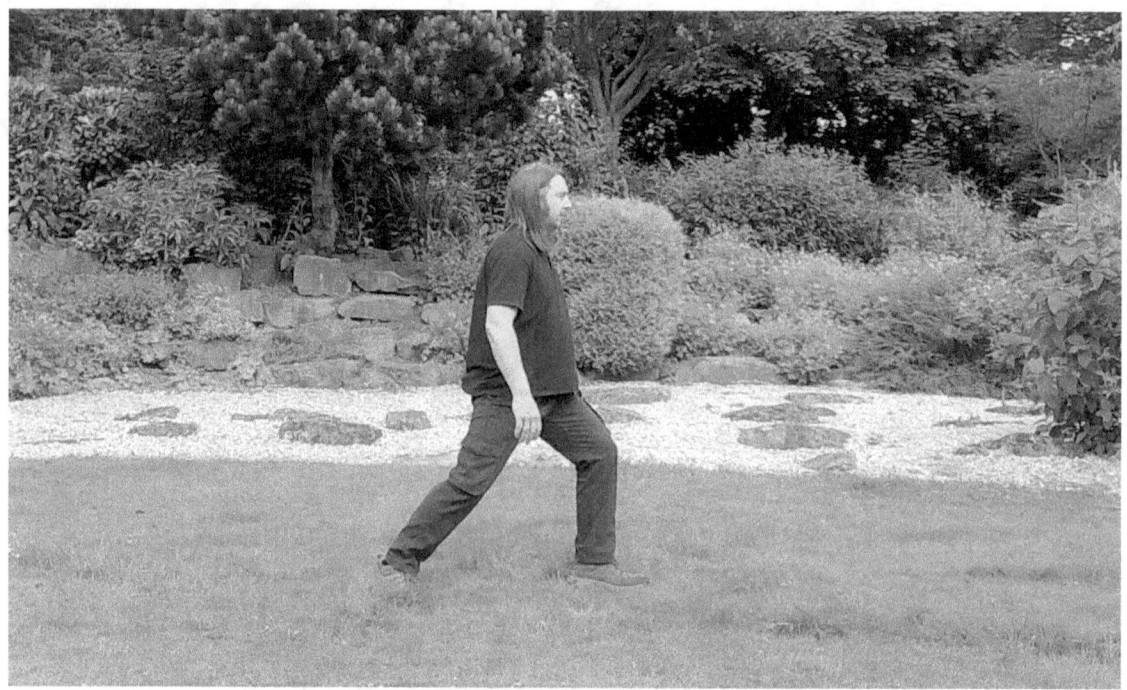

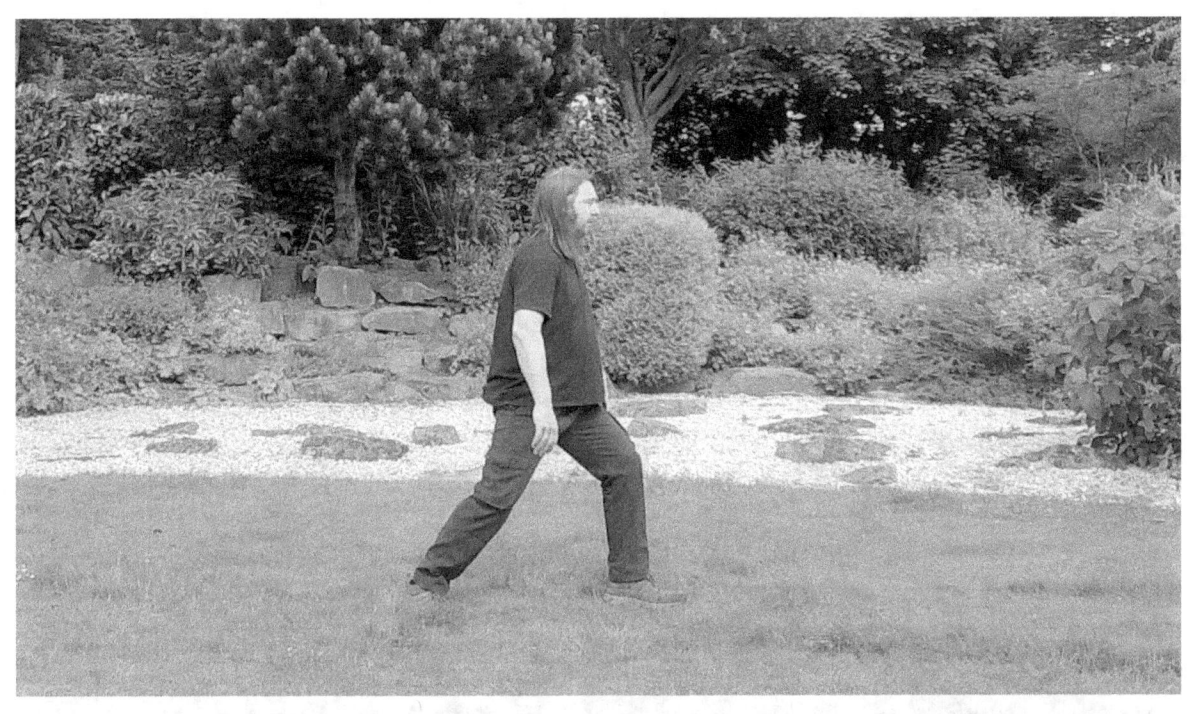

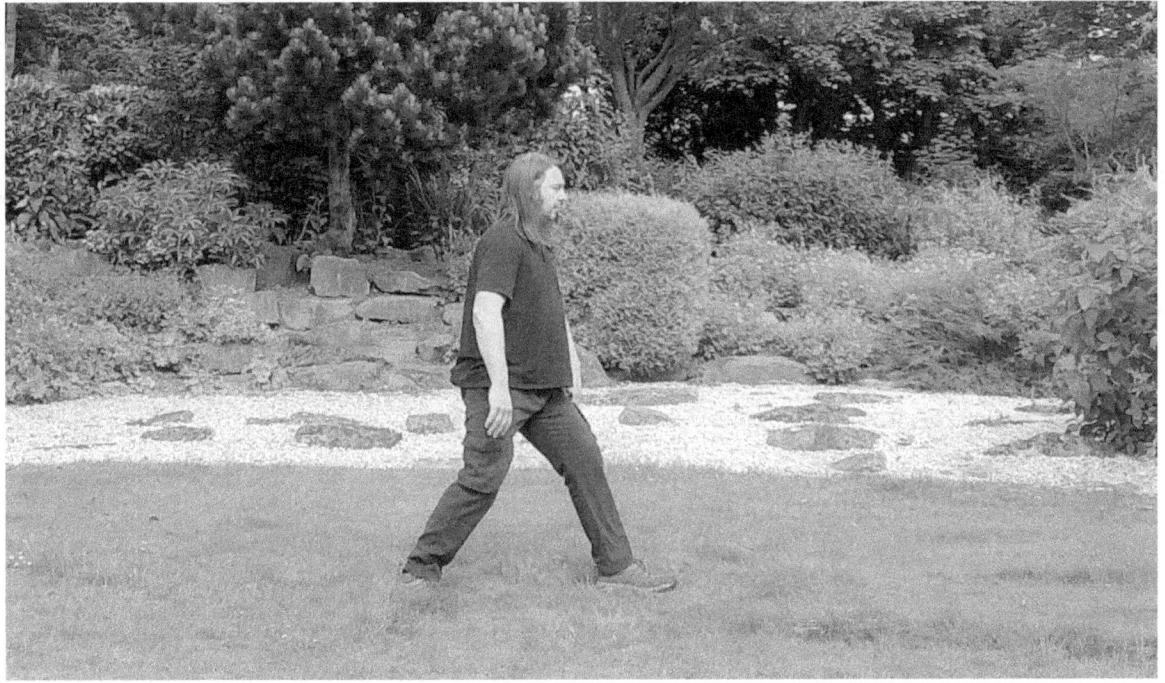

Repeat 20 times

Exercise Ten

This exercise helps you to experience how you can control the movement of your leg with your Dantien.
Stand in a small Cat stance with your left foot forward, shift your weight into your back leg and raise the toes of your right foot.

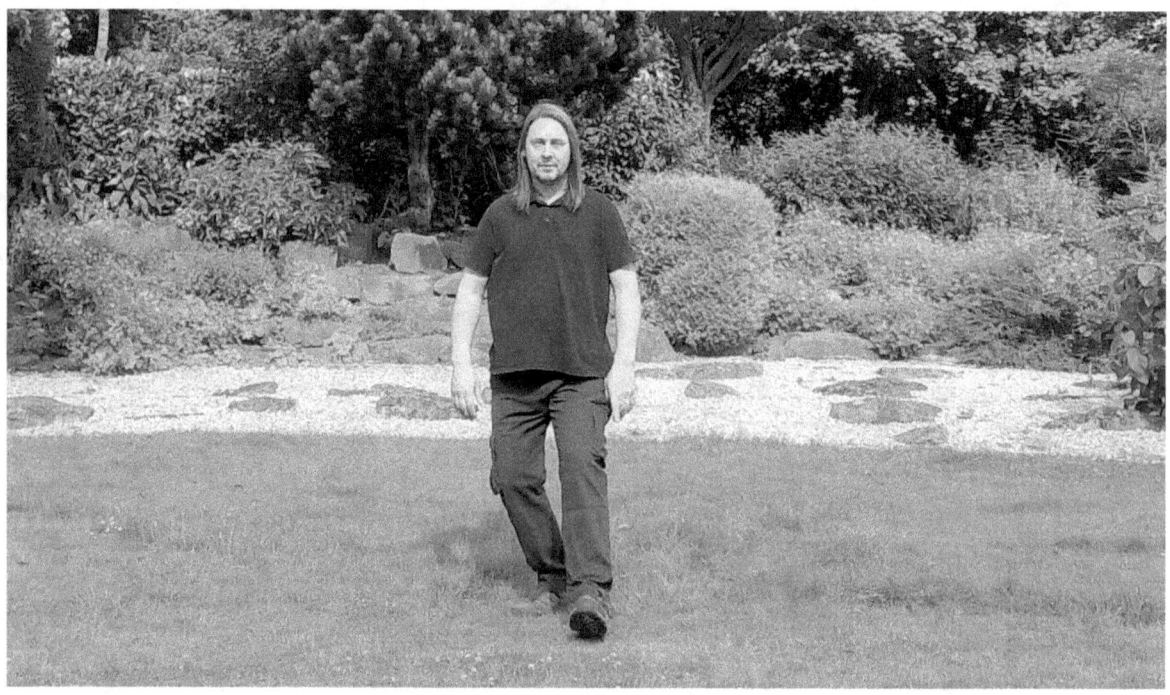

Turn your Dantien to turn your leg and foot to your right side, turn the toes (by pivoting on the heel) inwards twenty to thirty degrees.

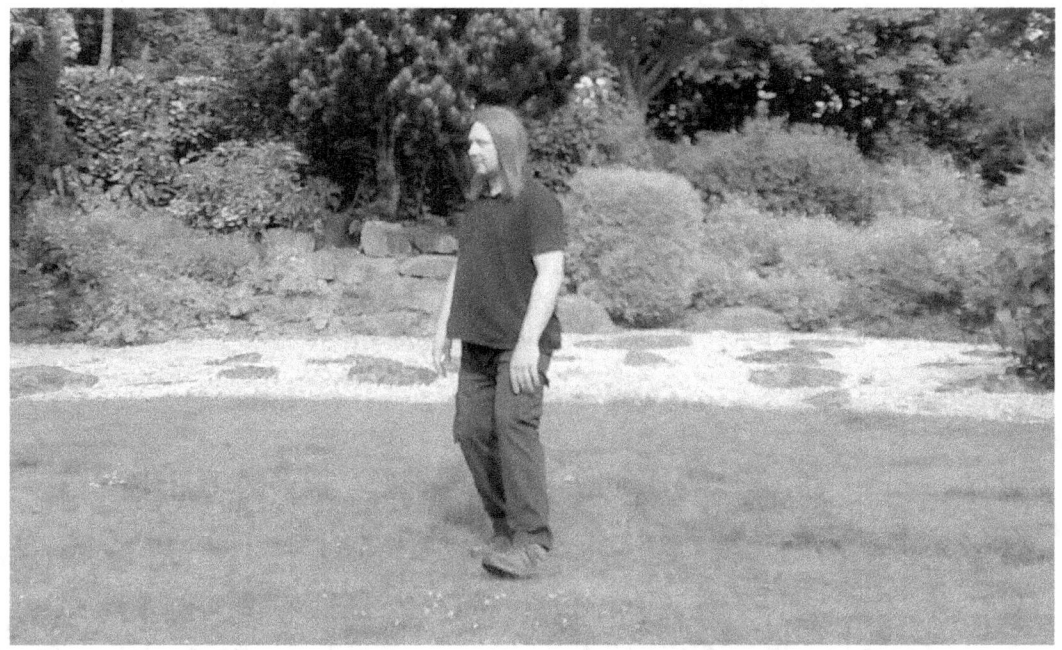

Turn left and turn the toes out twenty to thirty degrees. Change your legs over and repeat the movements.

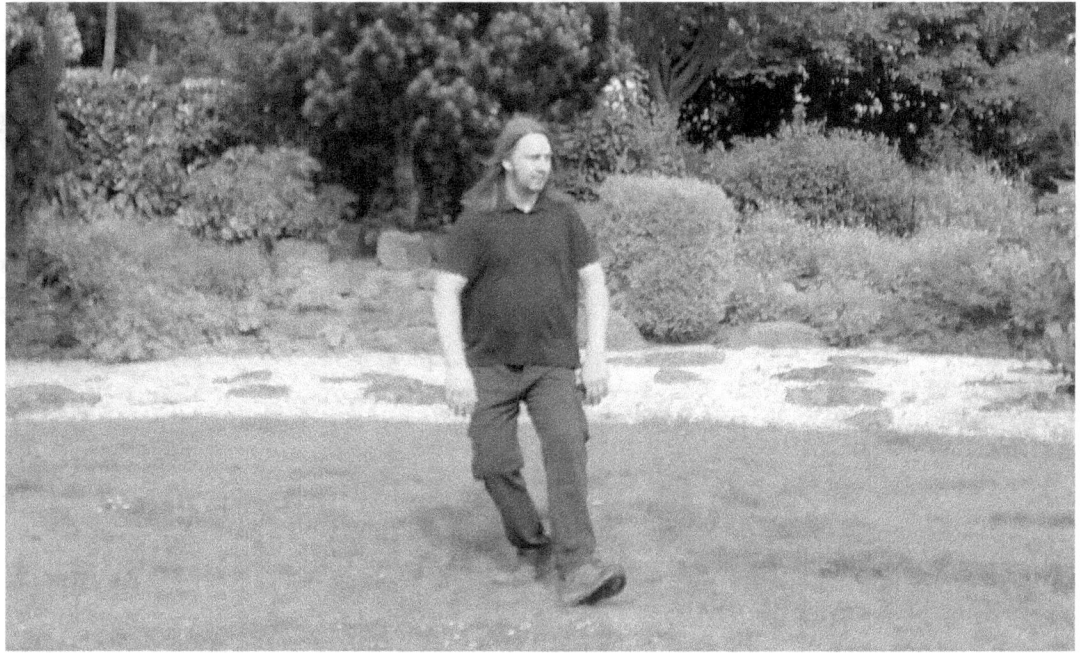

Repeat 20 times

Exercise Eleven

Stand in a forward Bow stance, with seventy percent of your weight in the front leg. Make a hold the ball shape in front of your upper chest.

Shift your weight back to the central fifty/fifty posture, pause and shift into a back weighted stance. Move forwards and backwards pausing in these three positions.

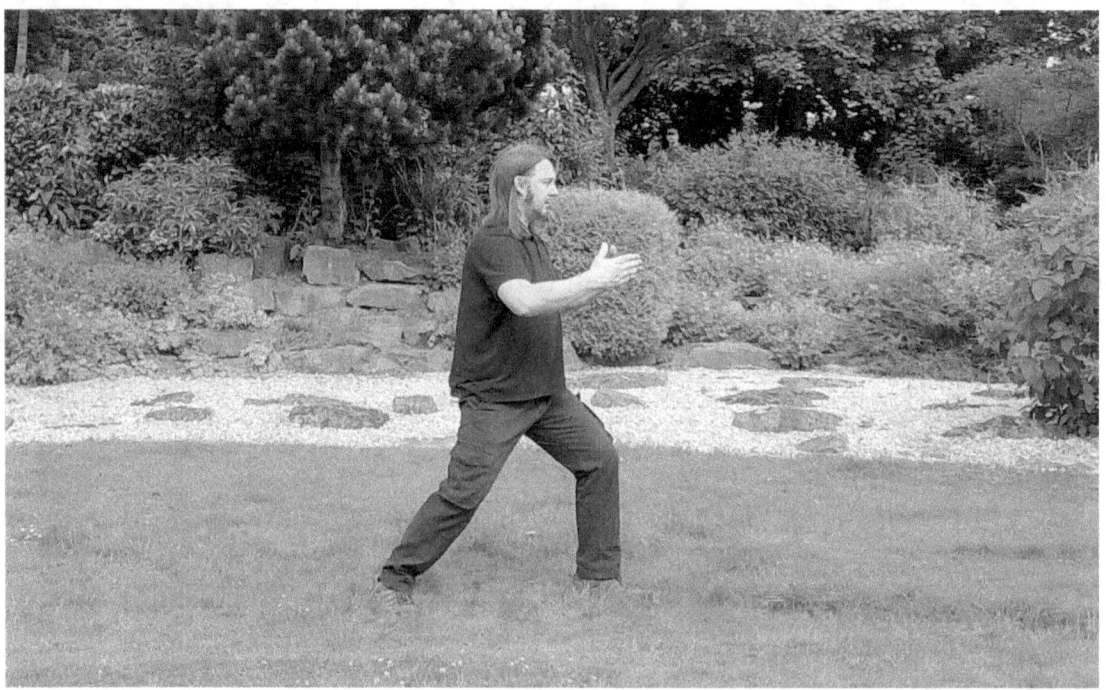

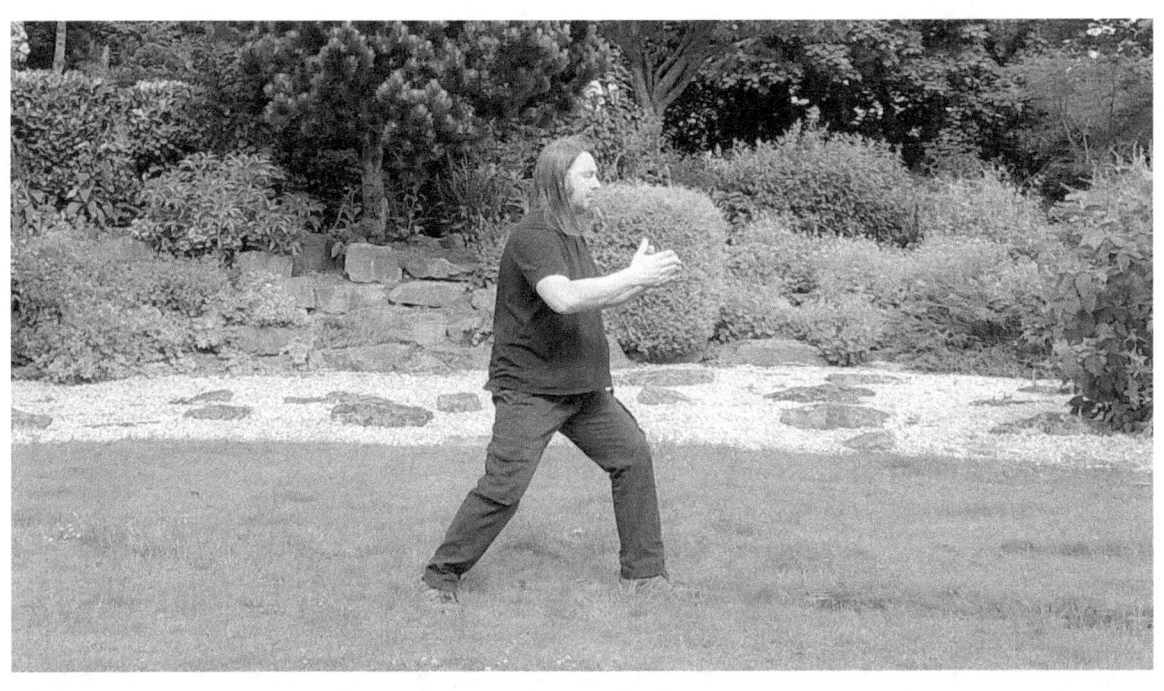

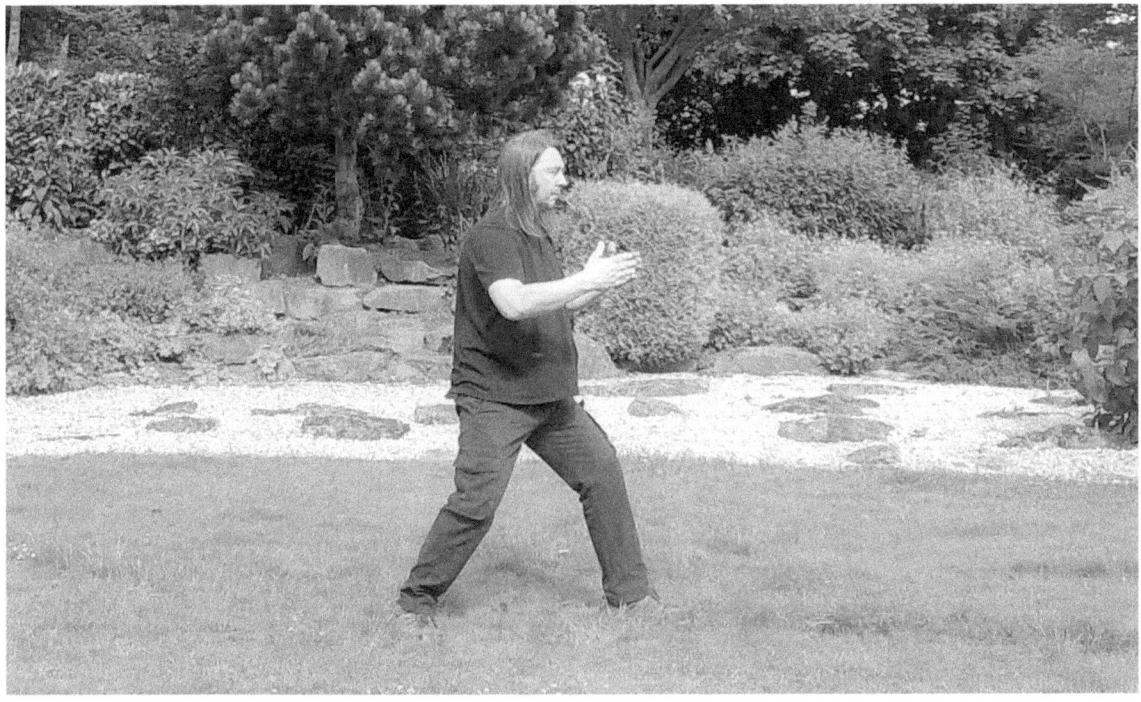

Repeat 20 times

Exercise Twelve

Repeat the previous exercise, this time move smoothly forwards, and back whilst holding the ball in position. (Be sure not to shift from side to side.)

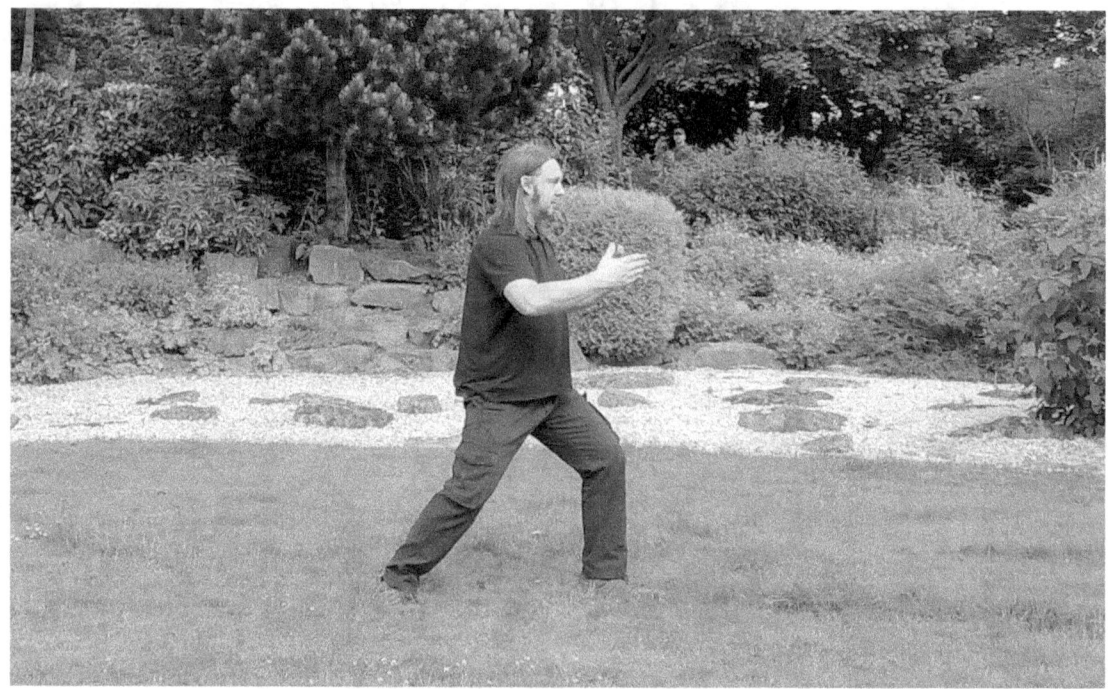

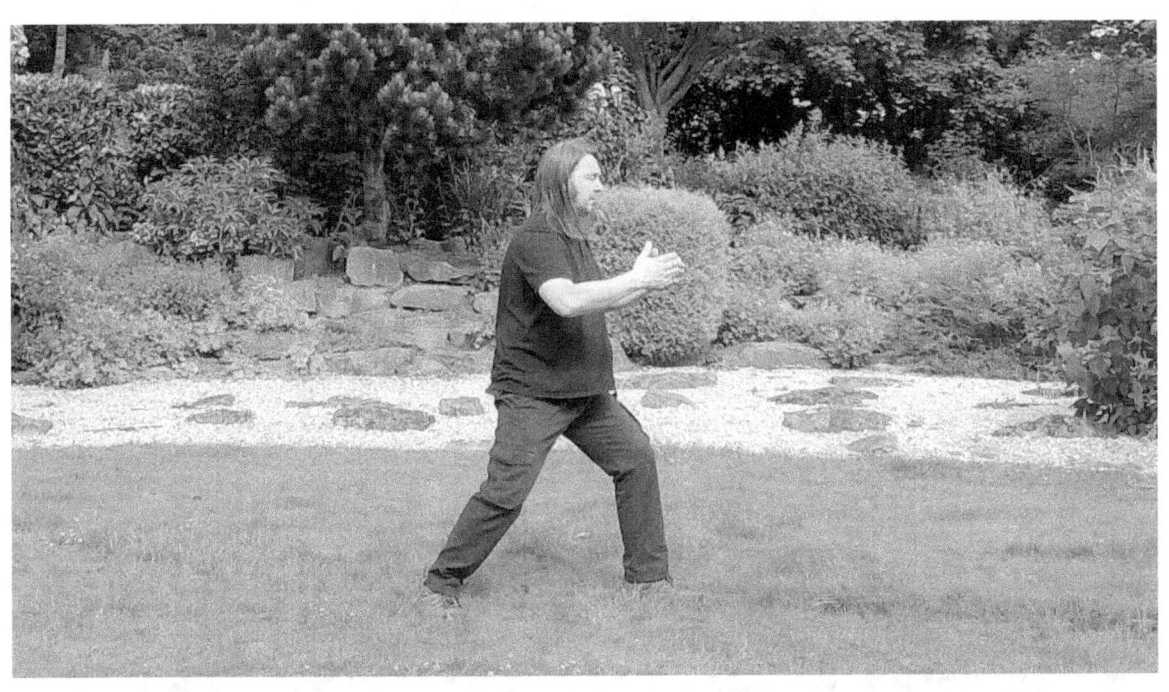

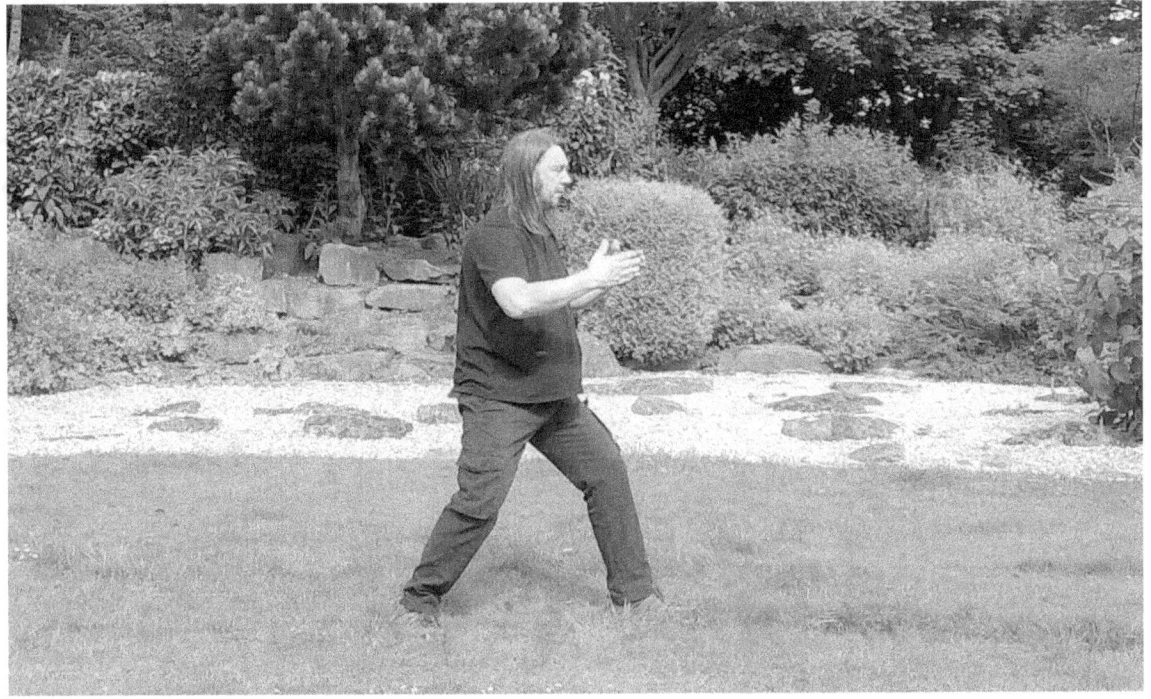

Repeat 20 times

Exercise Thirteen

The form movement, Waving Hands like Clouds can be very helpful when learning Tai Chi. It teaches you to turn around your centreline. It helps you to develop movement of the torso and arms from the lower Dantien and you can experience weight shifting in the legs without having to step.

Stand in a parallel stance, turn to your left side, and hold a ball with your left hand on top and right hand on the bottom.

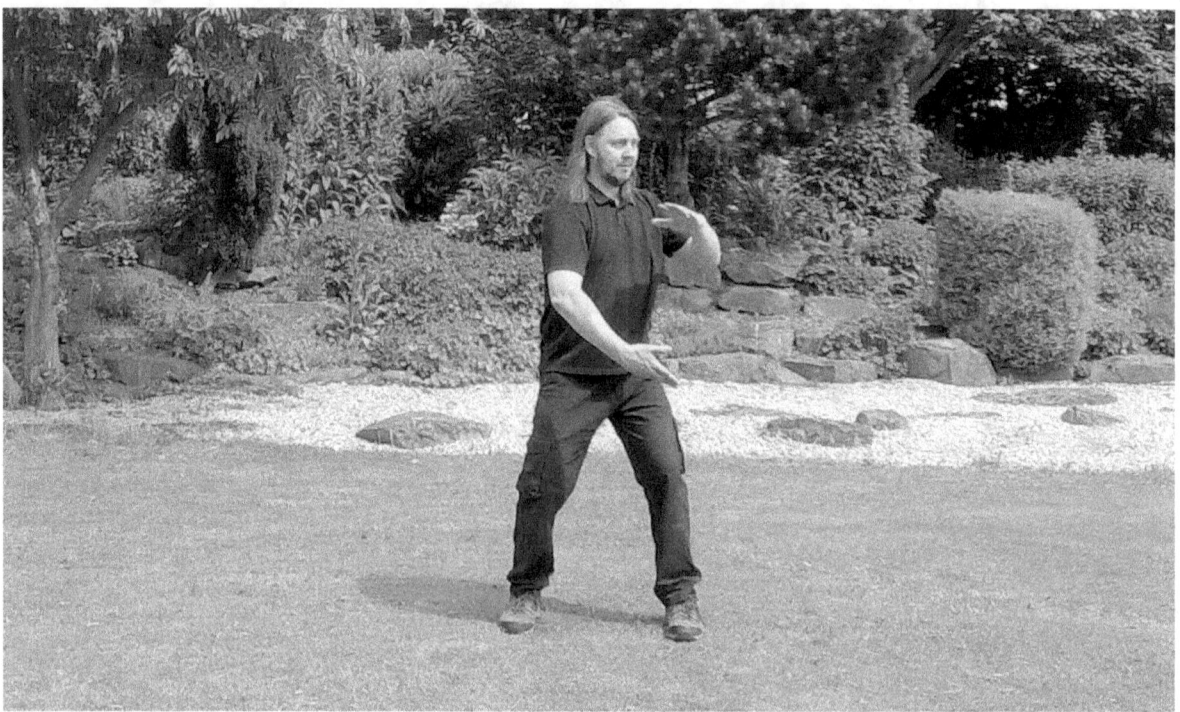

Turn to the centre while bringing your right arm up in a ward off shape and the left arm to your side in a scooping shape.

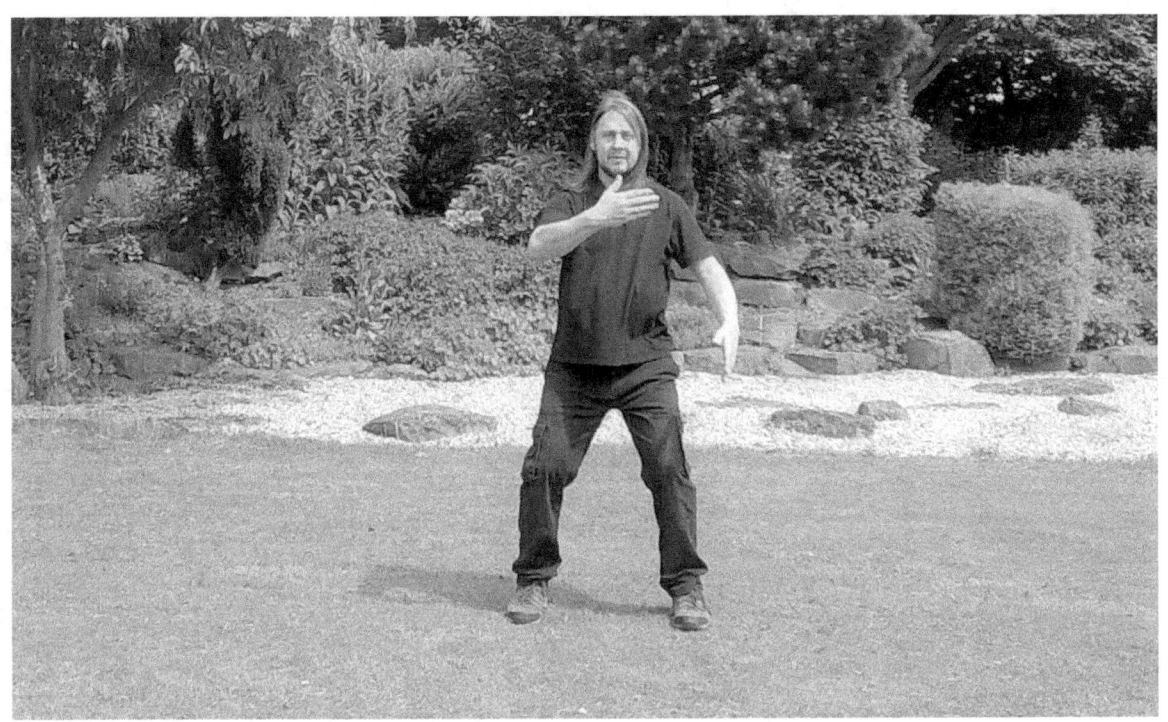

Turn to the right side and hold a ball with your right hand on top.

Once you are comfortable with this movement, repeat the exercise from right to left.

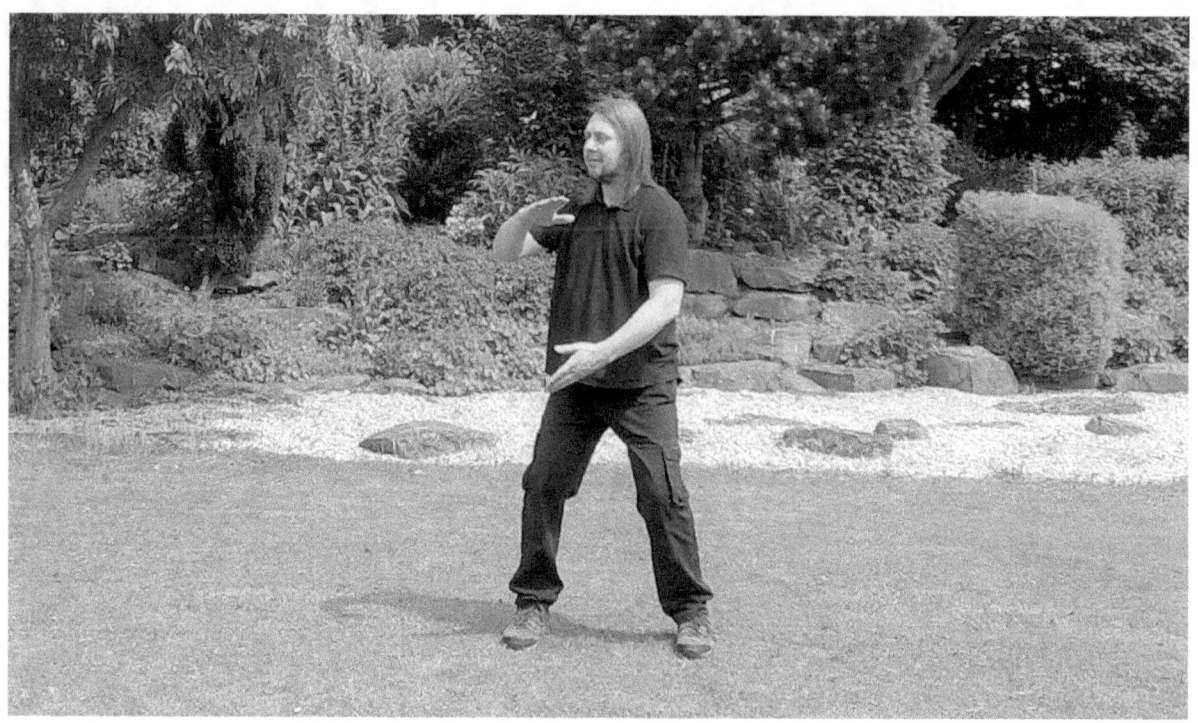

Repeat 20 times

Here are some other ways that you can experiment with Waving Hands like Clouds.

1) Experiment with Waving Hands, by moving from your centre.

2) Focus on your arm movements, making the arm changes, smooth, fluid, and circular.

3) Do the turns feeling your weight shift between your legs.

4) Do the exercise making sure that your head remains upright and level.

5) Focus on making sure that your shoulders remain level.

6) Focus on making sure that your hips remain level.

Chapter Eight: Meditation

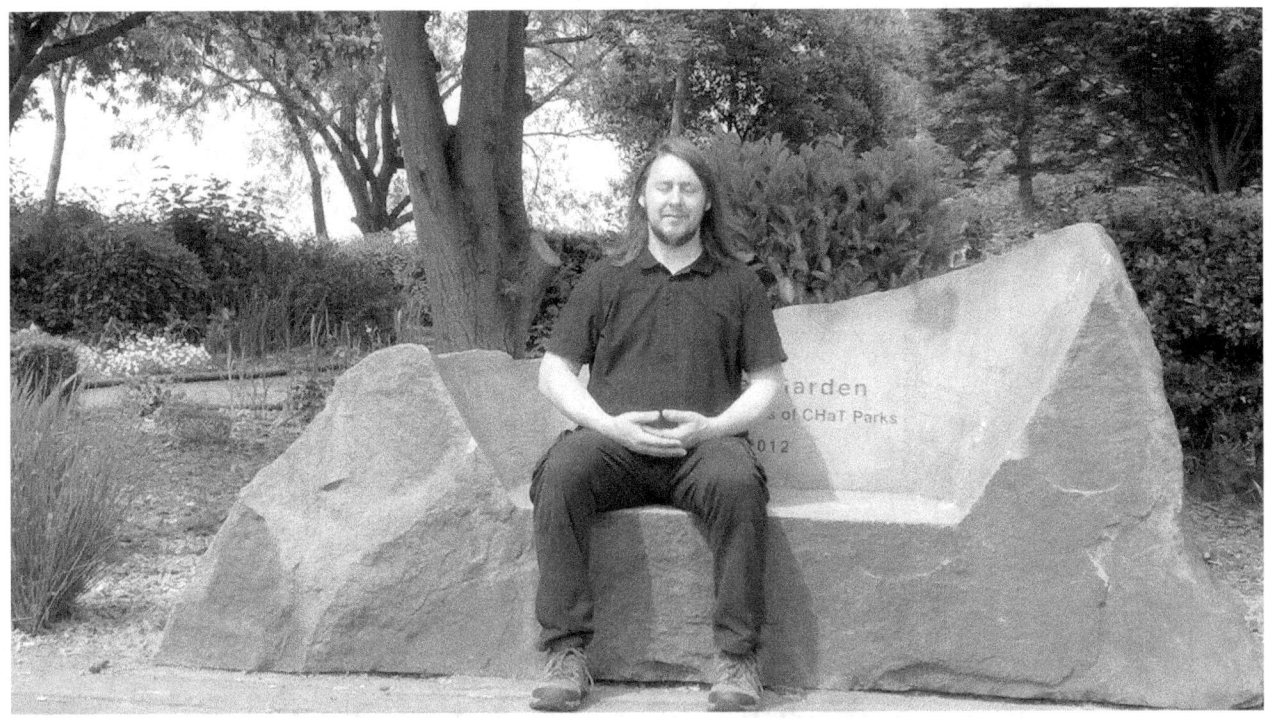

"Tai Chi, is meditation in motion"

Source: Harvard Medical School

 Meditation is an important aspect of your Tai Chi practice; as you perform the slow, flowing movements, you naturally develop a calmer, clearer, and more focused mind.

However, as a beginning student, you should try adding Sitting Meditation to your Tai Chi sessions to accrue the mental benefits faster.

Fortunately, you do not have to chant a mantra, or sit on the floor in the uncomfortable lotus position to get these benefits.

You just need to sit down on a chair for a few minutes and breathe.

"Imagine your mind is a glass of water. If you put some dirt (thoughts) into it and stir it up, the water will become turbulent and unclear, after a time (Meditation) the dirt will settle to the bottom of the glass and the water will become tranquil and clear."

To get the best result use these principles...

    1) Suspend the Crown Point
    2) Relax your shoulders and align them over your hips
    3) Hands palm up in lap for centredness

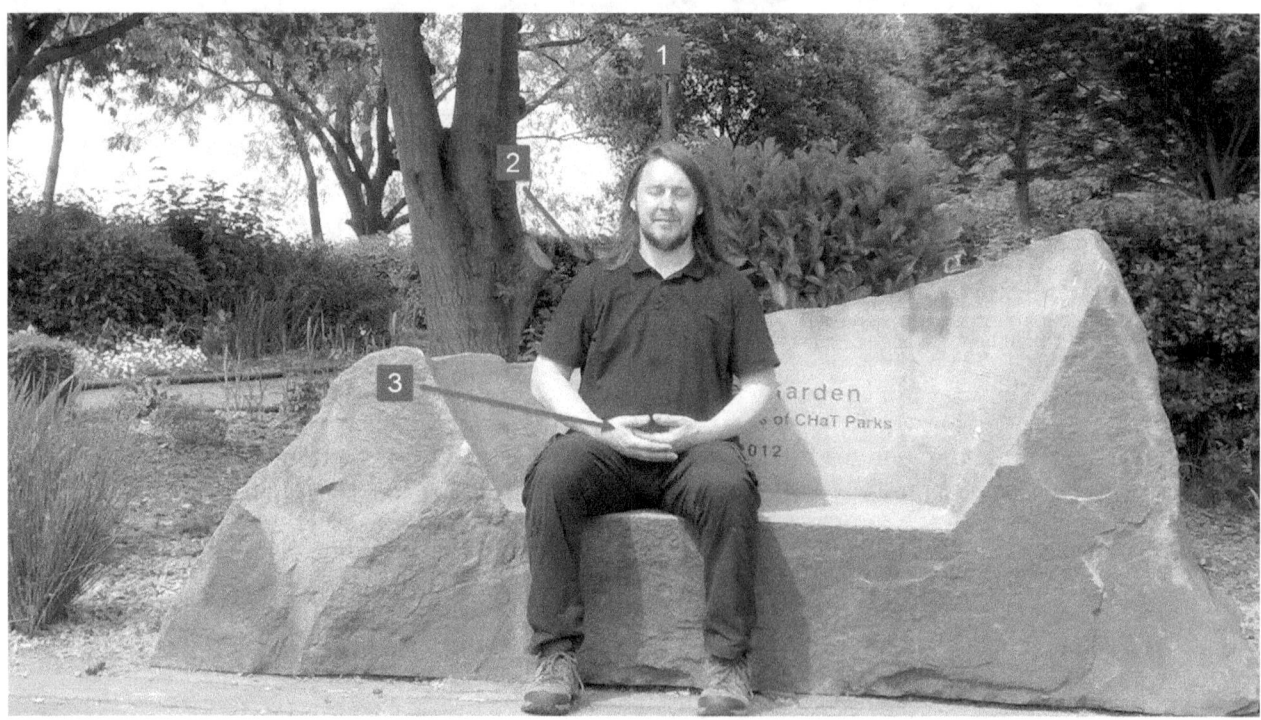

How to Meditate

Sit down on a chair and put the principles into place.

Next, close your eyes and put your attention on your breath, feel it at the tip of your nose as you breathe in and out.

Do this for one minute, then expand your awareness and follow the breath, as it flows from your nose into your body and follow it back out again.

Distracting thoughts will occur, that is natural, it is your job to notice when you are caught up in these thoughts, and bring your attention back to your breath.

As you sit and follow your breath, the distracting thoughts will slow down and your mind will start to become clearer, calmer, and more focused.

When you move on to your Tai Chi form practice after Meditation, you will be able to feel the internal more quickly and easily.

CHAPTER NINE: STANDING POST

Before practicing your Tai Chi form you should stand still for a few minutes, this will get your body and mind into the right state. The energy will flow more easily and your Tai Chi form will flow better.

Stand in a parallel stance and put your Tai Chi principles into place.

Next, relax as much as possible, all the way from the crown of your head all the way down to the soles of your feet. (Imagine a wave of warmth flowing downward and as it flows it carries the excess tension down and out of your body.)

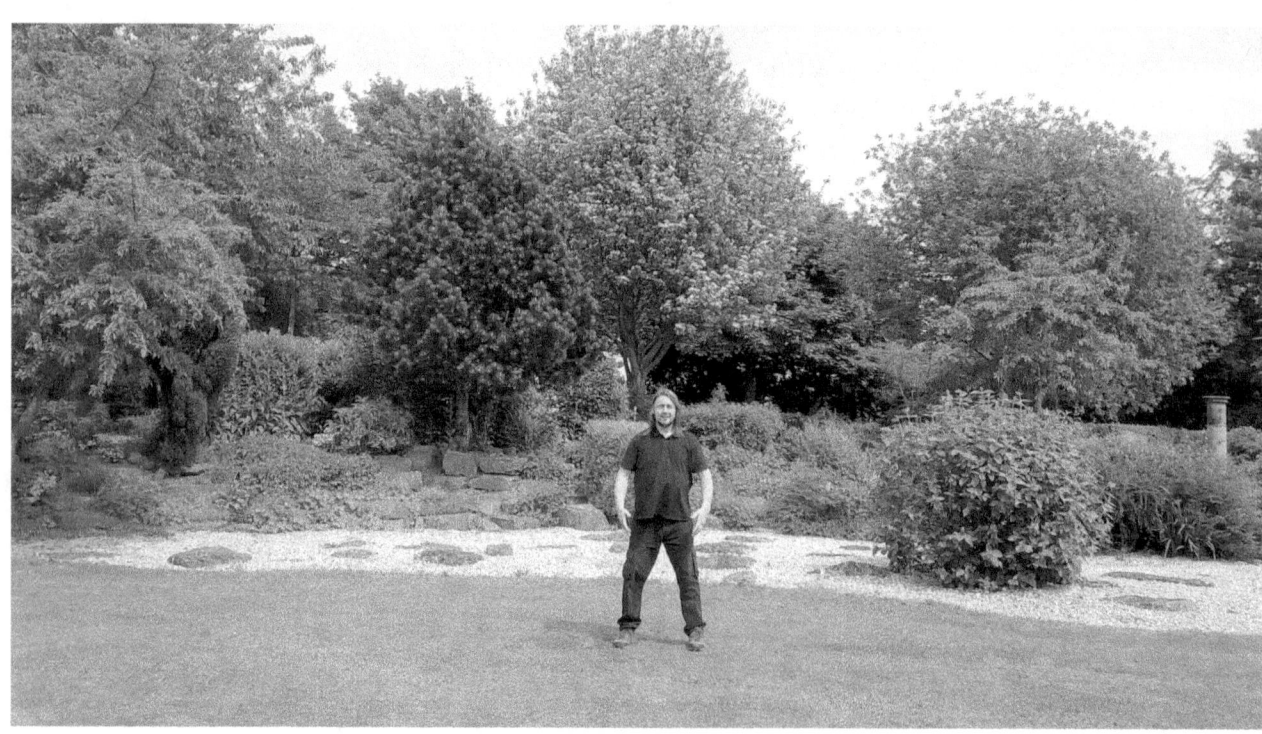

CHAPTER TEN: THE FORM MOVEMENTS DECODED

Wu Ji

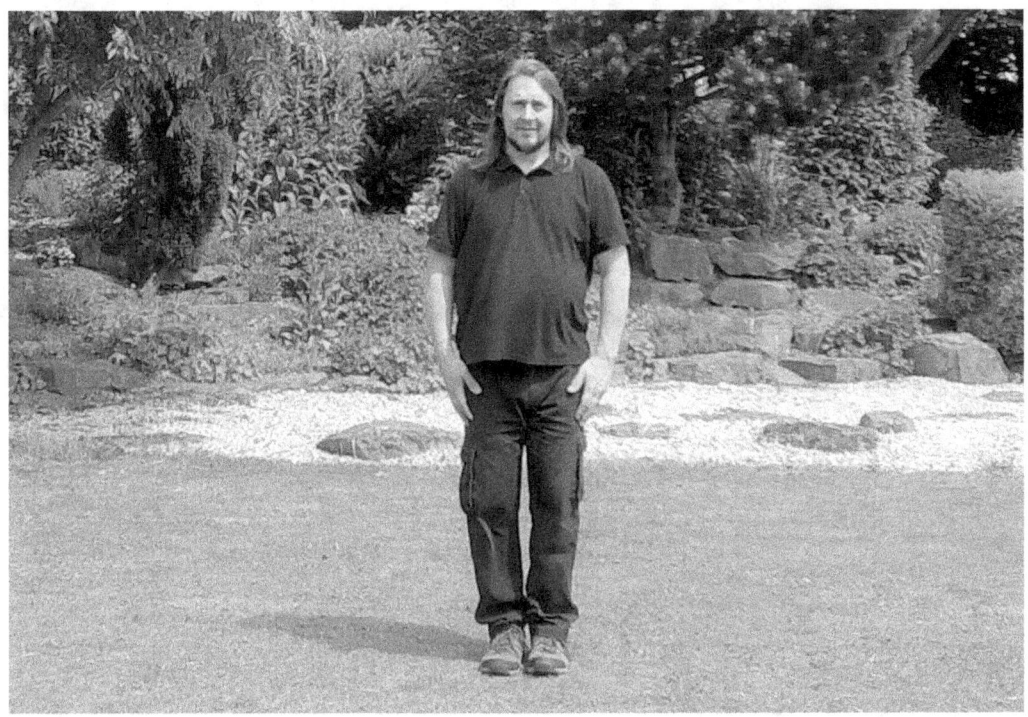

The first posture of the Tai Chi form is Wu Ji, this represents stillness and in Taoist cosmology, before Tai Chi there was Wu Ji. It is at this time you put the Tai Chi principles into place, quieting and calming your mind.

- Arms: Your arms face the corners of your torso.

- Body: In the Wu Ji posture your body is square to the front.

- Stance: Your feet are together in a V-stance.

- Weight: The weight is divided evenly between both feet.

Commencement

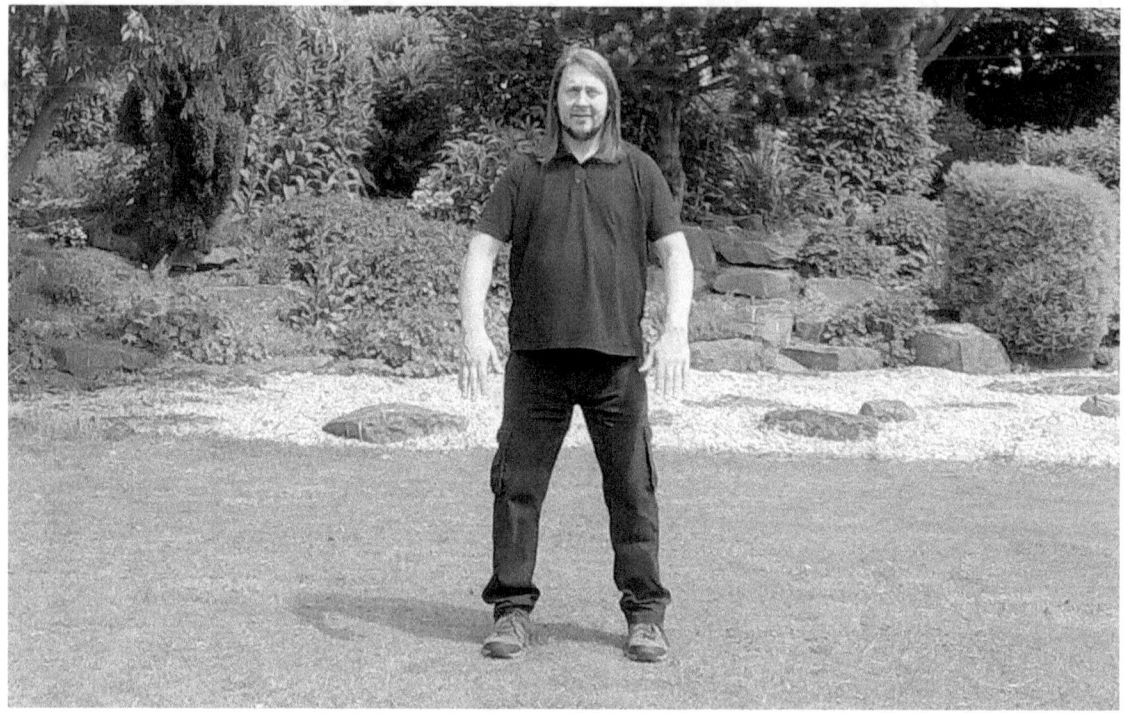

- Arm: The arms face the corners of the body and expand outward, making a small space under your armpits. Your elbow is roughly a fist distance from your ribs.

- Body: The body is square on to the front in this posture.

- Hands: The hands are in the Fair Maiden shape.

- Stance: Your feet are shoulder width apart.

- Weight: The weight is divided equally between the feet.

Heaven and Earth

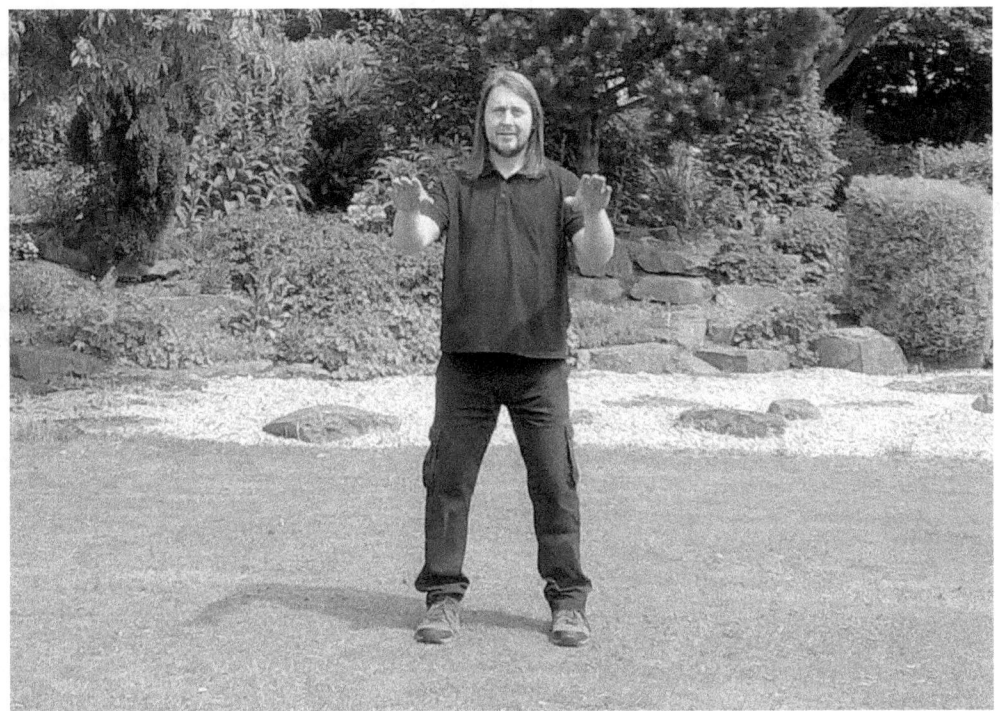

- Arms: The arms are raised up to shoulder height, and then lowered back down in this posture.

- Body: The body is square to the front.

- Hands: The hands are in the Fair Maidens hand shape.

- Stance: The stance is shoulder width and parallel.

- Weight: The weight is equal in each foot.

Ward Off Left

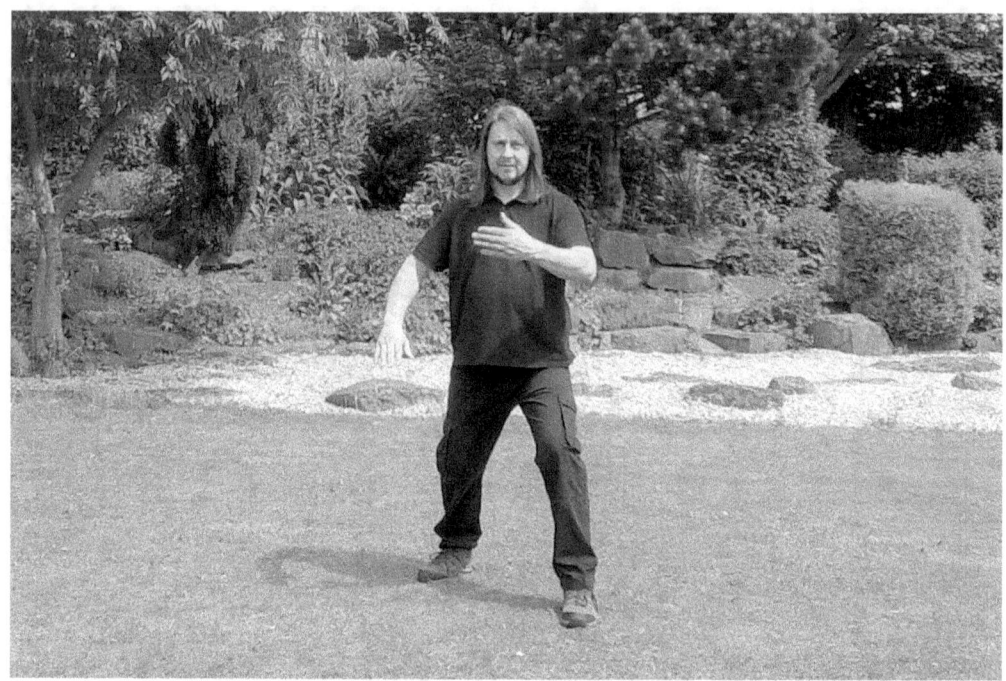

- Arms: The left arm is in front of the left upper chest, as if you are holding a large ball. The elbow is heavy and points down.

- Body: In the Ward off Left posture, the body, hips, shoulders, and torso are square.

- Hands: Both of your hands keep the Fair Maiden shape.

- Stance: Your stance in Ward Off Left is a left foot forward, Bow stance.

- Weight: This stance has seventy percent of the weight in the front foot and thirty percent in the back foot.

Ward Off Right

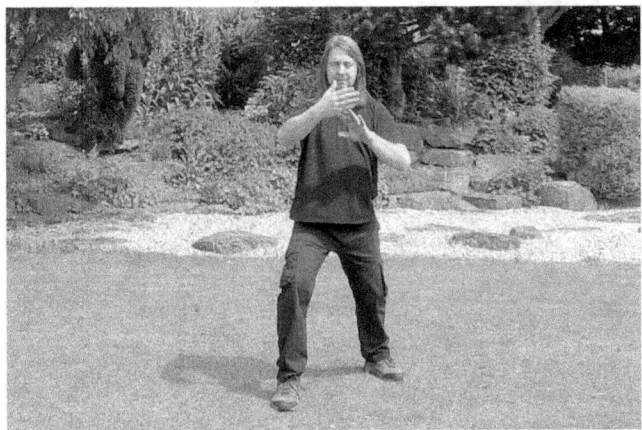

- Arms: The right arm is in front of the upper chest, at the eleven o'clock position. The left arm is in a lower position, pointing towards the left wrist.

- Body: The shoulders, torso, and hips are square to the front in this posture.

- Hands: In this posture, both of your hands keep the Fair Maidens shape.

- Stance: The stance is a right foot forward Bow stance.

- Weight: In this right Bow stance, the weight is seventy percent in the front foot and thirty percent in the back foot.

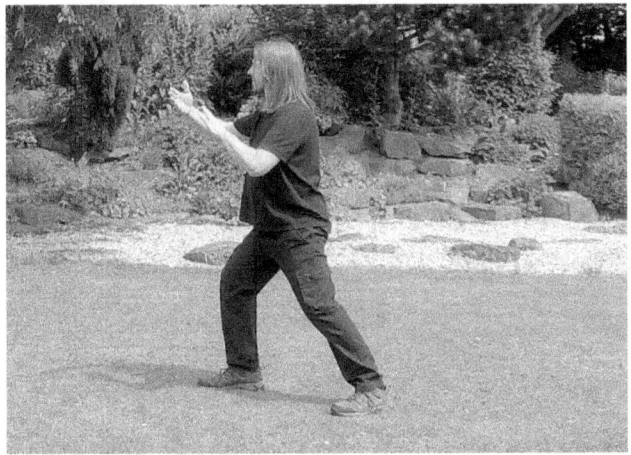

Rollback

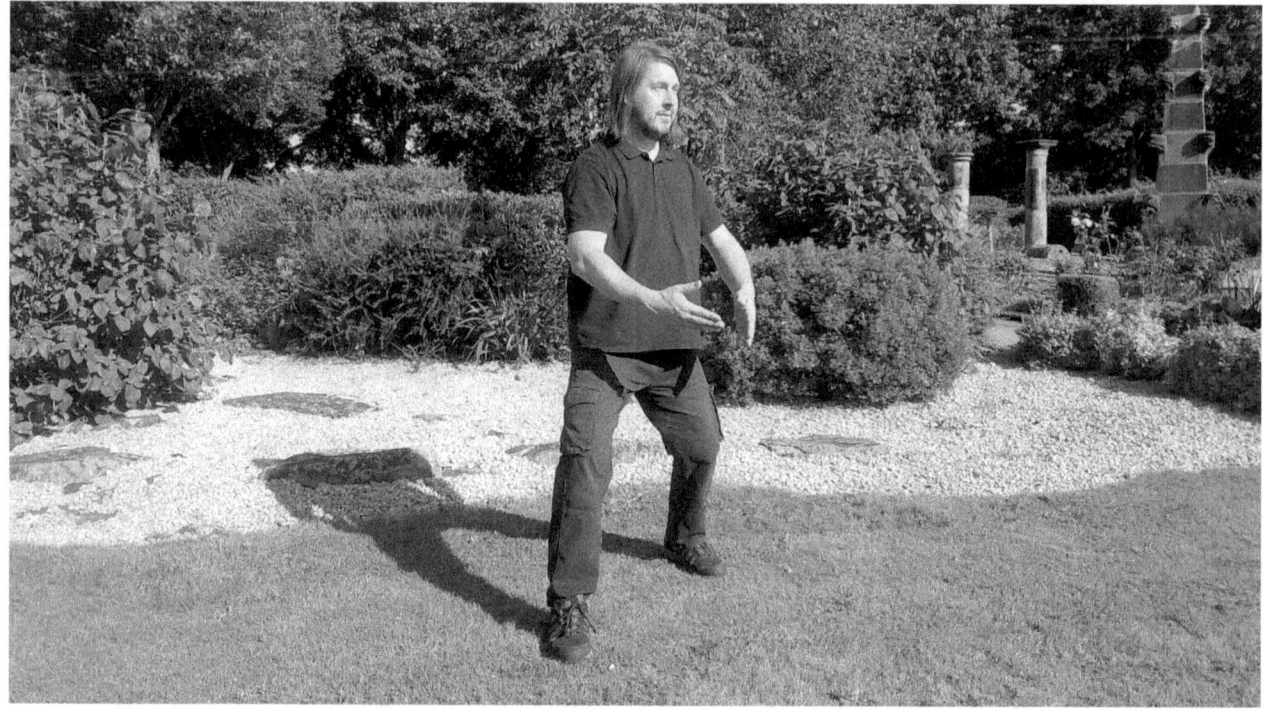

- Arms: The arms keep a rounded, ward off shape. The right arm moves down and to the left in front of your body and the left arm is out by your left side.

- Body: In the Rollback posture, you turn the body forty-five degrees to the left.

- Hands: In this posture, you keep the Fair Maidens hand shape.

- Stance: Your stance in Rollback is a right foot forward Bow stance.

- Weight: This time the weight is distributed seventy percent in the back foot and thirty in the front foot.

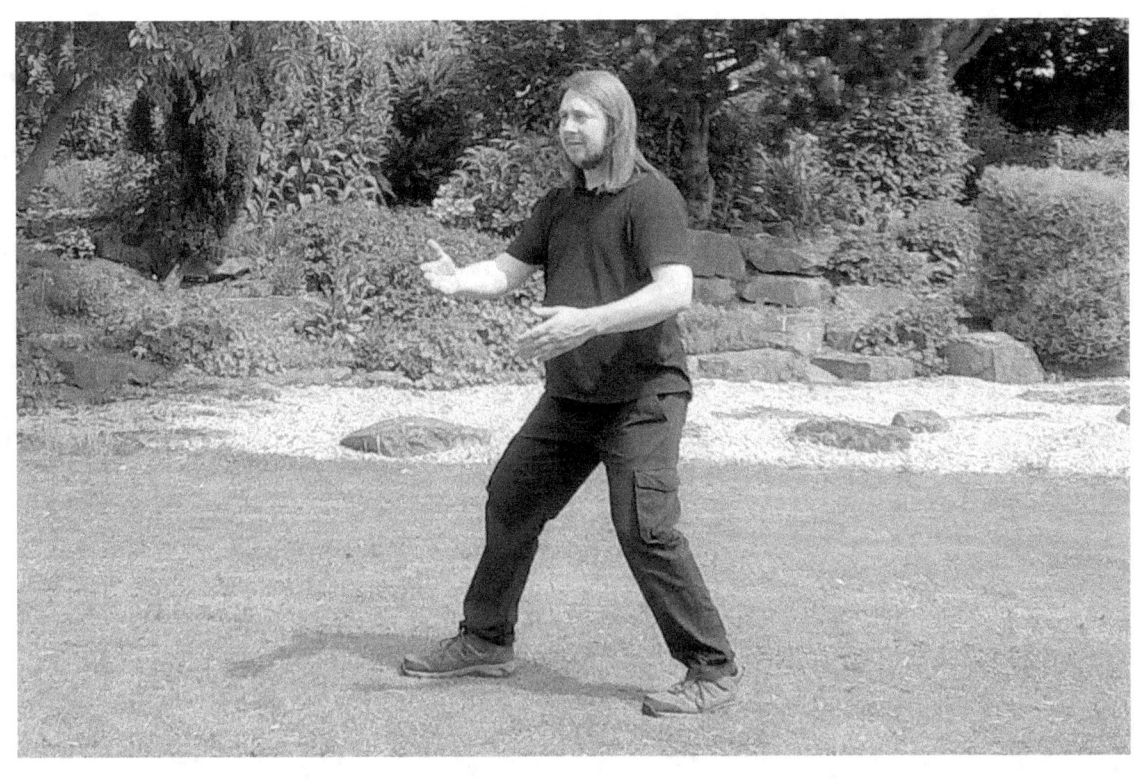

Press

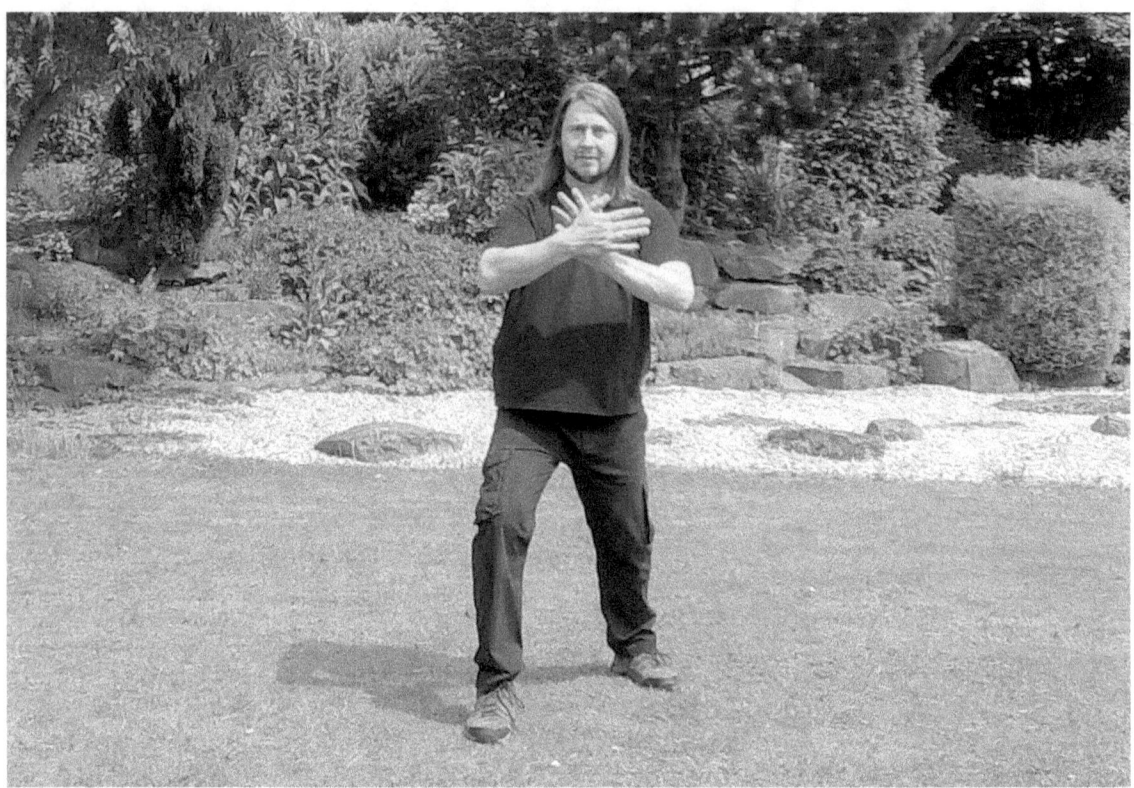

- Arms: Both arms form a triangular shape in front of the upper chest.

- Body: Your hips, torso, and shoulders are square to the front.

- Hands: In this posture, both hands keep the Fair Maidens hand shape.

- Stance: This stance is a right foot forward Bow stance.

- Weight: Your weight is seventy percent in the right front foot and thirty percent in the back foot.

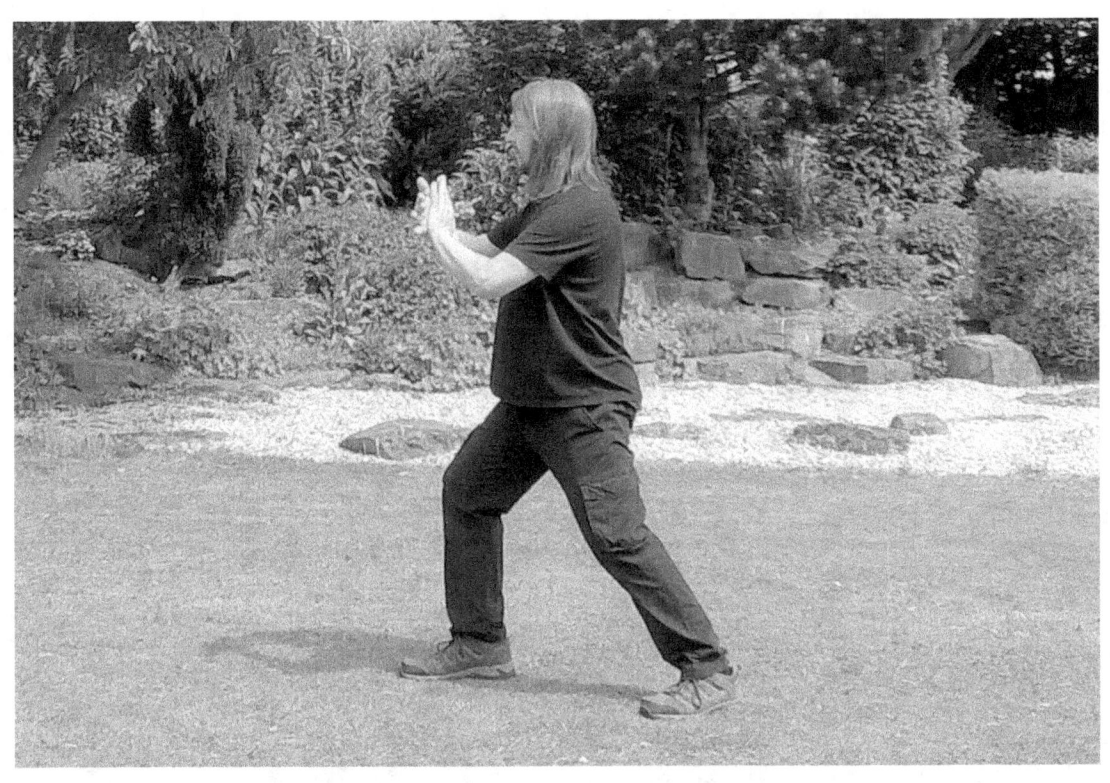

Push

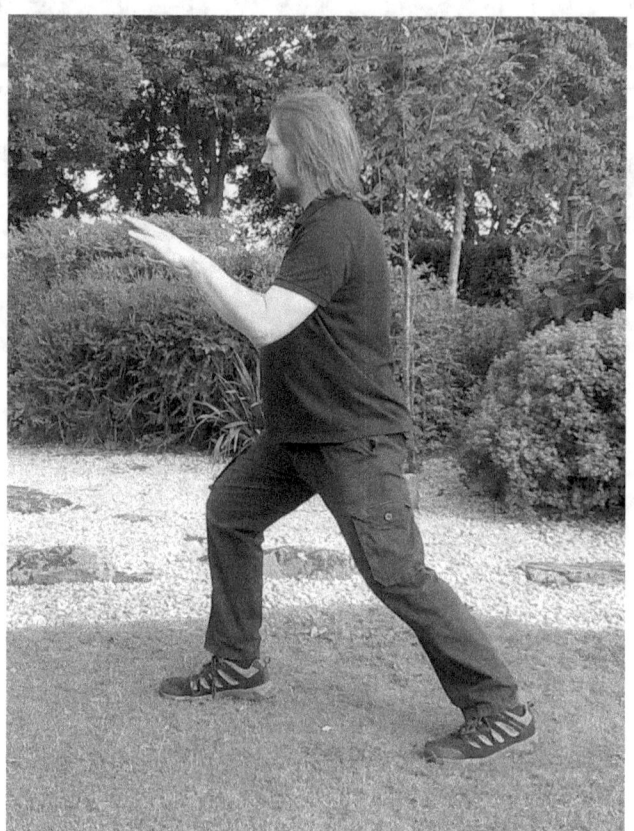

- Arms: The under arms face downward.

- Body: In this stance your body position is square.

- Hands: Your hands are in the Fair Maiden shape.

- Stance: The stance is a right forward Bow stance.

- Weight: In this posture the weight is seventy percent in the right foot and thirty percent in the left foot.

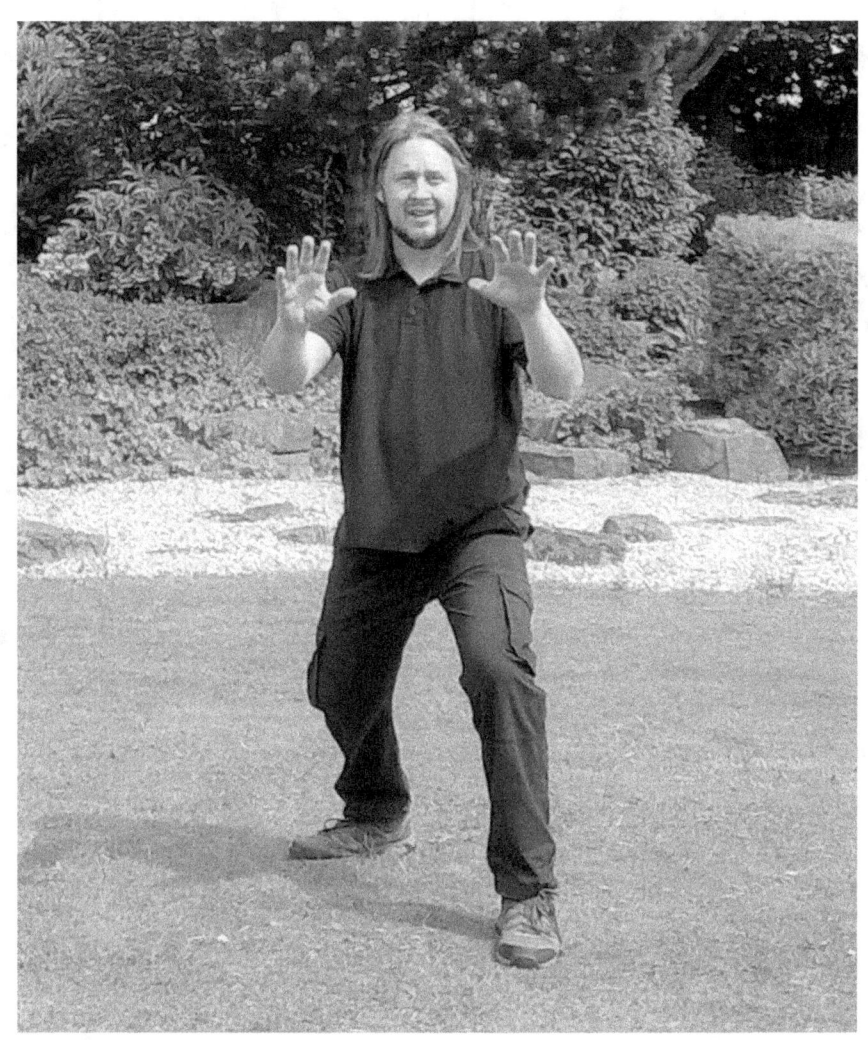

Single Whip

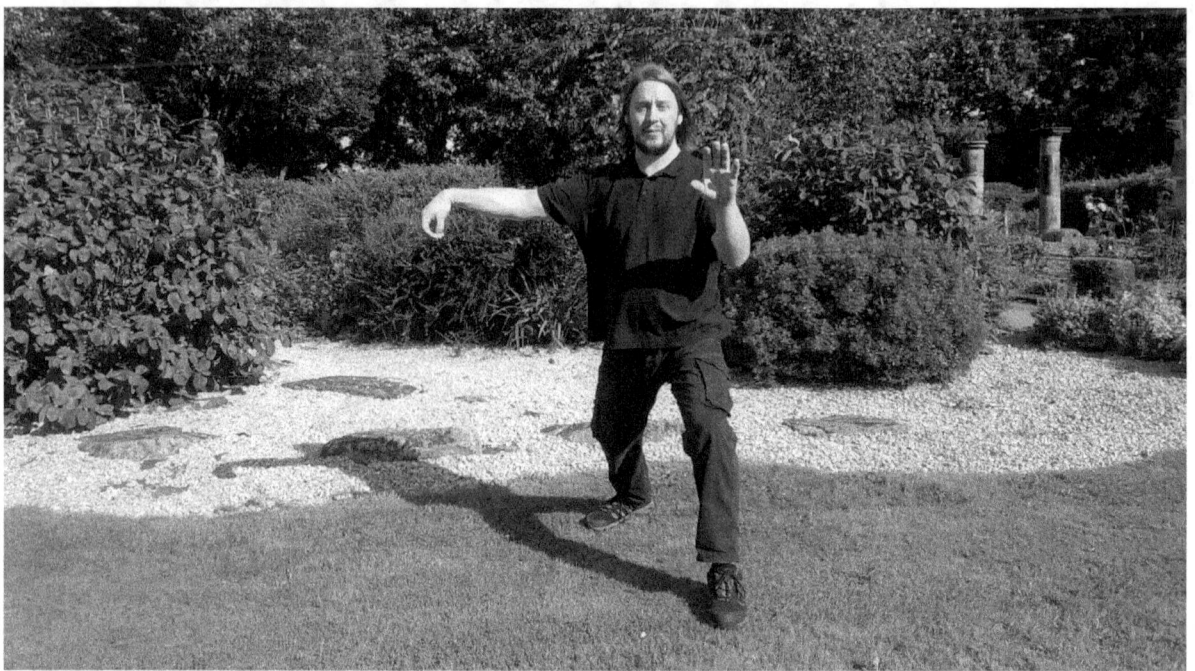

- Arms: The left arm is in front of the left side of the body. The right arm faces out from your right shoulder and is straight.

- Body: The position for your body is hips and shoulders turned slightly to the right. The central alignment of nose, chest, and navel is maintained in this posture.

- Hands: In the Single Whip posture, your right hand is in a Fair Maiden shape, in front of your left shoulder. Your left hand forms a beak, the thumb drops down and the fingertips close around it.

- Stance: This stance is a left foot forward Bow stance.

- Weight: Single Whip has seventy percent of weight in the front foot and thirty percent in the back foot.

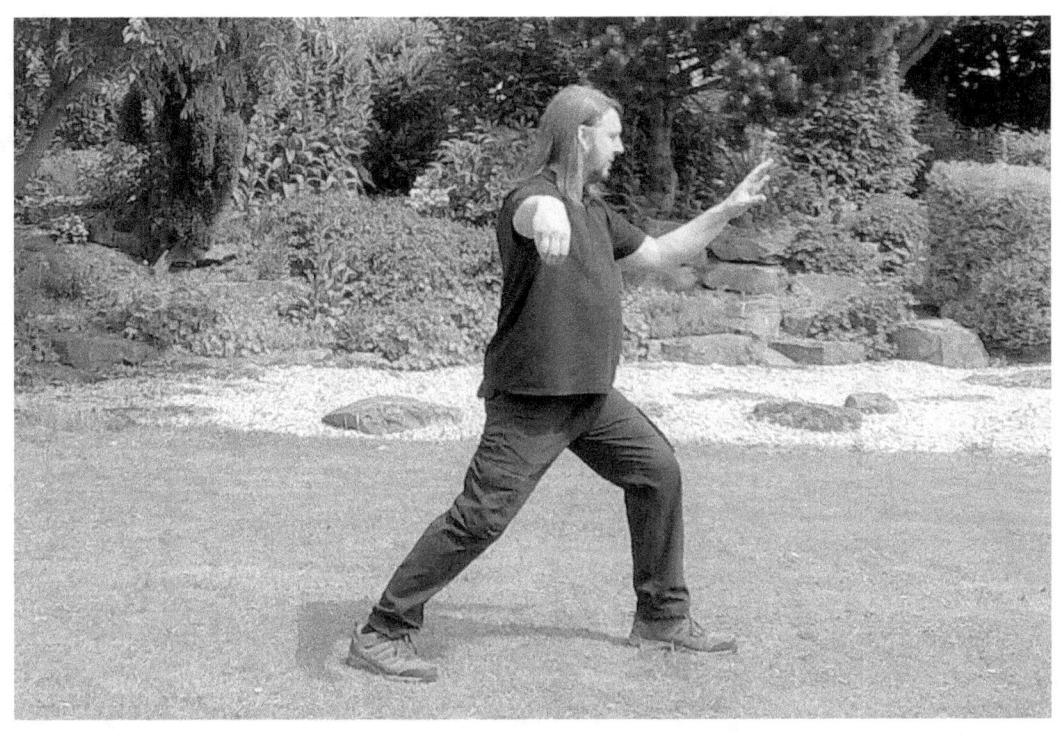

Lift Hands/Play Guitar

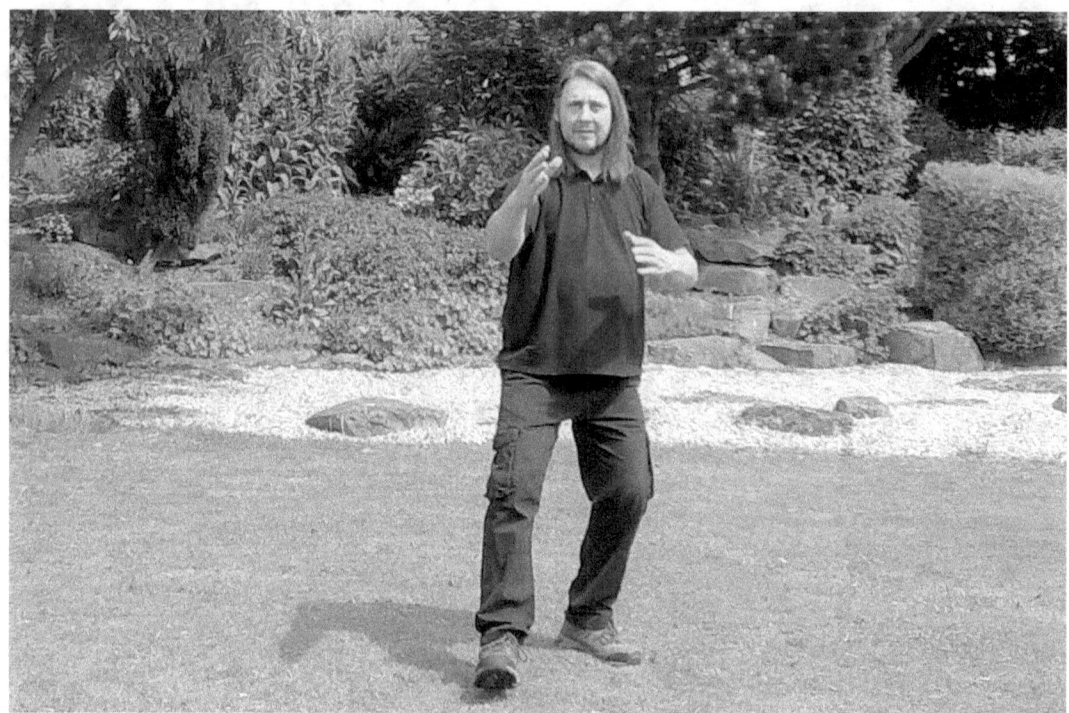

- Arms: The arms both have a rounded shape. The right forearm rising towards shoulder height, the left arm is a few inches lower.

- Body: The body is turned to your left corner with the centre of your chest and navel aligned.

- Hands: The left and right hands are in the Fair Maiden shape.

- Stance: The stance is a Cat stance.

- Weight: In the Lift Hands posture, the weight is ninety percent in the back foot and ten per cent in the front foot.

Pluck

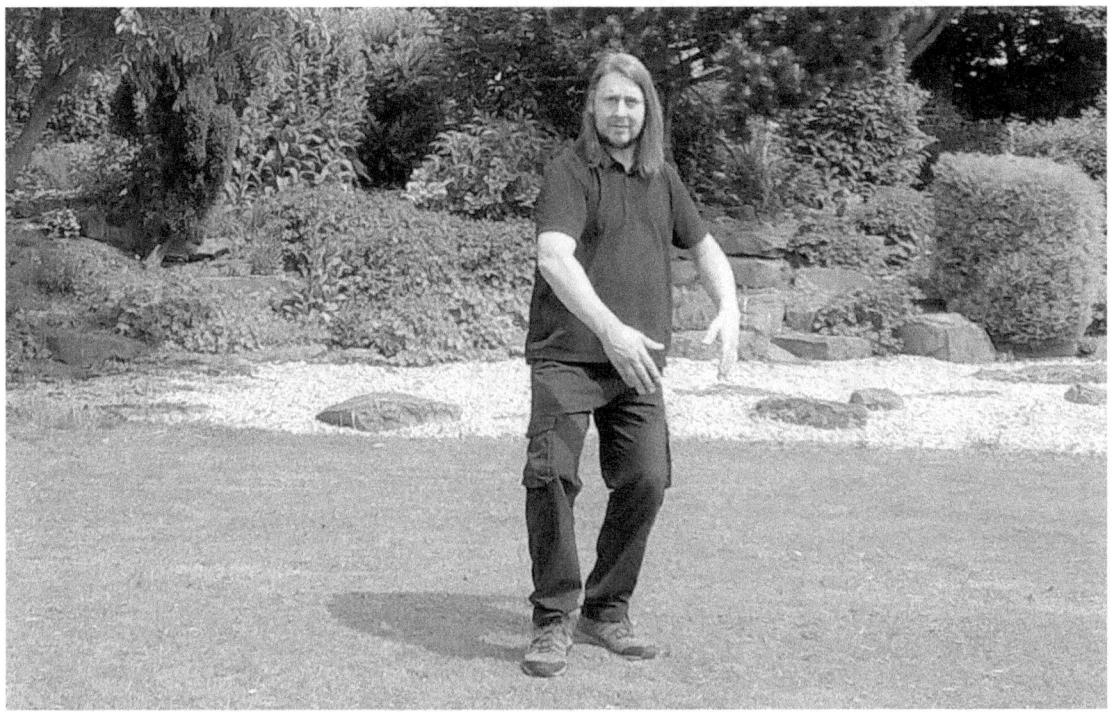

- Arms: In the Pluck posture, your right forearm is in front of your lower abdomen and the left arm is by your left hip.

- Body: Your body is diagonal.

- Hands: The hands keep the Fair Maidens hand shape.

- Stance: The stance is a Cat stance.

- Weight: Ninety percent of the weight is in the left foot and ten percent is in the front foot.

Elbow/Shoulder Stroke

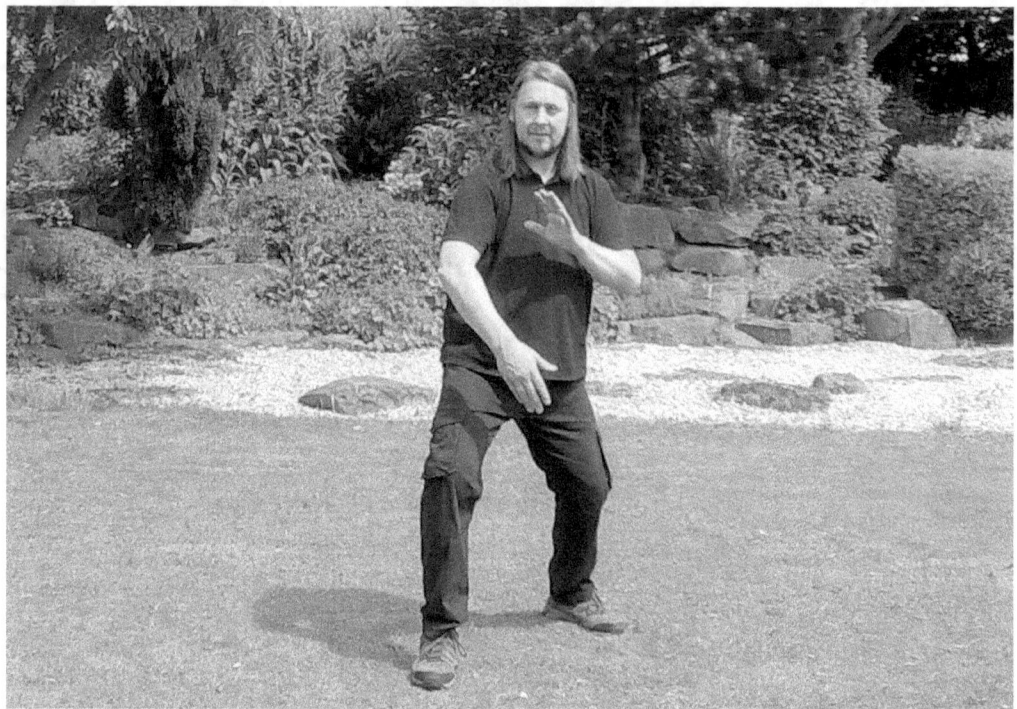

- Arms: The right arm points down and is in front of the right side of the body and the left arm is in front of the left side.

- Body: The body is diagonal throughout this movement.

- Hands: When performing Elbow/Shoulder Stroke both hands are in the Fair Maidens shape.

- Stance: The stance for Elbow/ Shoulder Stroke is a right foot forward Bow stance.

- Weight: In this posture, the front foot has seventy percent of the body weight in it and the back foot has thirty percent.

White Crane Spreads its Wings

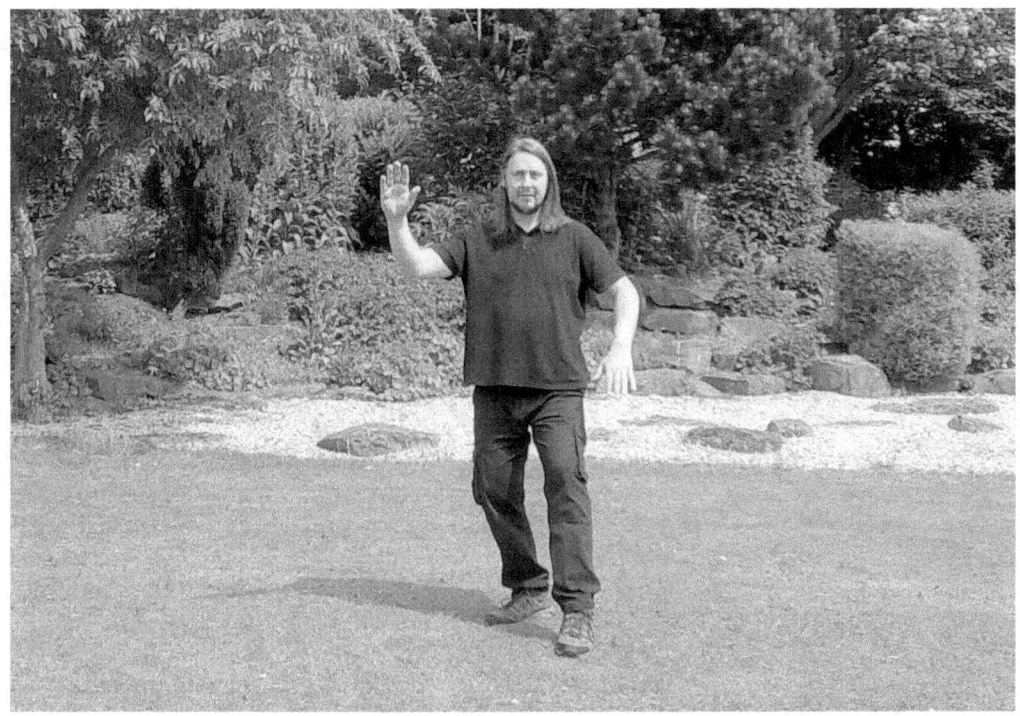

- Arms: In this posture, the right arm is at forehead height and out to the right side. The left forearm clears the left leg and points to the floor.

- Body: The body is square to the front, shoulders, torso, and hips aligned.

- Hands: In, White Crane spreads its Wings; the hands are in the Fair Maidens shape.

- Stance: This posture is a left foot forward Cat stance.

- Weight: Ninety percent of the weight is in the right rear foot and ten percent is in the left front foot.

Brush Knee and Push

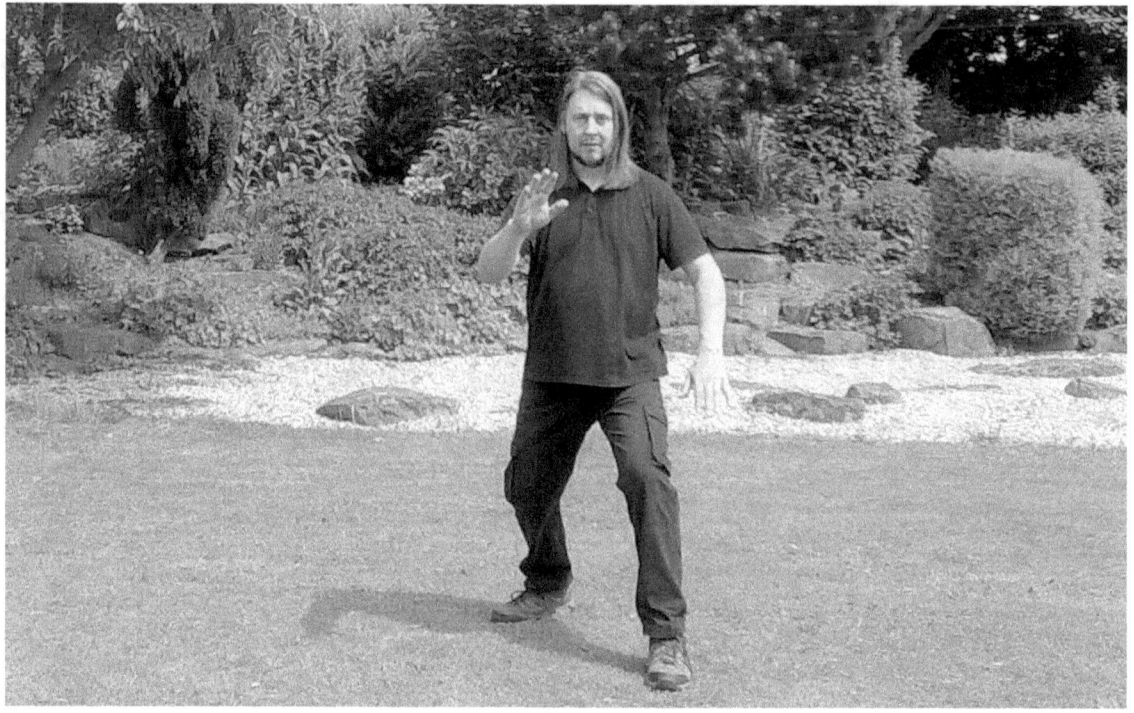

- Arms: In Brush Knee and Push the right arm is in front of chest, the left arm rests at the outside edge of the left leg.

- Body: The body alignment is square to the front.

- Hands: In this posture, both hands are in the Fair Maidens hand shape.

- Stance: The stance for this movement is a left foot forward Bow stance.

- Weight: In Brush Knee and Push, the weight is seventy percent in the front foot and thirty percent in the back foot.

Parry and Punch

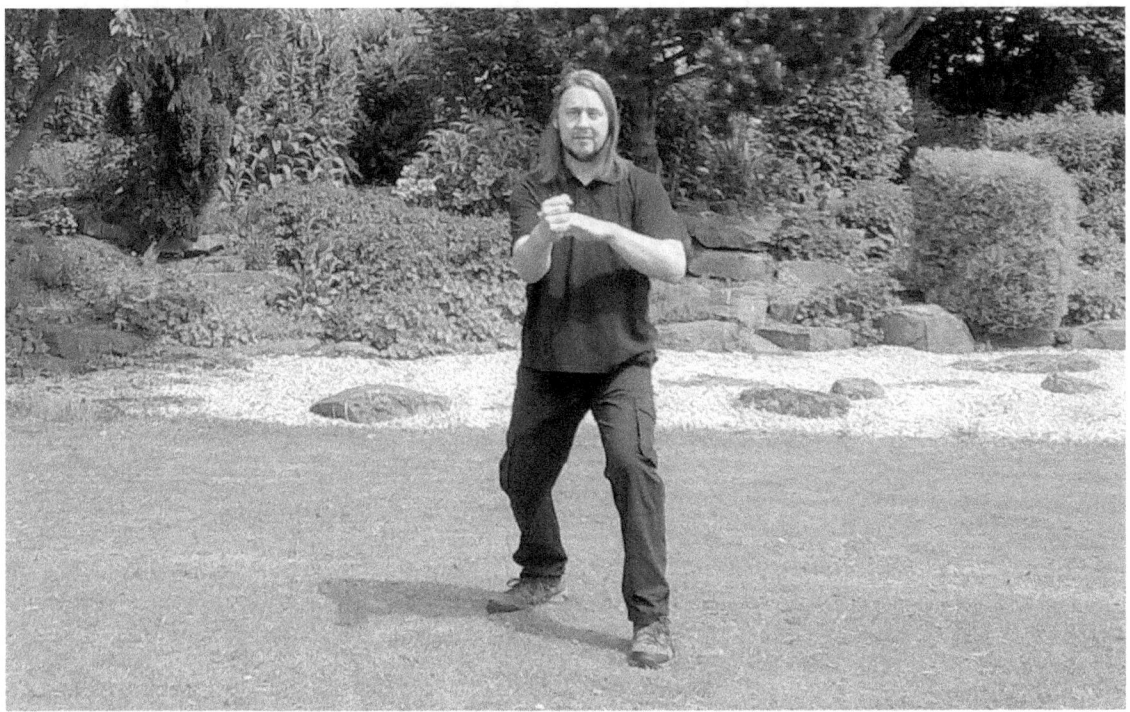

- Arms: The left and right arms are in front of the centreline of your body.

- Body: In this posture, your hips, shoulders, and torso are square.

- Hands: The left hand has a Fair Maiden palm shape; the right hand forms a relaxed fist.

- Stance: Your stance is a right foot forward, Bow stance.

- Weight: The weighting for this form movement is seventy percent in the left foot and thirty in the right foot.

Apparent Close Up

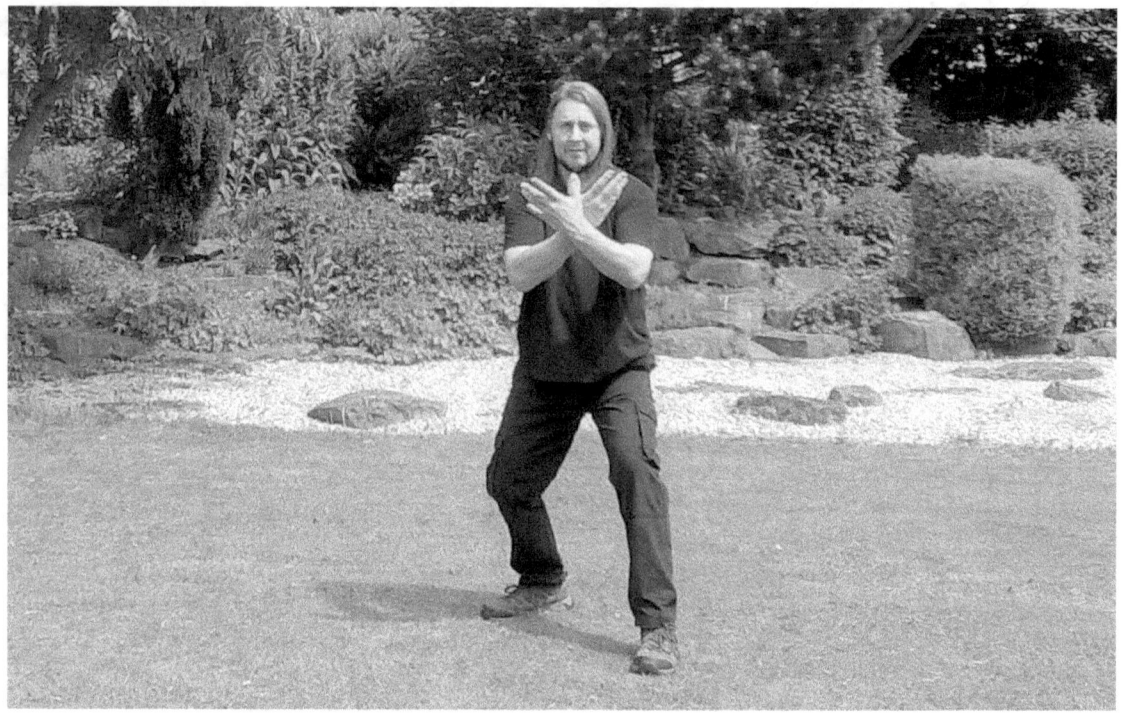

- Arms: Both of your arms cross at the wrists in front of the upper chest. Your left arm is on the outside of the right arm and the outsides of the forearms face forward.

- Body: When in Apparent Close Up, your body is square to the front.

- Hands: The hands keep the Fair Maiden shape in this posture.

- Stance: The stance for Apparent Close Up, is a left foot forward Bow stance.

- Weight: In this form movement, the body weight is thirty per cent in the left foot and seventy percent in the right foot.

Seal the Knot

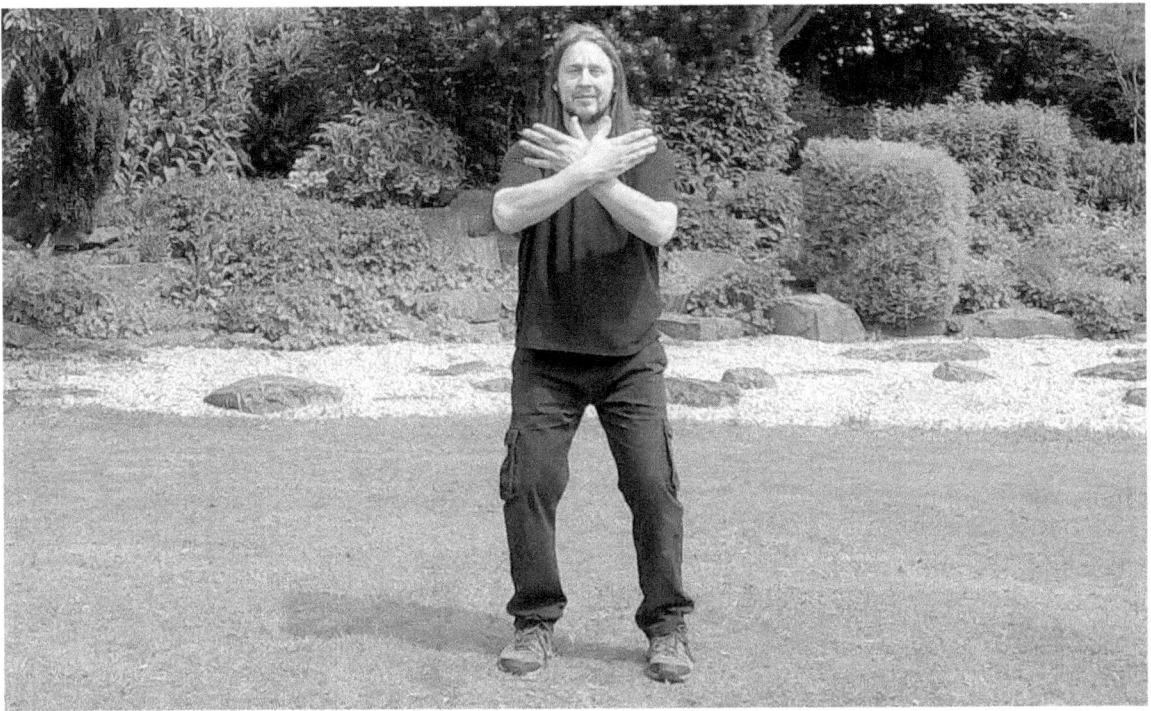

- Arms: Your arms cross at the wrists, forming a triangle in front of the upper chest; your right arm is on the outside and the tops of the forearms face forward.

- Body: The position of the body is square, hips, torso and shoulders in alignment.

- Hands: You should keep your hands in the Fair Maiden shape in this posture.

- Stance: This form movement is a parallel stance.

- Weight: In close up the weight is equal between the feet.

Fist Under Elbow

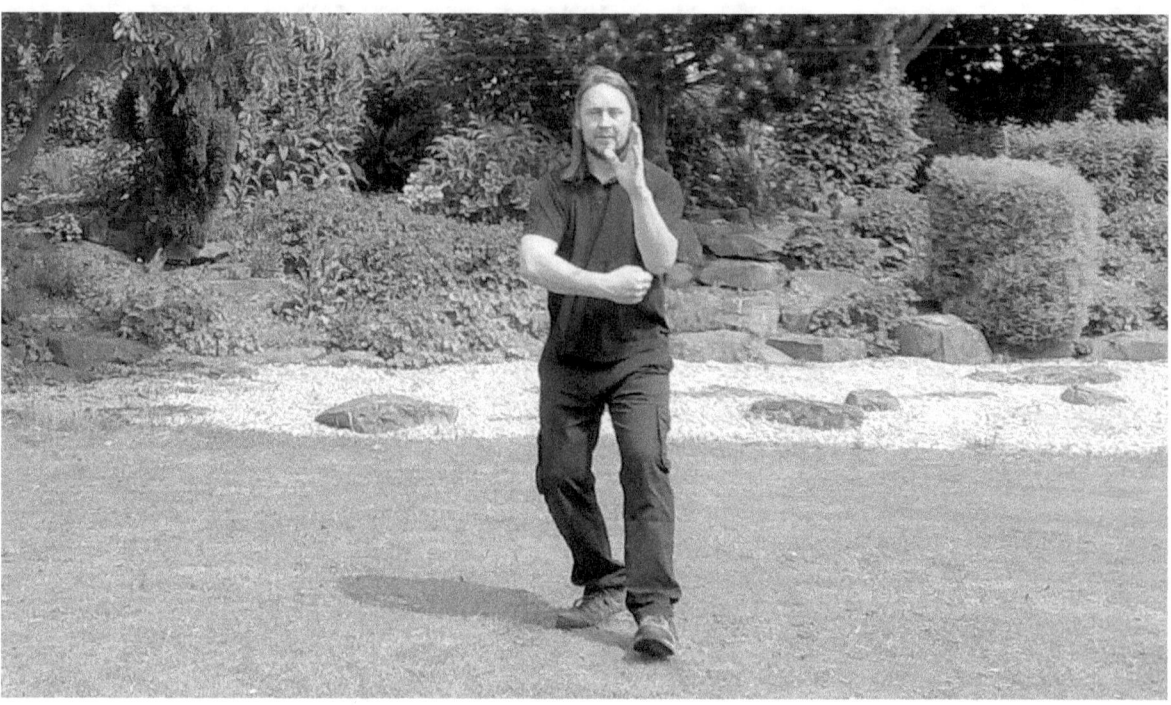

- Arms: The left arm points upwards and the right arm is in a horizontal position across the body.

- Body: In this posture, the body position is square to the front.

- Hands: When in Fist Under Elbow, the left hand keeps the Fair Maidens shape and the right hand forms a relaxed fist.

- Stance: The form movement of Fist Under Elbow, has a toes up Cat stance.

- Weight: In this Cat stance, your weight is ninety percent in the right foot and ten percent in the left foot.

Repulse Monkeys

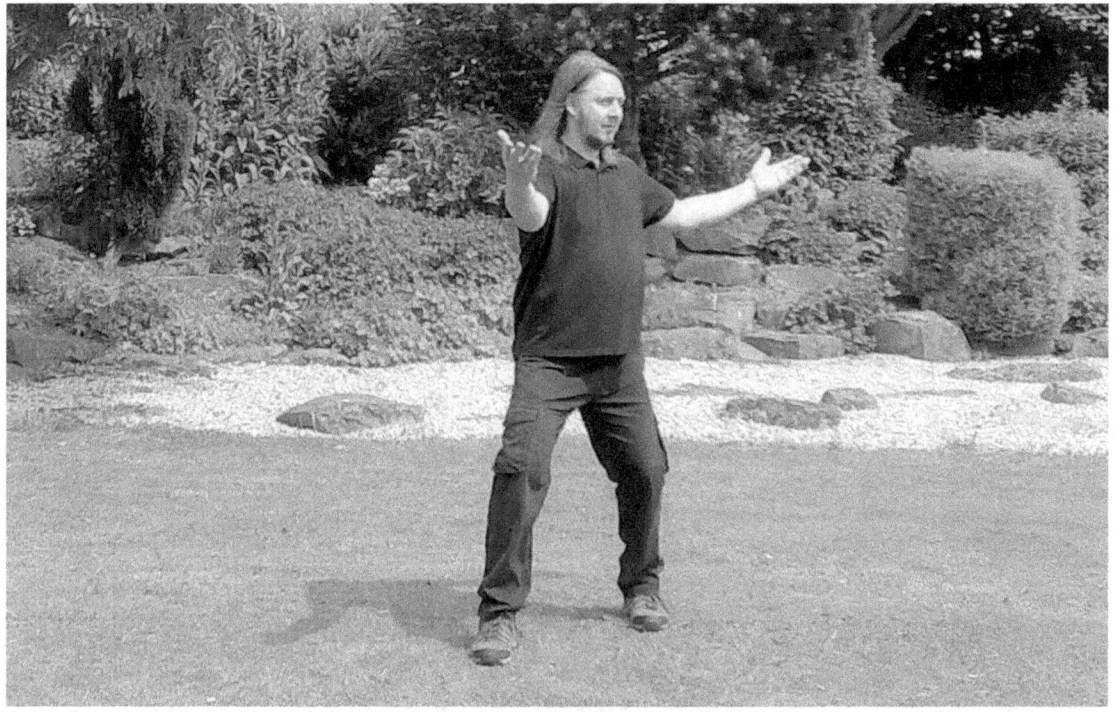

- Arms: The arms in this posture are pushing forwards and pulling back.

- Body: The body alternates between square to the front and diagonal.

- Hands: Fair Maidens palm.

- Stance: Back, Bow Stance.

- Weight: Your weight is seventy percent in the back foot and thirty percent in the front foot.

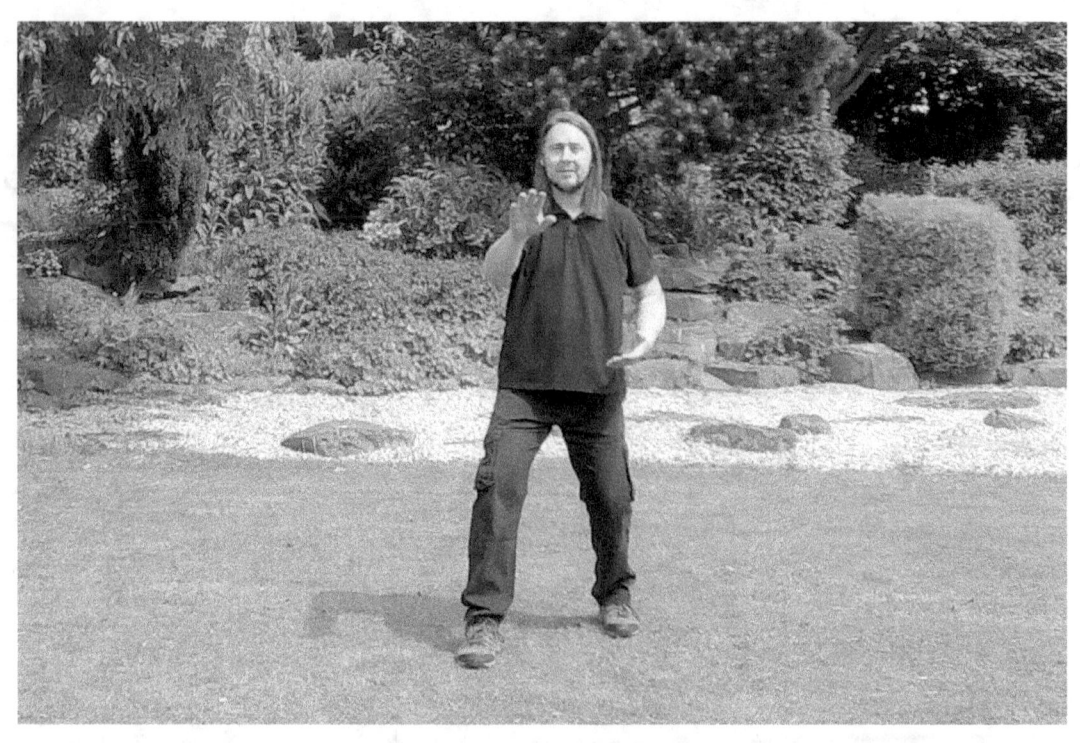

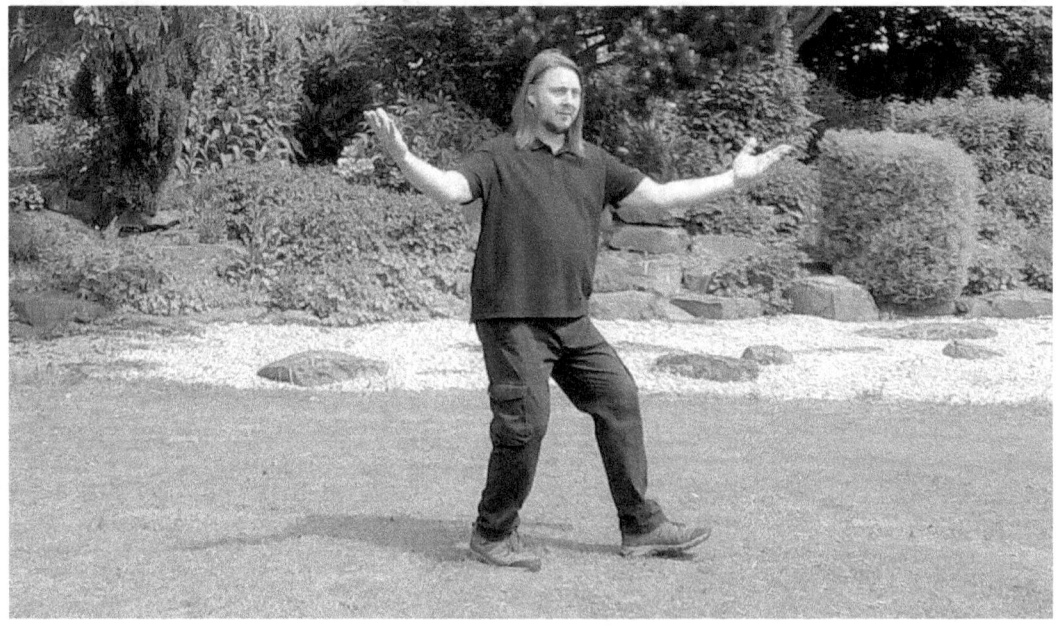

Diagonal Flying

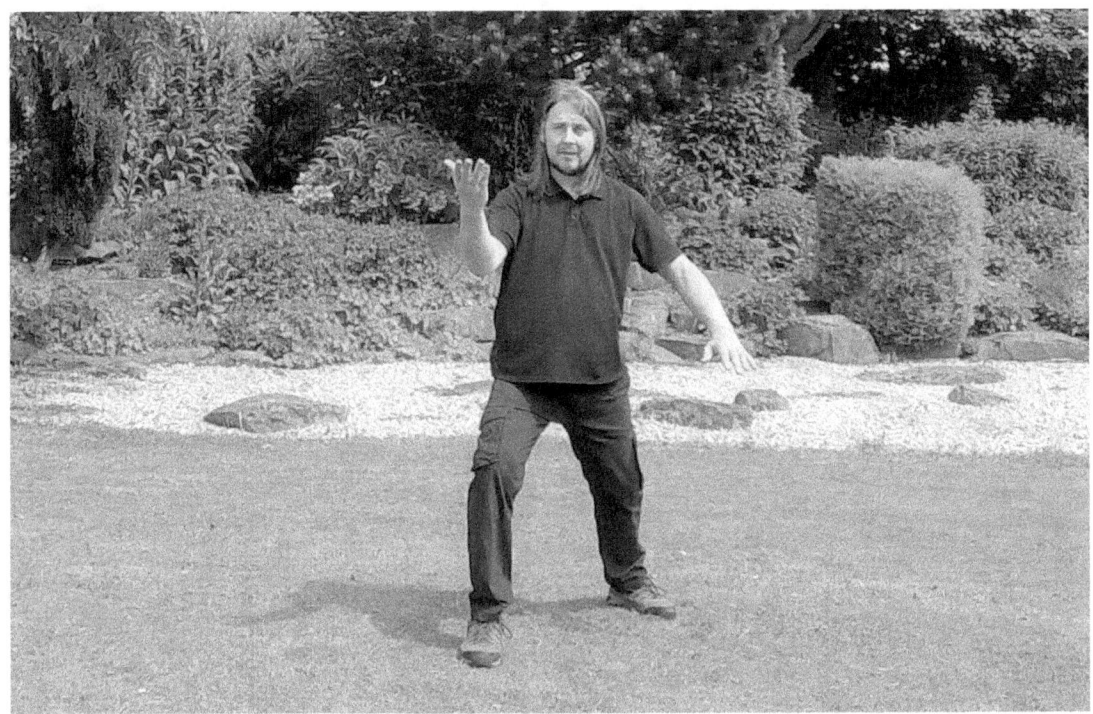

- Arms: The left arm is at the left side of the hip.

- Body: The body is square to the front.

- Hands: The hands are in the Fair Maidens shape, the right hand palm up and the left hands palm facing down.

- Stance: The stance is a right foot forward Bow stance.

- Weight: The body weight is seventy percent in the right foot and thirty percent in the left foot.

Wave Hands Like Clouds

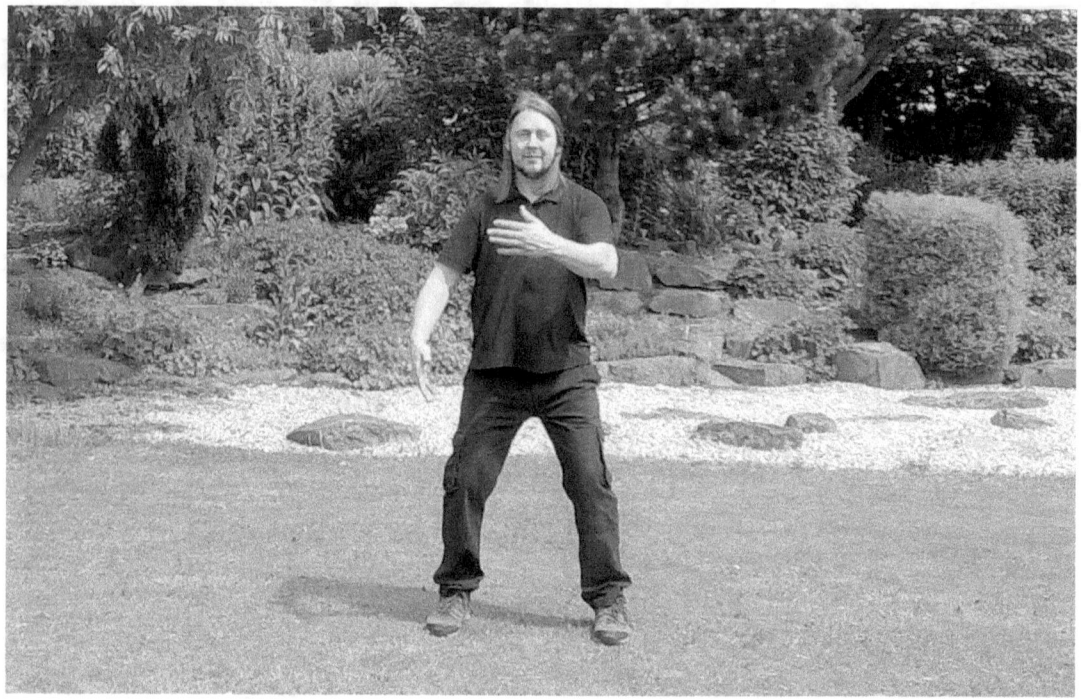

Waving Hands Like Clouds is a parallel feet stance. Turn your body from corner to corner, while keeping your centreline. Your hands make a Warding Off shape with the upper hand and scooping shape with the lower hand, when facing forward. When your body is turned to the side, you make a hold the ball shape.

- Arms: Ward Off, scooping and hold the ball.

- Body: Square and diagonal.

- Hands: Fair Maiden.

- Stance: Feet parallel.

- Weight: Your weight shifts fully from one leg to the other as you turn from side to side in Wave Hands.

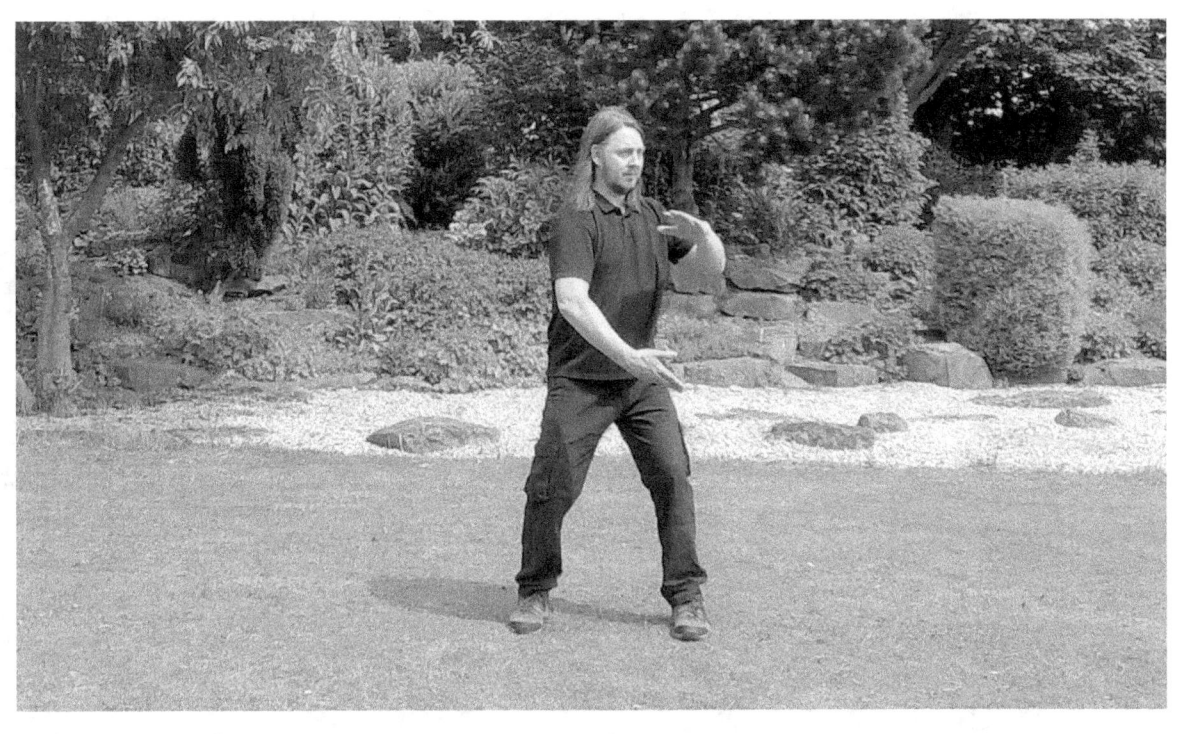

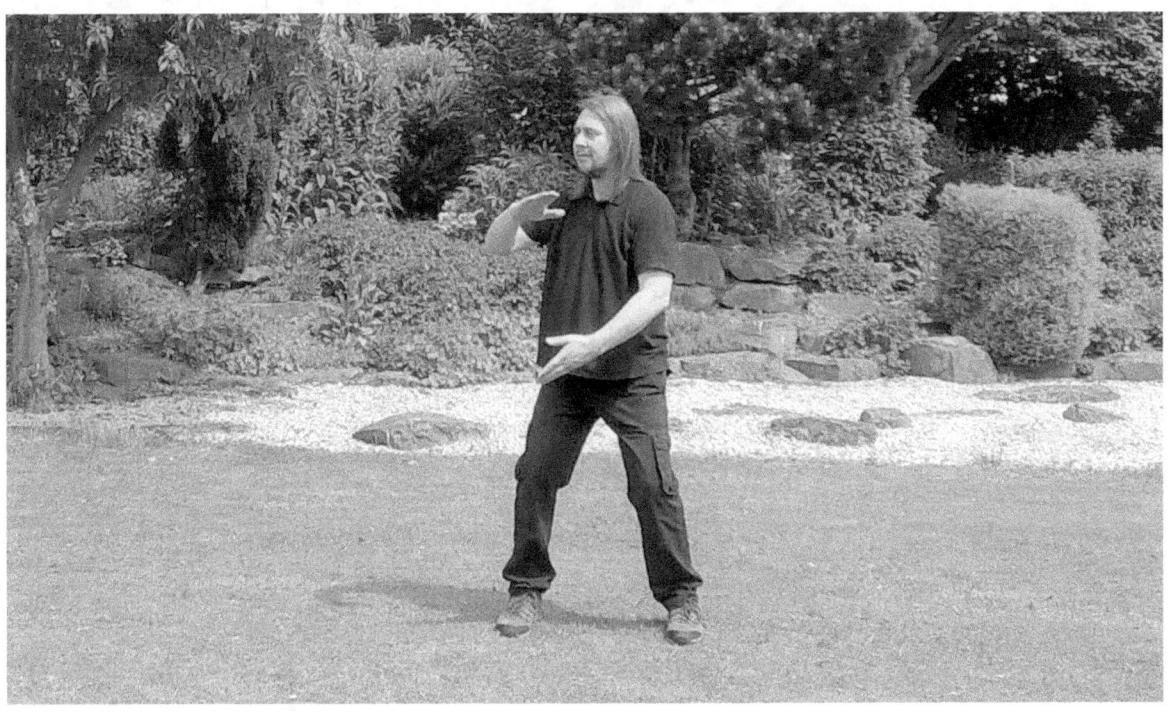

Snake Creeps Down

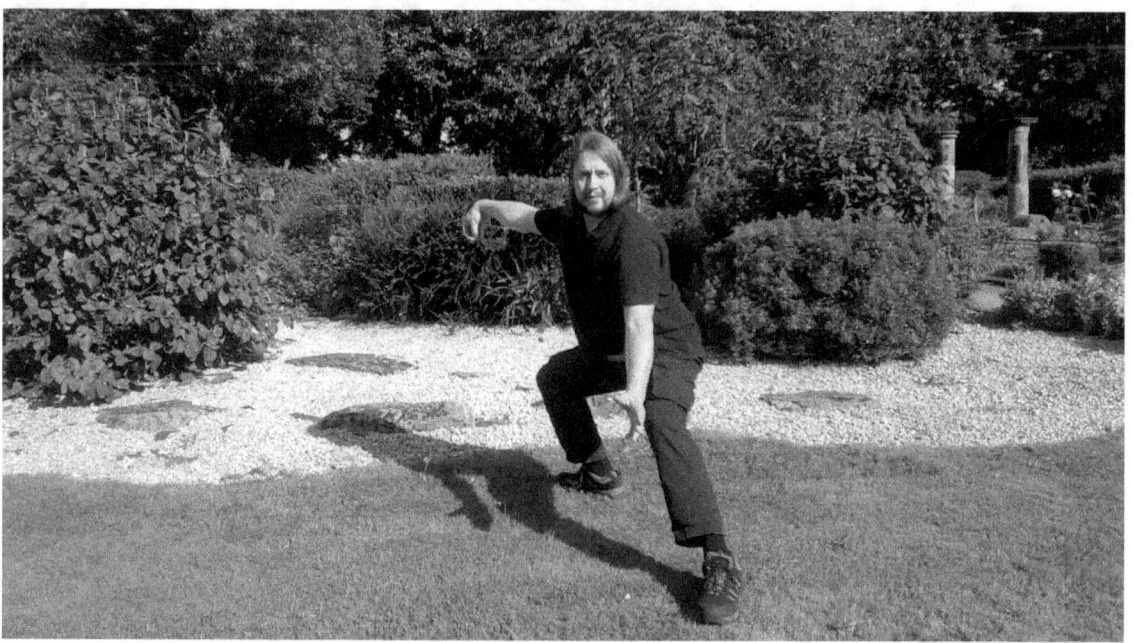

- Arms: The right arm is straightened, but unlocked at the elbow.

- Body: The body is diagonal; you must maintain your alignment of the center of the chest and navel.

- Hands: In Snake Creeps Down, the right hand makes a beak shape and the left hand is in the Fair Maidens hand shape.

- Stance: Starting in a left foot forward Bow stance, it changes to left toes in and right toes turned out.

- Weight: In this posture, the weight changes from seventy percent of the weight in the front foot. It changes to the back foot.

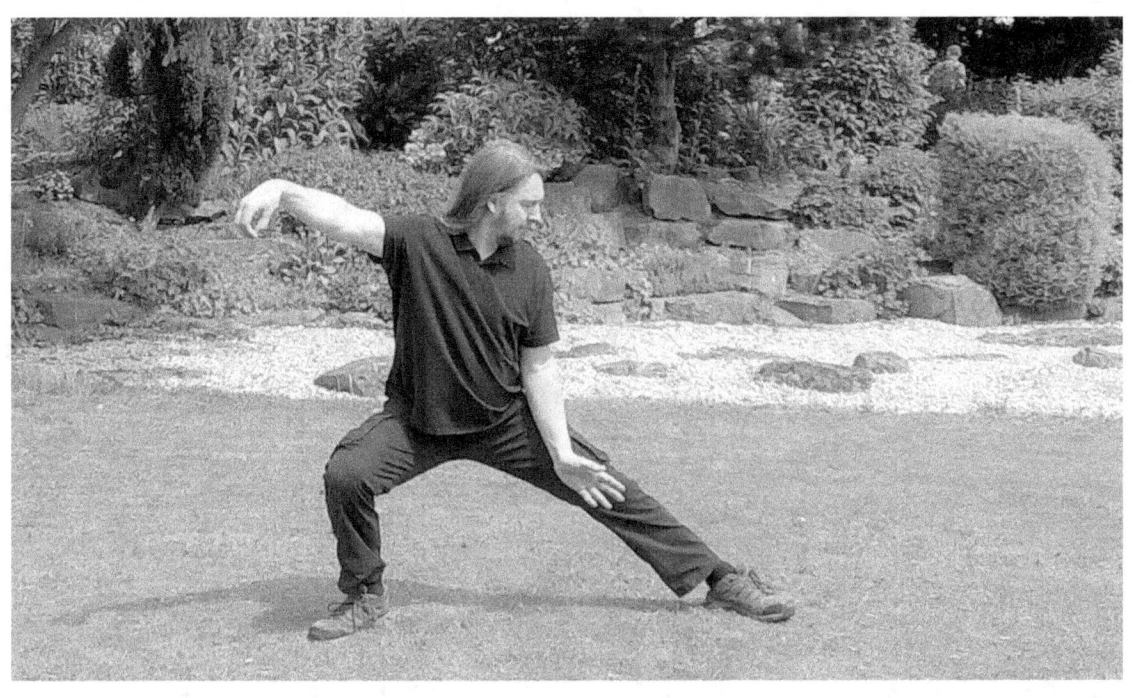

Golden Phoenix Stands on Left and Right Legs

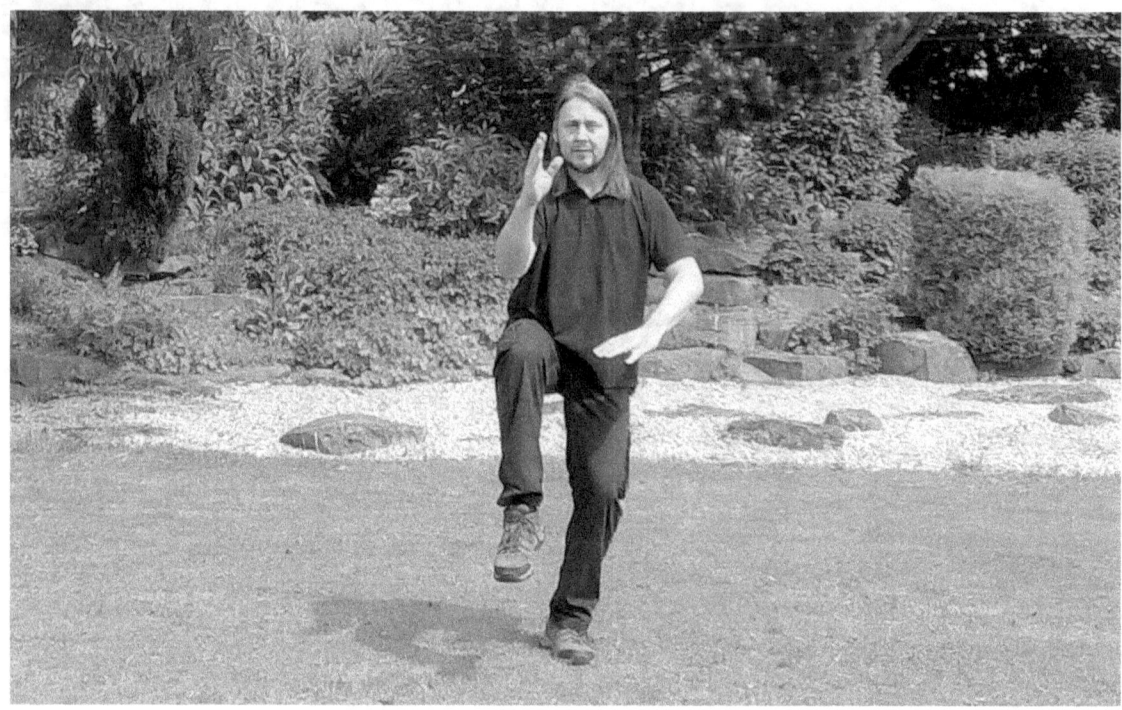

- Arms: In Golden Phoenix Stands on the Left Leg, the right arm points upwards, and the left arm curves in and down across the front of the left hip.

   In Golden Phoenix Stands on Right Leg the left arm points upwards and the right arm curves in and down across the front of the right hip.

- Body: The body, hips, shoulders, and torso are all square.

- Hands: The hands are in the Fair Maidens shape.

- Stance: This is a single legged stance.

- Weight: The weight is one hundred percent in your left leg in Golden Phoenix Stands on left leg and one hundred percent in the right leg in Golden Phoenix stands on right leg.

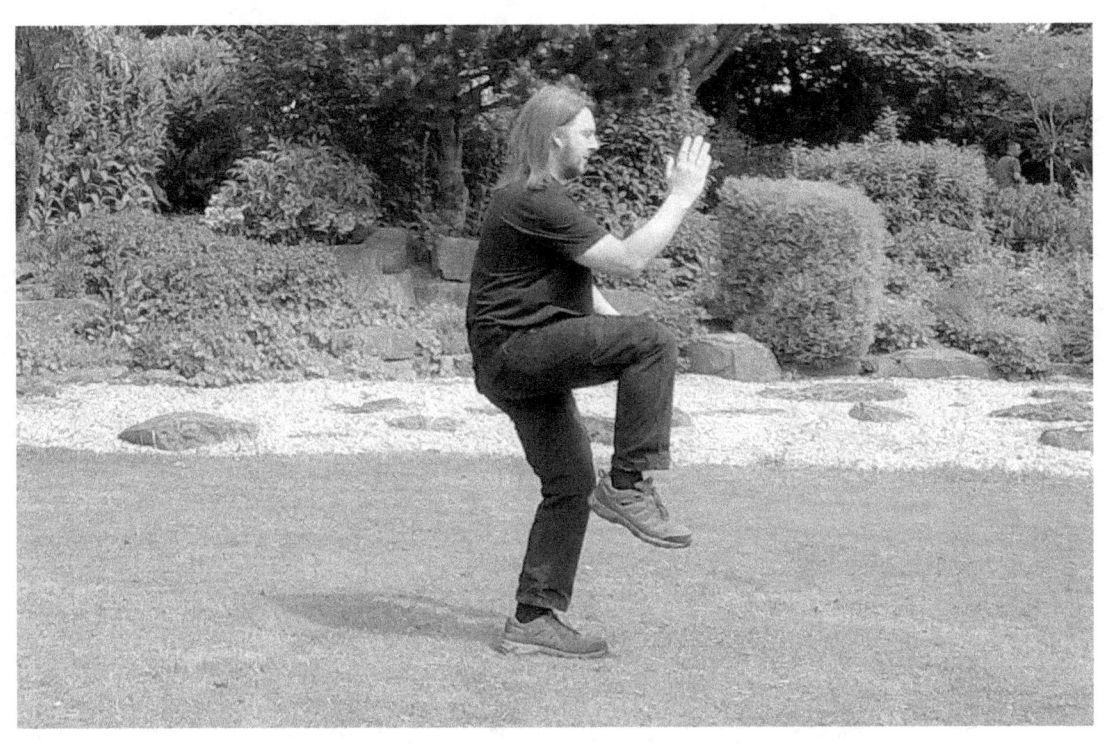

Separate and Kick with Right Foot and Left Foot

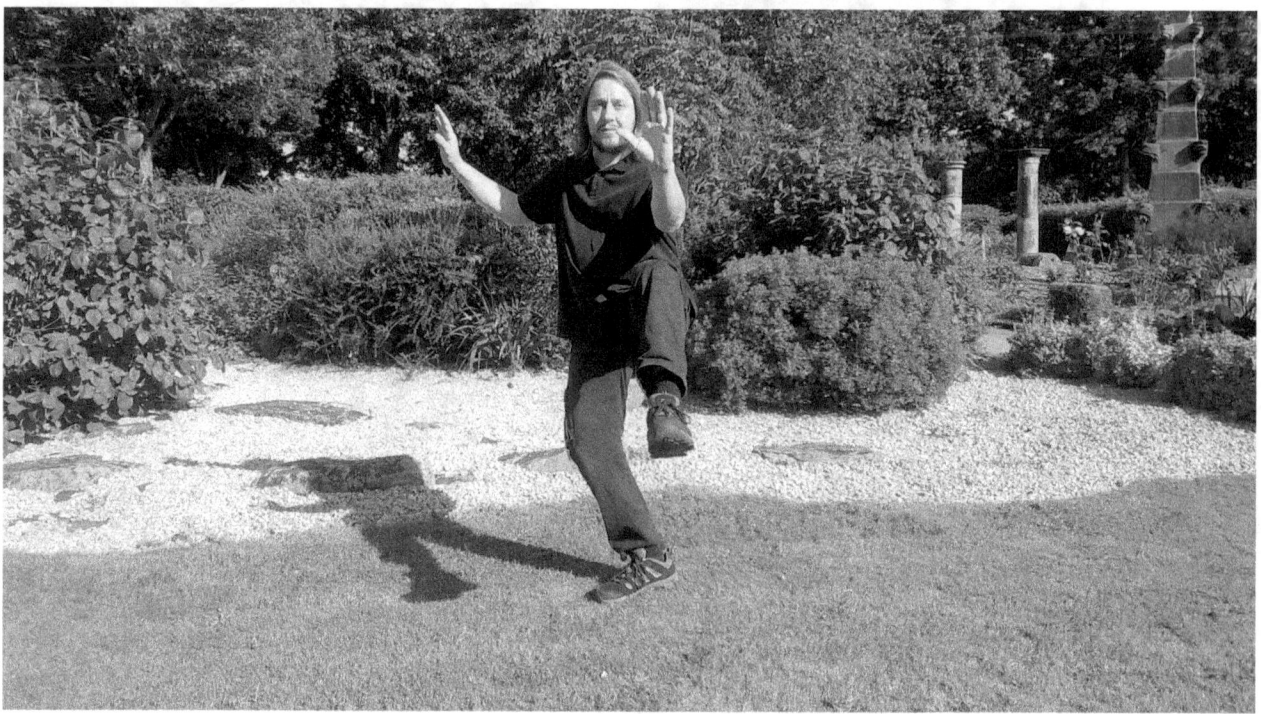

- Arms: Both of your arms opened out to the side and the forearms point upward.

- Body: The body position for this posture is diagonal.

- Hands: The fingers point upward in this posture and are in the Fair Maiden's hand configuration.

- Stance: Separate and Kick is a single legged stance.

- Weight: The weight is one hundred percent in the supporting leg.

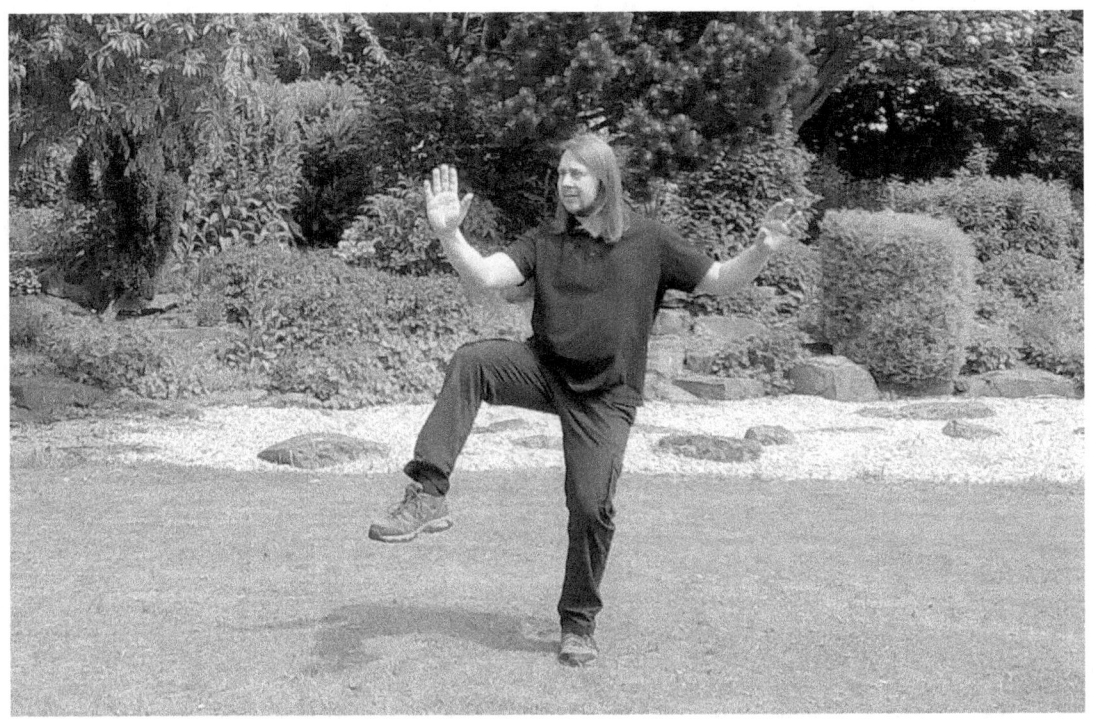

The instructions for the form movement Separate and Kick with right foot are the same as for the left foot.

Turn and Kick with Heel

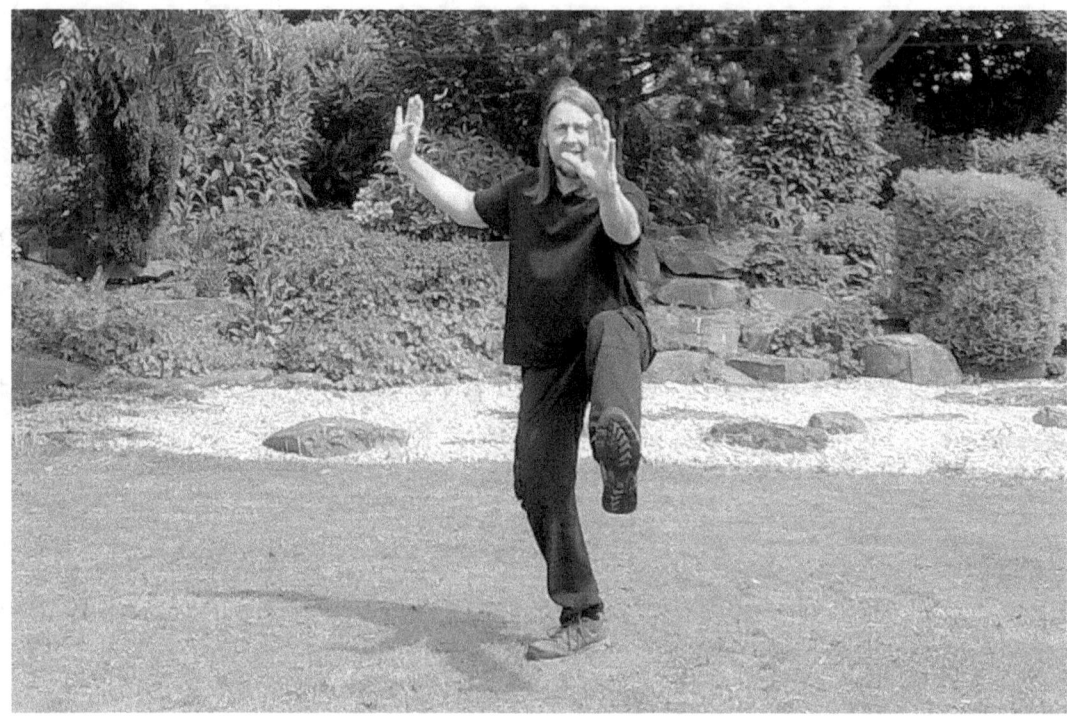

- Arms: The arms make a bow shape and are opened out to the right and left sides of the body. Both forearms point out and upward.

- Body: For this posture, your body is diagonal.

- Hands: The hands must point upward in this posture and are in the Fair Maiden's hand shape.

- Stance: Turn and Kick with Heel is a single legged stance.

- Weight: The weight is one hundred percent in the right leg.

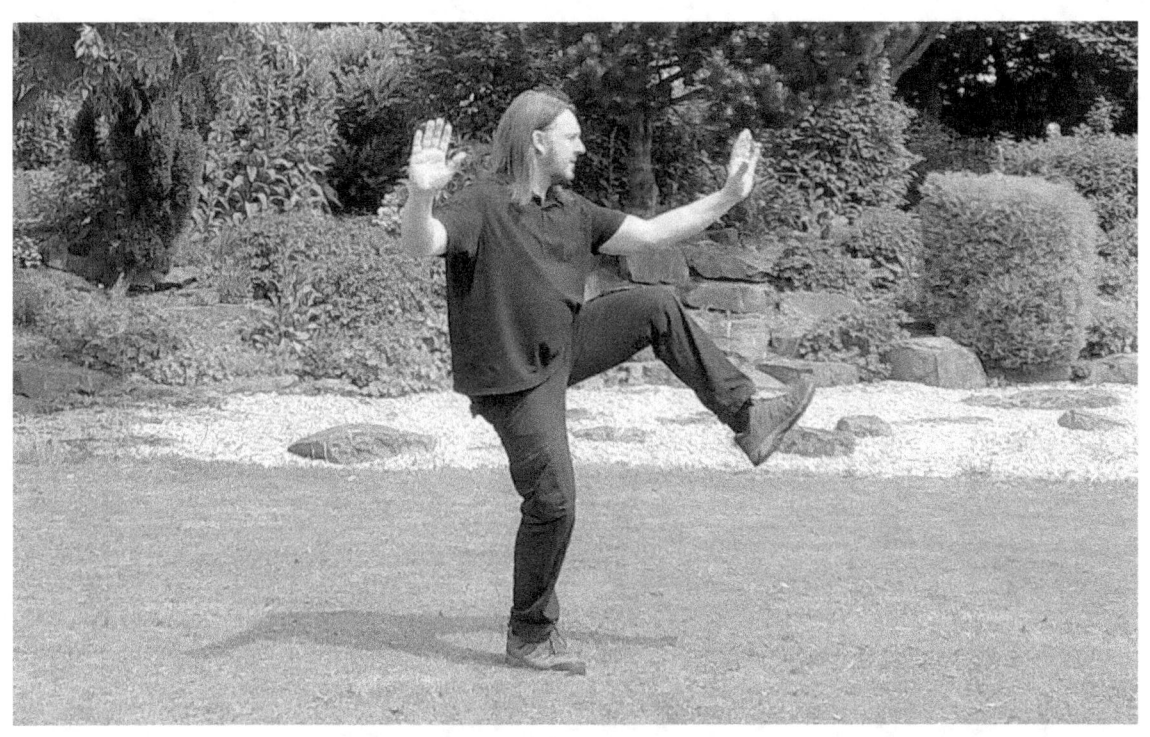

Punch to Groin

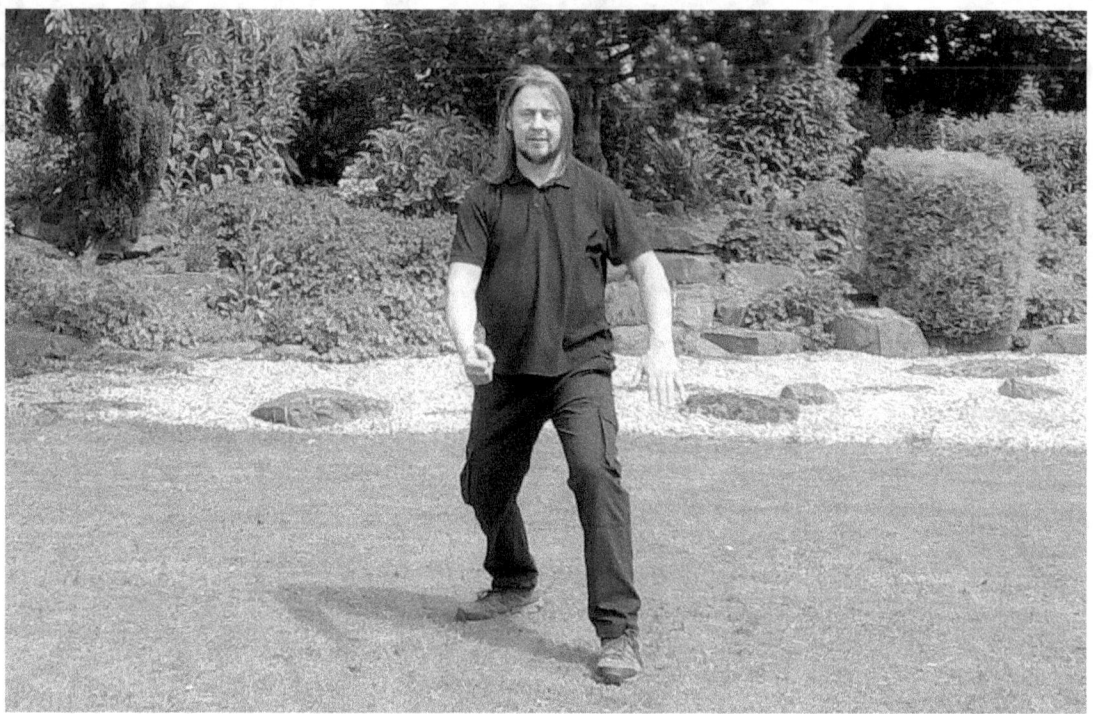

- Arms: In Brush Knee and Punch to Groin, the right arm is in front of the lower abdomen, the left arm is at the outside edge of the left leg.

- Body: Body alignment is square to the front.

- Hands: In this posture, the right hand is in a soft fist and the left hand keeps the Fair Maidens shape.

- Stance: The stance for this form movement is a left foot forward Bow stance.

- Weight: When you make this forward Bow stance, the weight is divided seventy percent in the right foot and thirty percent in the back foot.

Fair Lady Works at Shuttles

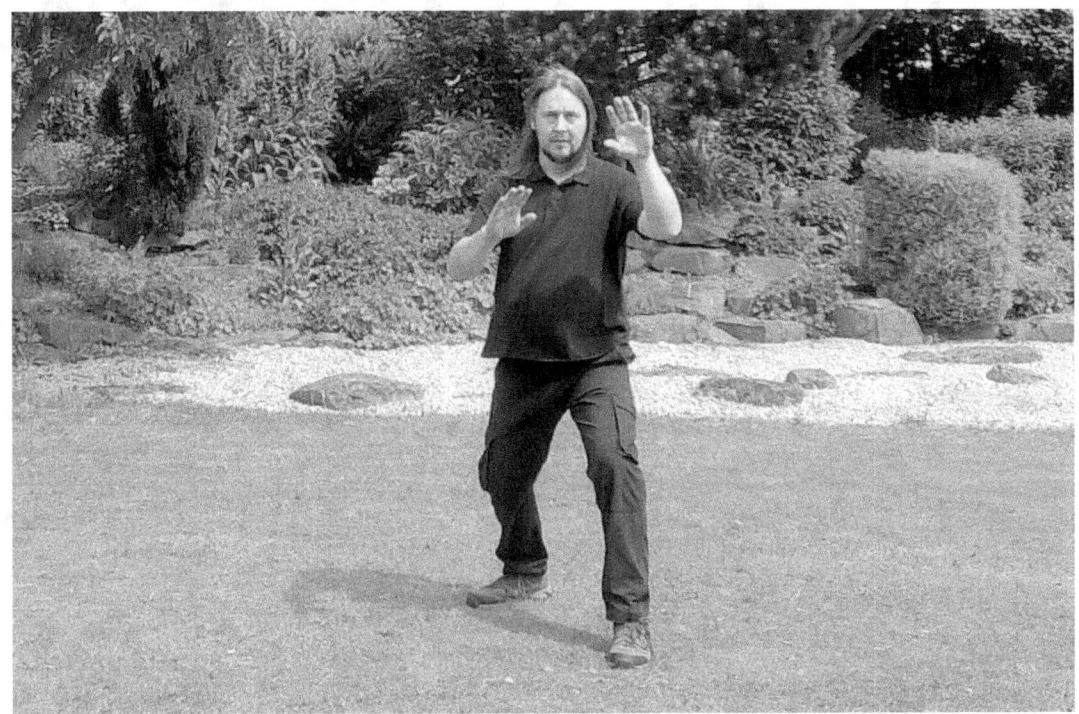

- Arms: In Jade Maiden Works the Shuttles, one arm is at the height of your forehead and moved out past its outside edge by a few inches. The other arm is in front of your centre line.

- Body: Your body alignment is square to the front.

- Hands: For this posture, the right, and left hand are in the Fair Maidens hand shape, and both palms face outwards.

- Stance: The stance for this form movement is a left foot forward Bow stance.

- Weight: When you are in this forward Bow stance, the weight is seventy percent in the front foot and thirty percent in the back foot.

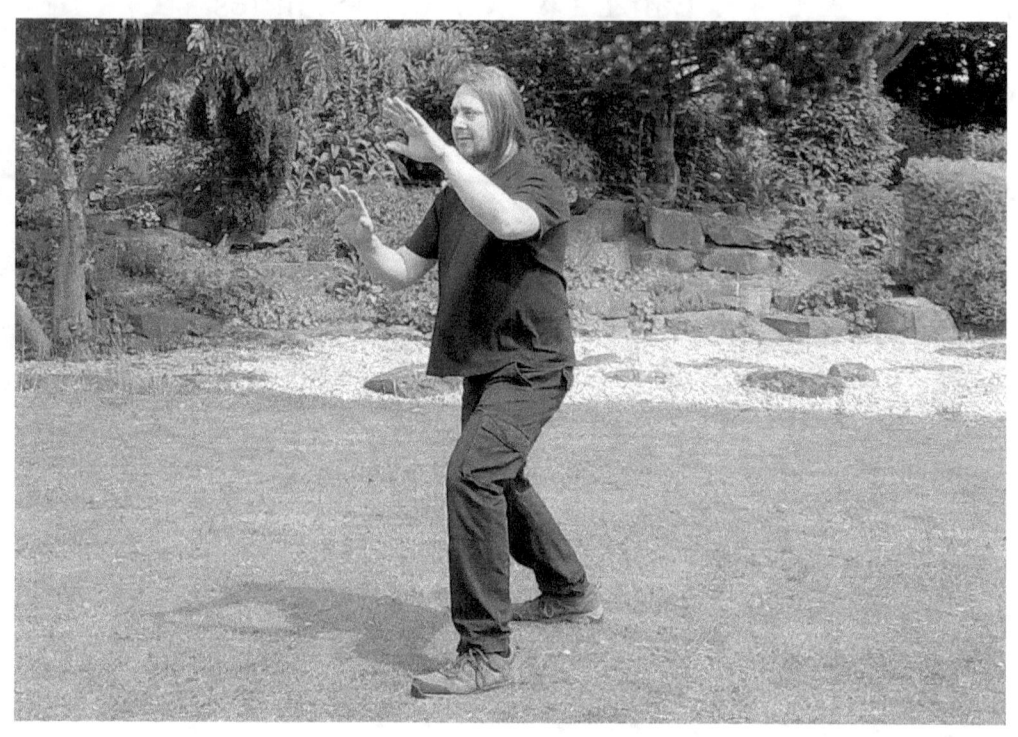

Step Up to Seven Stars

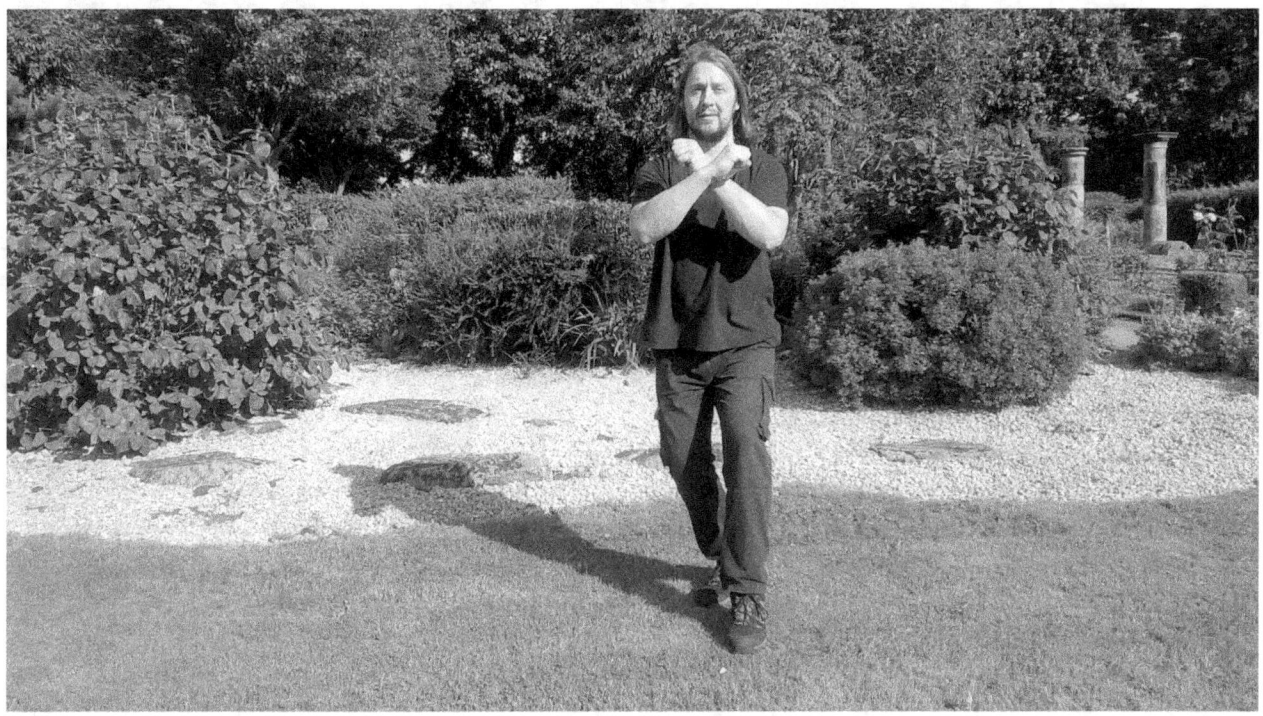

- Arms: When you practice this posture, your arms cross at the wrists in front of your upper chest, they form a triangular shape, and the outside edges of the forearms face forward.

- Body: The body should be square and aligned to the front.

- Hands: In this movement the hands form relaxed fists.

- Stance: This is a Cat stance.

- Weight: Ninety percent of your weight is on the left foot and ten percent is on the right foot.

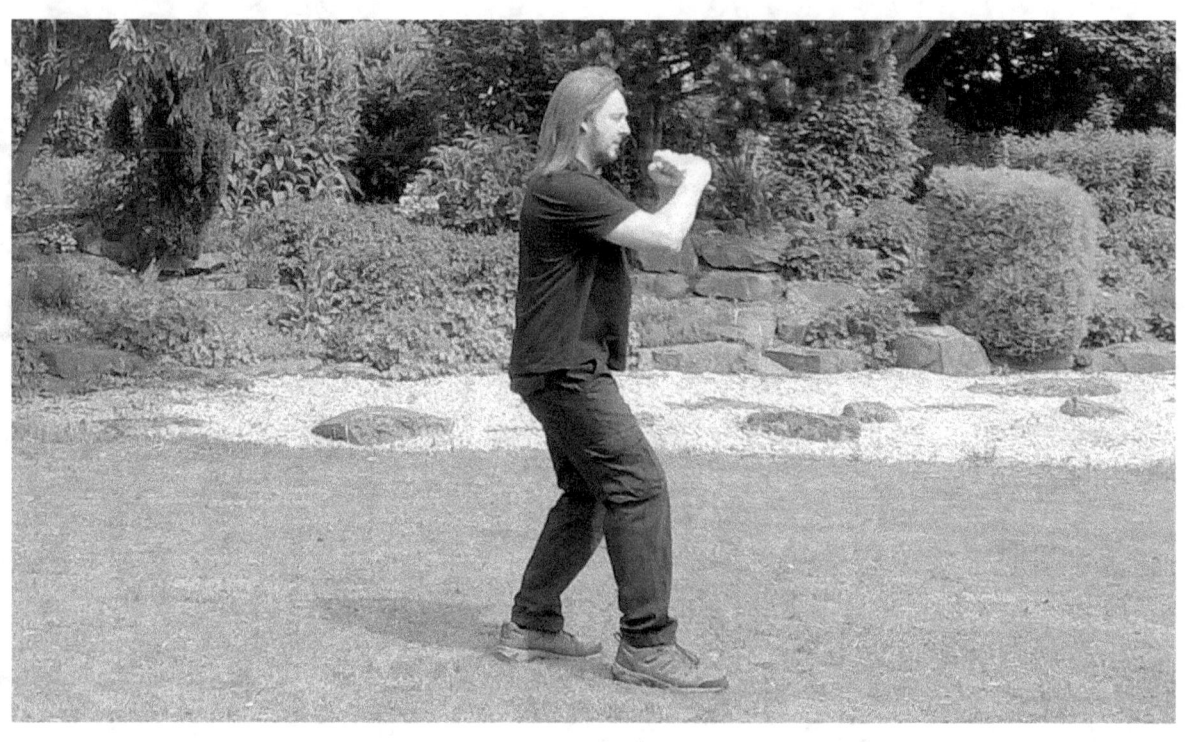

Step back and Ride the Tiger

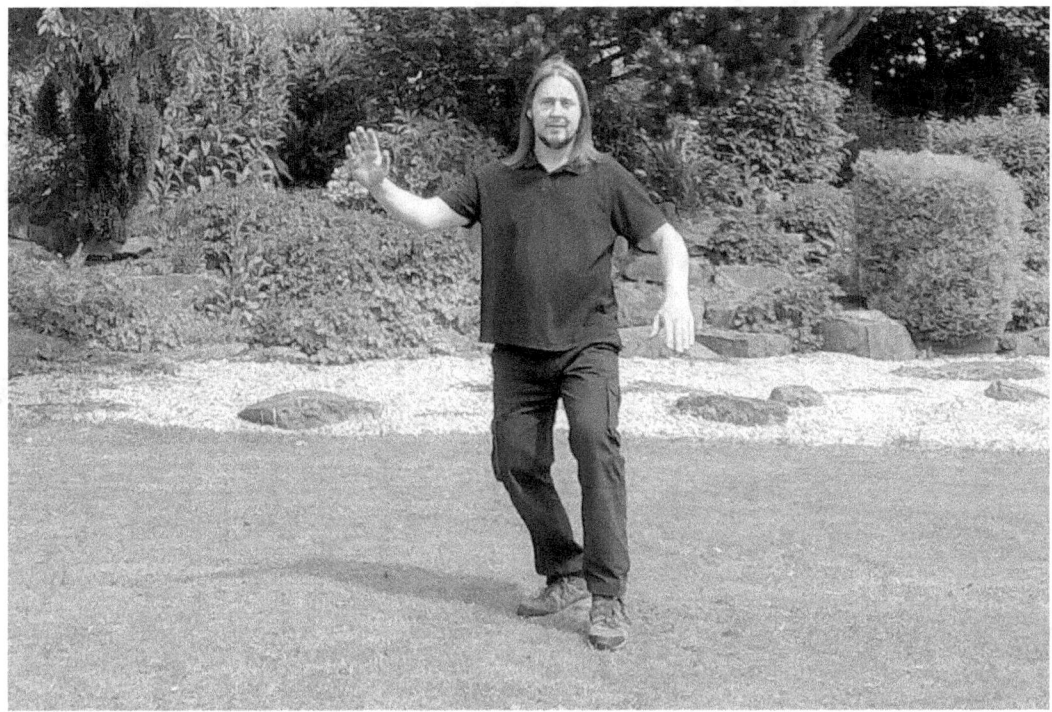

- Arms: In this posture, the arms open out to the sides of the body with the right forearm pointing up and out, the left forearm pointing down.

- Body: Your body is square in this posture.

- Hands: Both hands are in the Fair Maidens hand posture.

- Stance: This stance is a back weighted, Cat stance.

- Weight: The weight sits mainly on the left rear leg, the weight distribution is ninety percent in the left leg and ten percent in the right leg.

Turn and Sweep Lotus with Leg

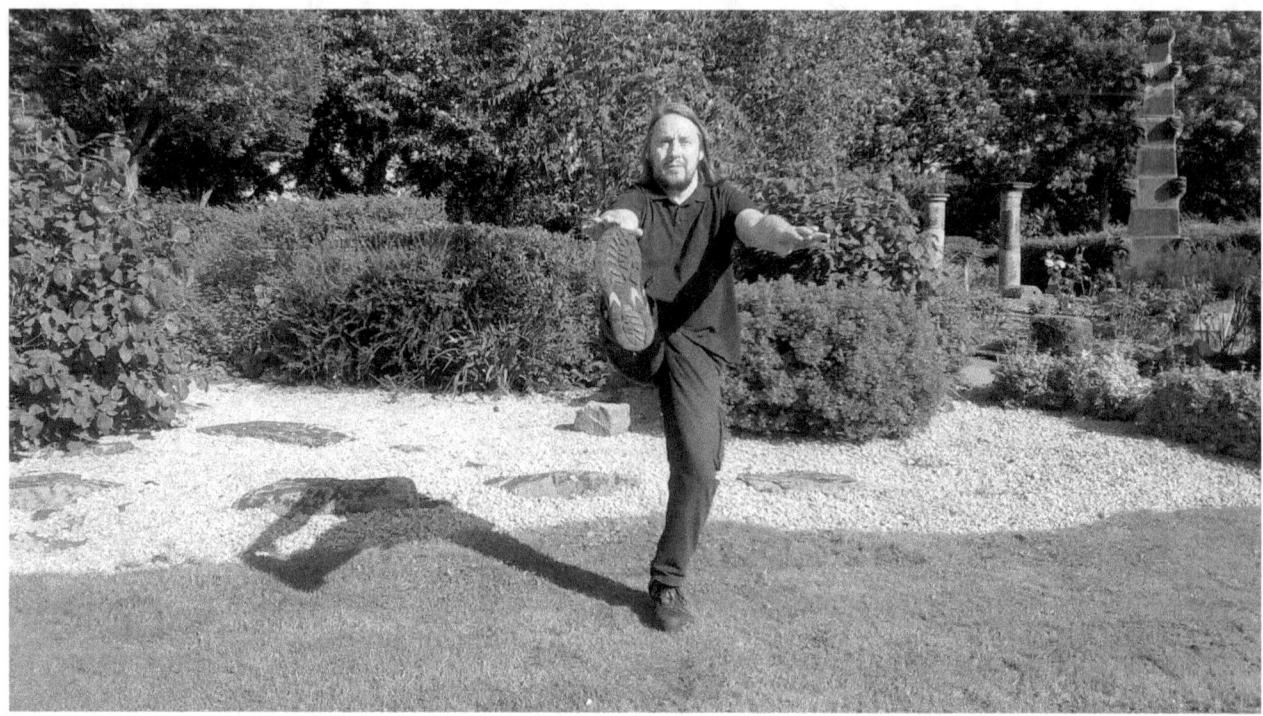

- Arms: Both arms are in front of the body at shoulder height

- Body: The body is square to the front.

- Hands: The hands are in the Fair Maidens shape and the palms face downward.

- Stance: This is a single legged, kicking posture.

- Weight: All of the body's weight is one hundred percent on the left leg.

Bend Bow to Shoot the Tiger

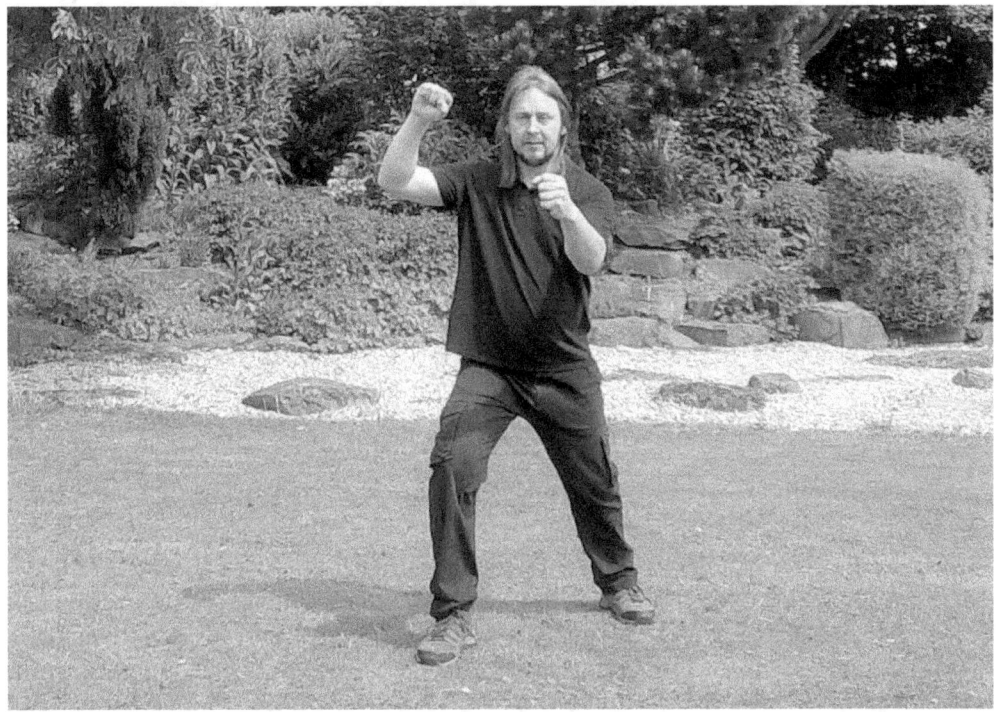

- Arms: The right arm is to the outside of the forehead and your left arm is in front of your upper chest.

- Body: The body turns slightly to the right, but keeps its alignment.

- Hands: In this posture, both hands make relaxed fists.

- Stance: This is a right foot forward bow stance.

- Weight: When performing the posture Bend Bow to Shoot a Tiger, the weighting is seventy percent in the right foot and thirty percent in the left rear foot.

CHAPTER ELEVEN: THE 37 STEP TAI CHI FORM MOVEMENTS

1. Heaven and Earth

2. Ward Off

3. Grasp Sparrow's Tail, Ward Off, Roll Back, Press and Push

4. Single Whip

5. Play Guitar

6. Shoulder Press

7. White Crane Spreads Wings

8. Brush Knee and Push

9. Play Guitar

10. Brush Knee and Push

11. Parry and Punch

12. Seal the Knot

13. Embrace Tiger and Return to Mountain (Diagonal Brush Knee and Push, Grasp Sparrow's Tail, Roll Back, Press, Push, Diagonal Single Whip)

14. Fist Under Elbow

15. Repulse Monkeys x 3

16. Diagonal Flying

17. Wave Hands in Clouds

18. Single Whip

19. Snake Creeps Down

20. Golden Phoenix Stands on One Leg (Left and right leg.)

21. Separate and Kick with Right Foot and Left Foot

22. Turn and Kick with Left Heel

23. Brush Knee and Push (right hand), Brush Knee and Push (left hand)

24. Punch to Groin

25. Grasp Sparrow's Tail, Roll Back, Press and Push

26. Single Whip

27. Fair Lady works at Shuttles (to four corners)

28. Ward Off

29. Grasp Sparrow's Tail, Roll back, Press and Push

30. Single Whip

31. Snake Creeps Down

32. Step Up to Seven Stars

33. Step Back and Ride the Tiger

34. Turn and Sweep Lotus with Leg

35. Bend Bow to Shoot the Tiger

36. Parry and Punch

37. Seal the Knot

CHAPTER SIX: THE 37 STEP TAI CHI FORM WITH INSTRUCTIONS

Note: When performing the Tai Chi Form movements everything moves into place at once, in these descriptions the movements are of necessity sequential, but should be performed as a continuous whole.

A Tai Chi Form is actually a series of transitions and Form movements, the transitions link the Forms together and are equally as important as the Forms themselves. In this part of the book I describe the Cheng man Ch'ing Tai Chi Form, from start to finish, including the transitions and the Forms.

Commencement

Stand with your feet together, with your arms by your sides and your hands touching the corners of your thighs.

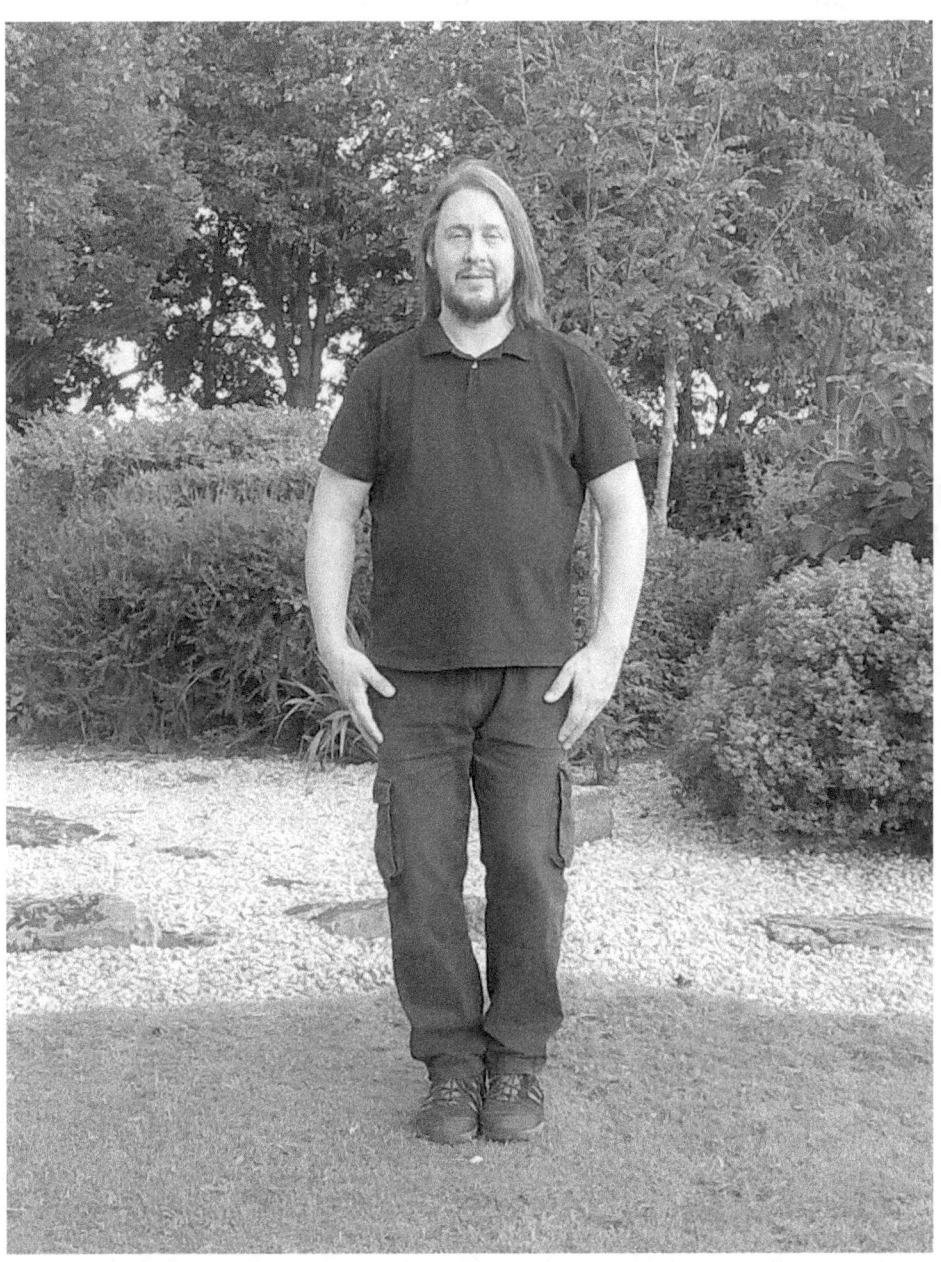

1) Heaven and Earth

Sit down, as if you are sitting on a tall barstool. Move your weight fully onto your right leg, and step out with the left foot into a shoulder width stance.

Place the heel down first and then roll the rest of your foot down onto the floor. Once this is accomplished, shift your weight across, until you have fifty percent of your weight in each foot.

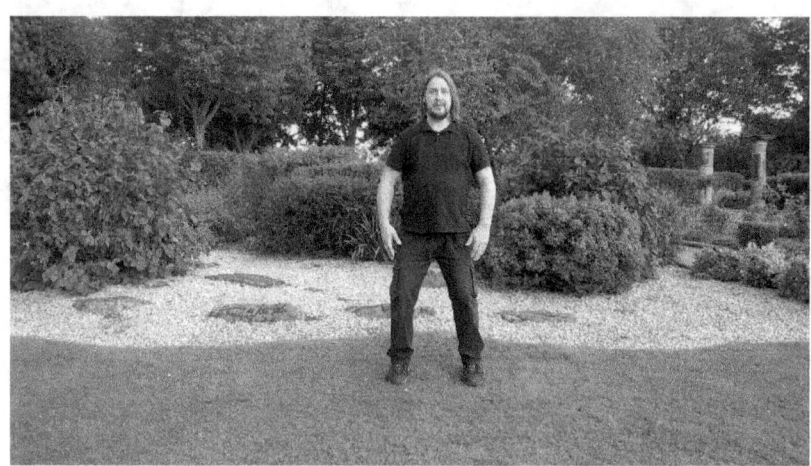

Turn the backs of your hands forwards and raise them up to the height of your shoulders.

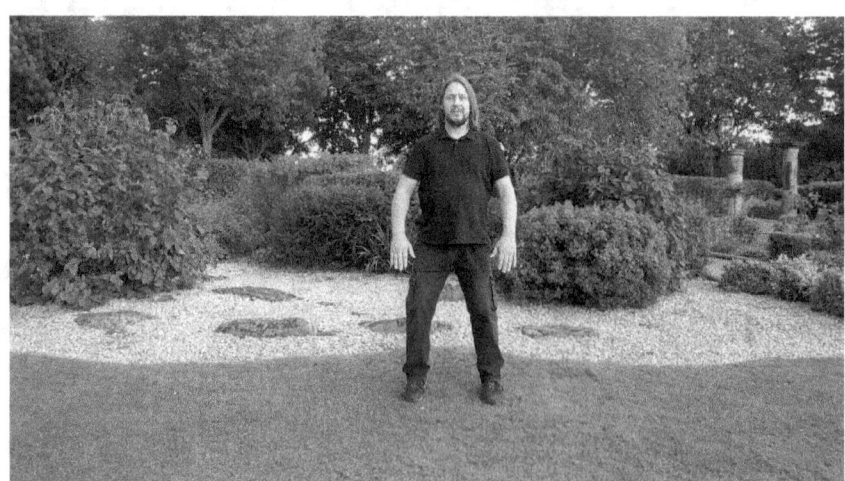

Once your hands reach shoulder level, pull them back towards you and downwards (as if rolling them over the top of a ball), before returning them to their starting position.

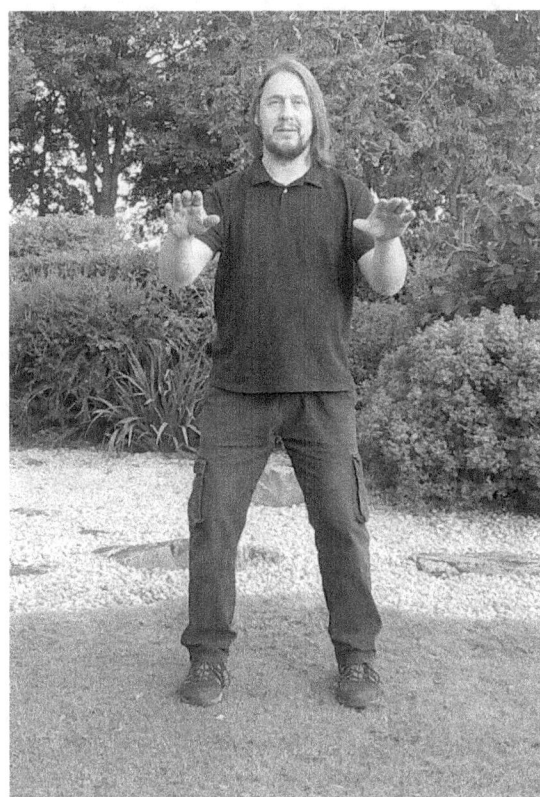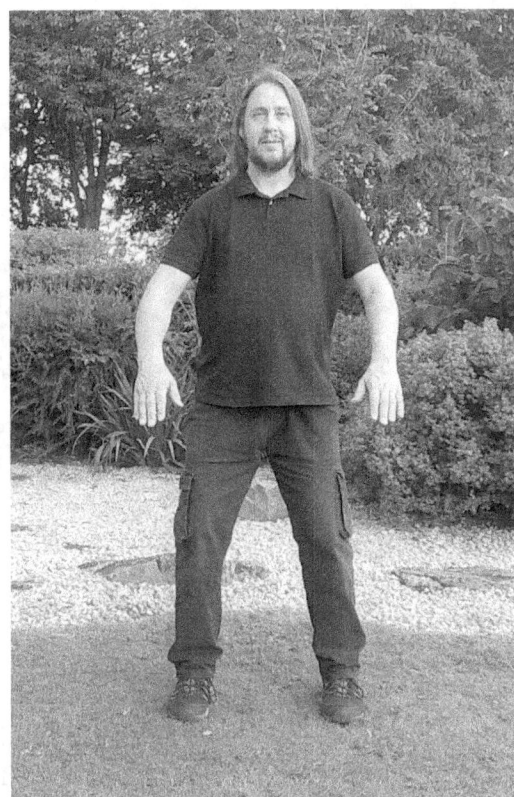

2) Ward Off Left

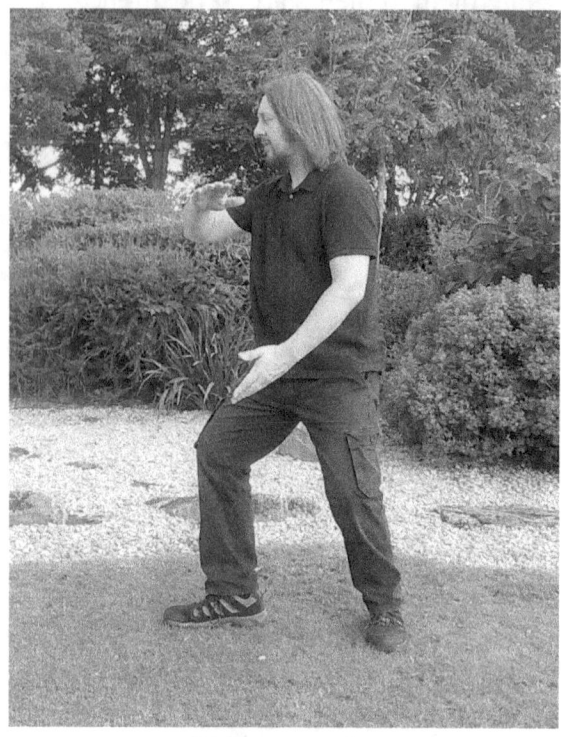 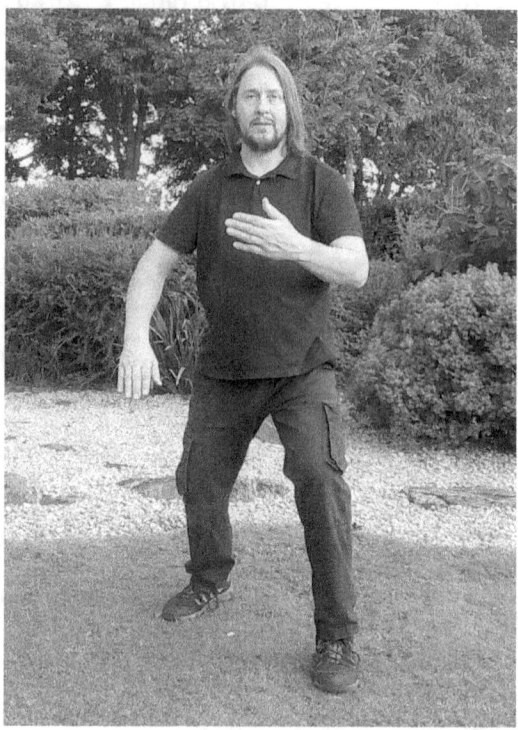

Hold an imaginary ball in front of the centre of your body. Your right hand is palm down on top of the ball and the left palm faces up. (You will use this hold the ball shape many times during this Tai Chi form)

At the same time, shift your weight to the left leg, lift the toes of your right foot, and turn your body to your right side, this turns the right foot out to a forty-five degree angle.

Shift your weight into your right leg and sit fully on that leg.

(Keep a shoulder width space between your feet.)

Step forward with your left foot, place the heel down first, and then roll the rest of the foot down.

Transfer seventy percent of your weight into the left leg and bring your left forearm up in an arc in front of your upper chest.

At the same time, lower your right hand, with the palm facing down beside your right hip, it must be slightly forward of your body.

3) Grasp the Sparrows Tail

Ward Off Right

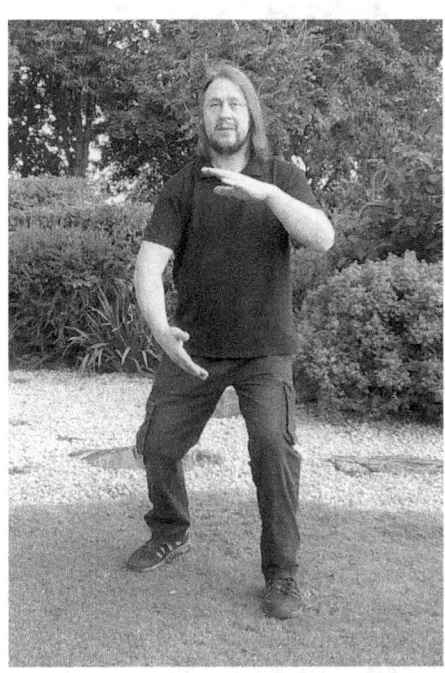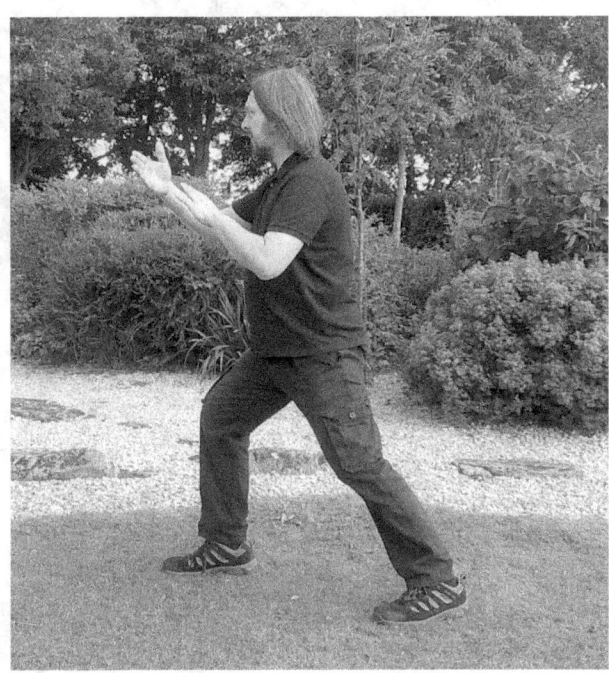

Hold the ball, and shift your weight backwards into the right leg. Turn your Dantien to your right side, raise your left toes, and pivot on the heel to your right. Shift gradually into your left leg. Then lift up your right heel and turn on the right toes until you face square again.

Step straight forward with the right foot into a Bow stance. (Keep a shoulder width space between your legs).

Leave the left hand in front of your chest and roll your right hand upwards in a curve to the 11 o'clock position in front of your right upper chest. The fingers of your left hand point to your right wrist and your elbows are heavy.

Rollback

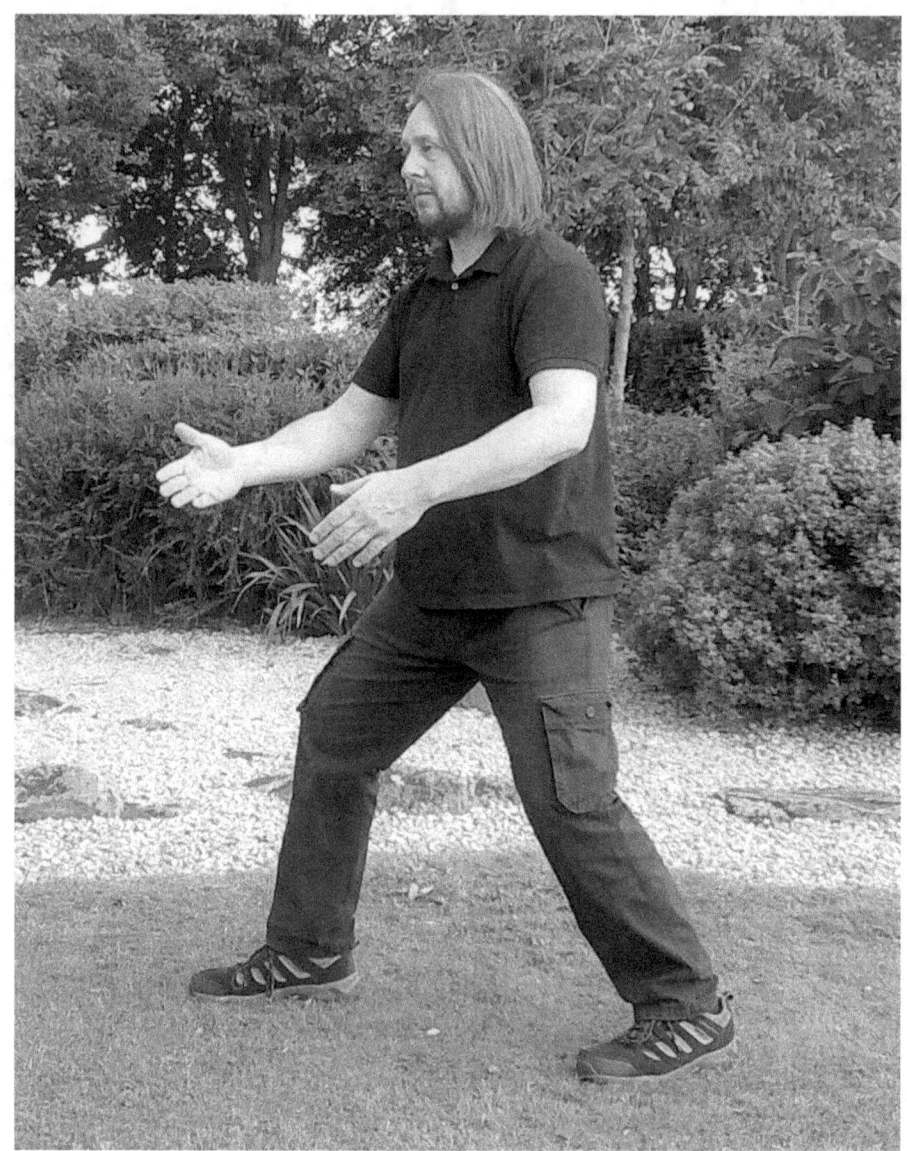

Slowly, lower your arms, keeping a space between the arms and your body. At the same time move into your left leg and turn your body towards your left corner. Keep your centreline aligned.

Press

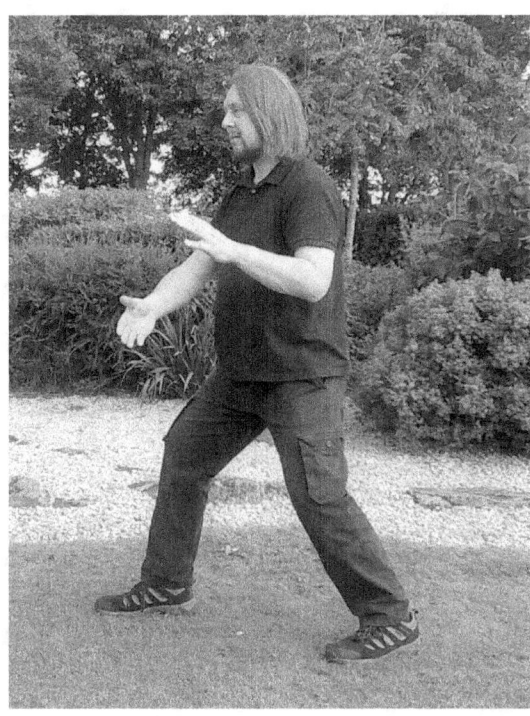 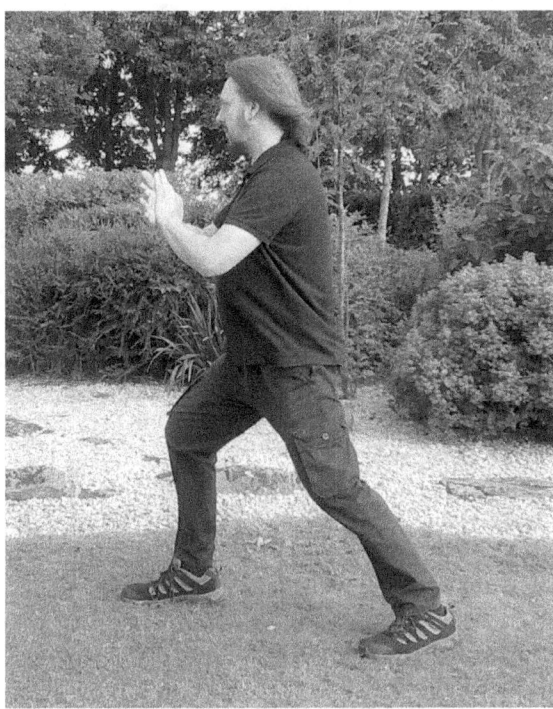

Circle your left hand round and place your palm on your right inner wrist. Turn your body to square again and move your weight forward from the left leg into a seventy percent front weighted, right bow stance.

At the same time, bring your connected hands up in front of your chest, (your arms form a triangle shape) and press them forward.

Separate Hands

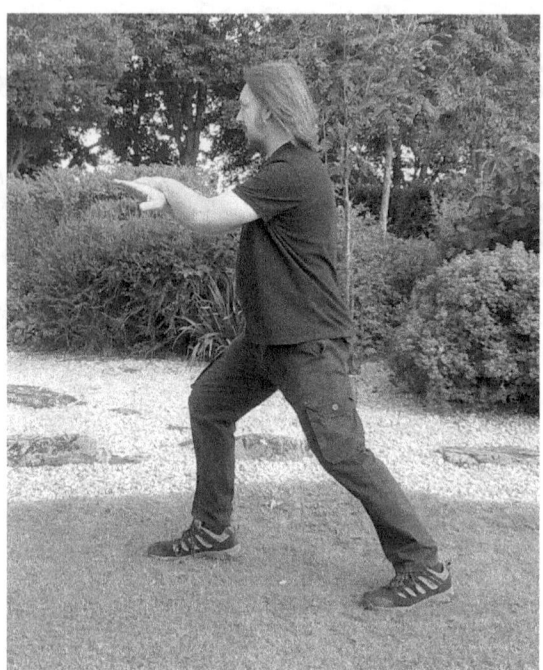 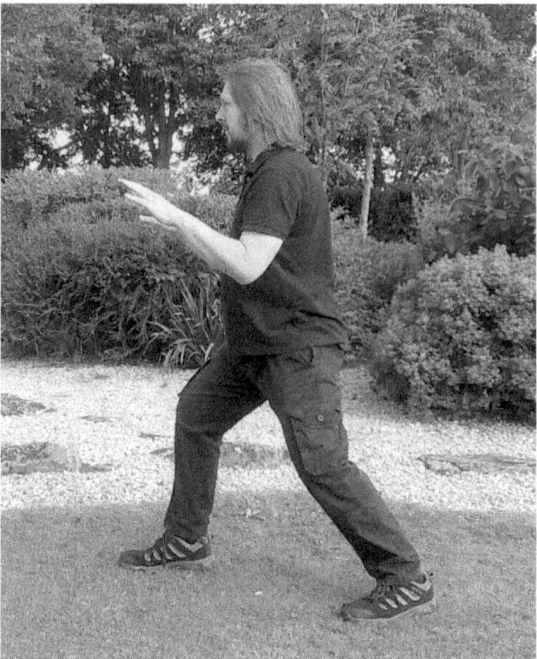

Rotate your hands to palms down and at the same time cross your wrists with the left hand on top. Immediately uncross your wrists and separate your hands to shoulder width. At the same time, move backwards until you have seventy percent of your weight in your left leg.

Push

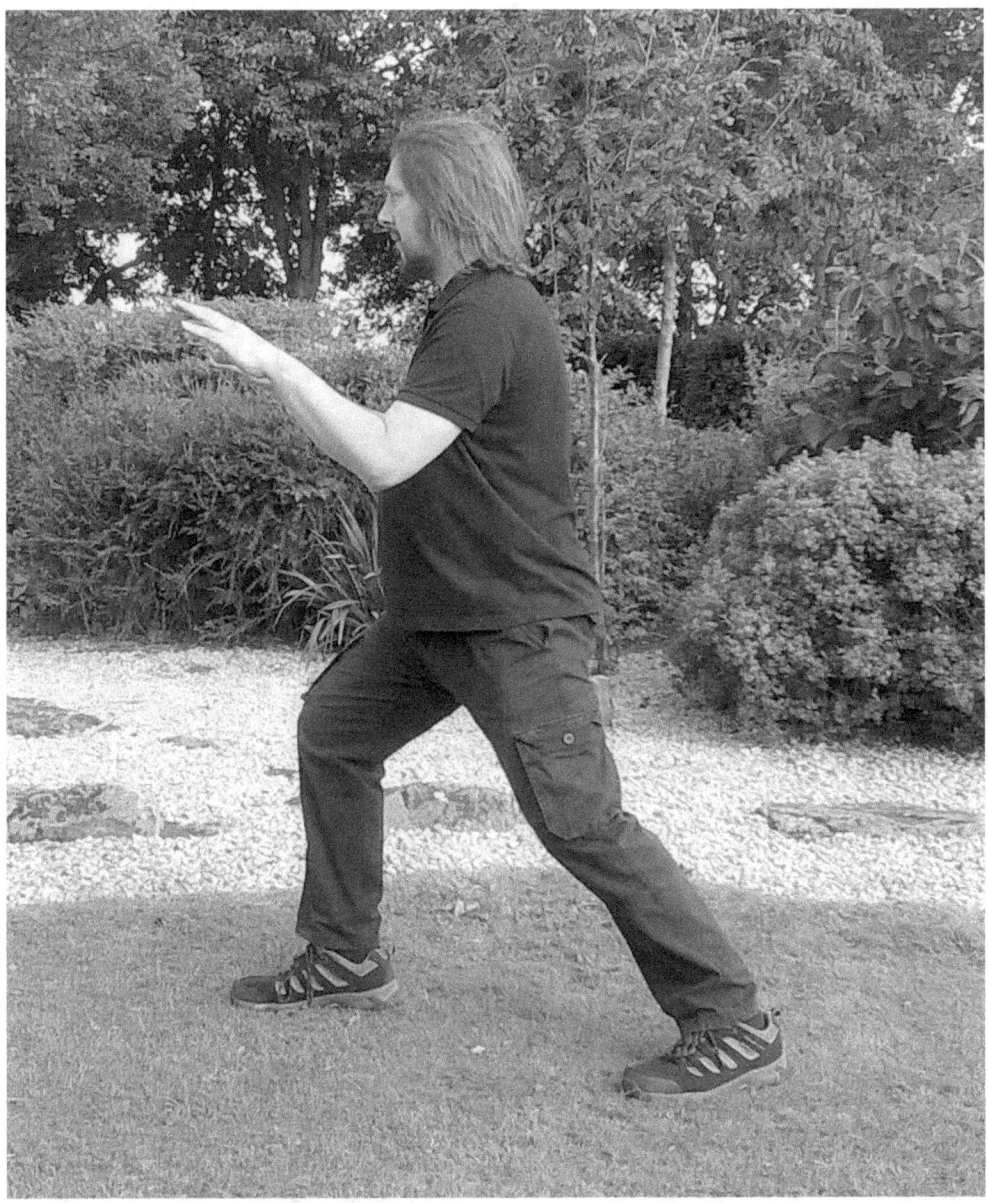

Separate your hands to either side turn them until the palms face down and push forward into a left bow stance.

4) Single Whip

Slowly shift backwards into your left leg.

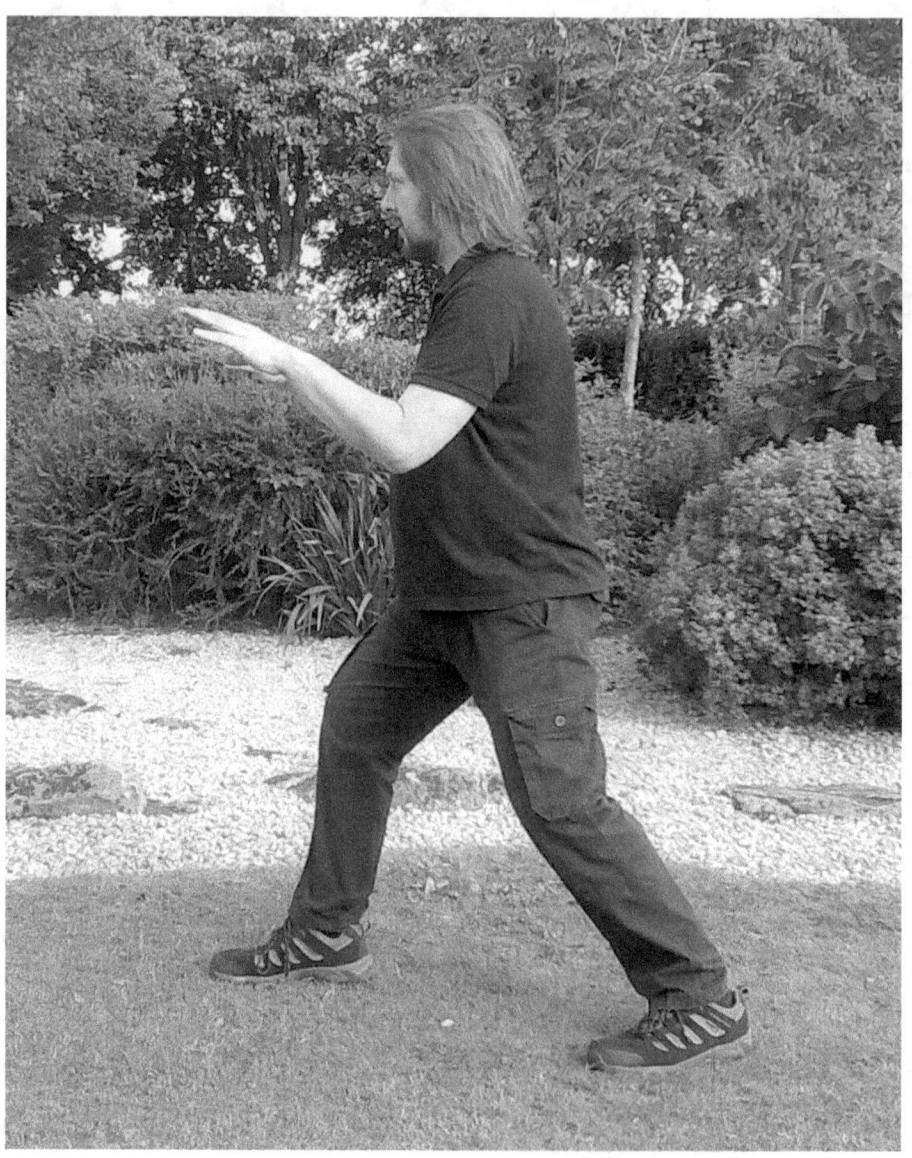

Raise the toes of you right foot. Turn your Dantien to the left corner; your hands remain in front of your shoulders as you turn your body.

Pivot on your right heel, turning the toes in to your left side.

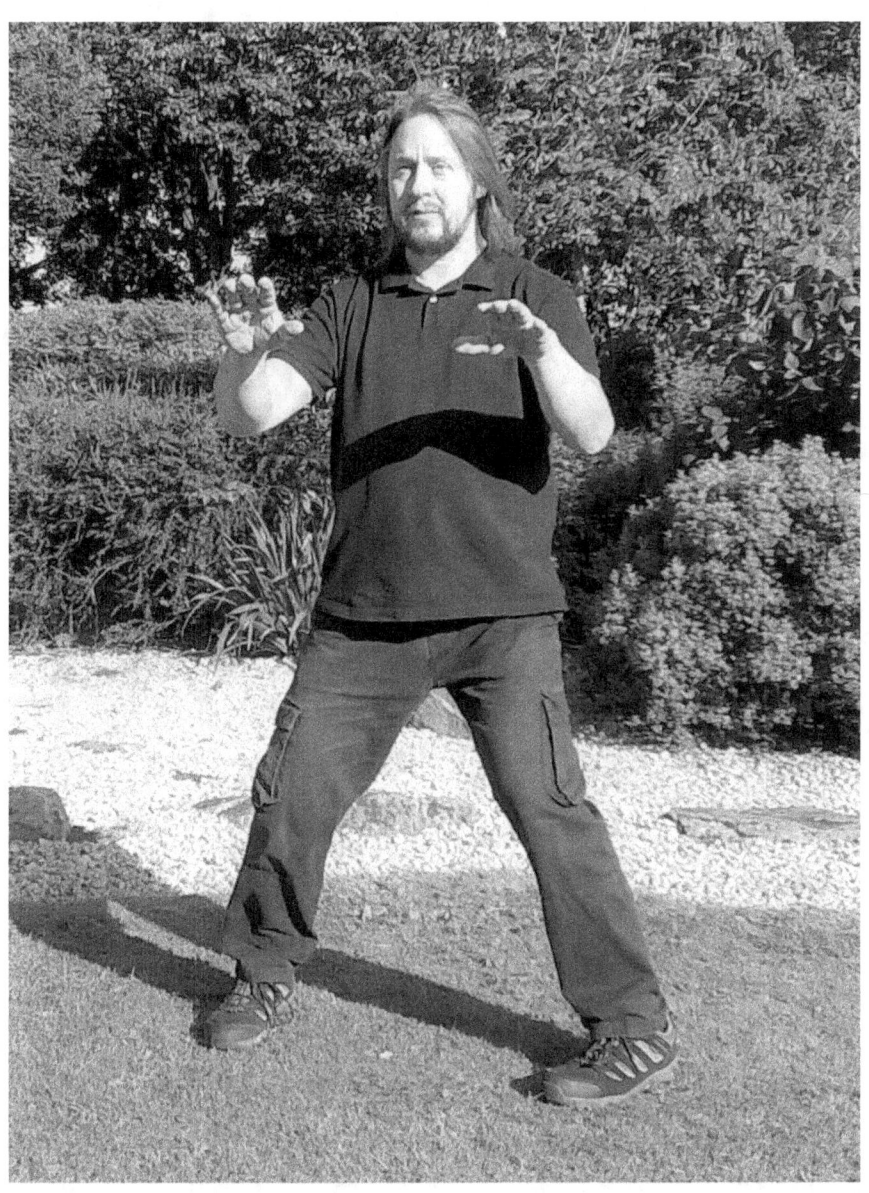

Turn your body fully to the left; make a hold the ball shape, with the right hand on top, the left hand palm upward in front of your Dantien.

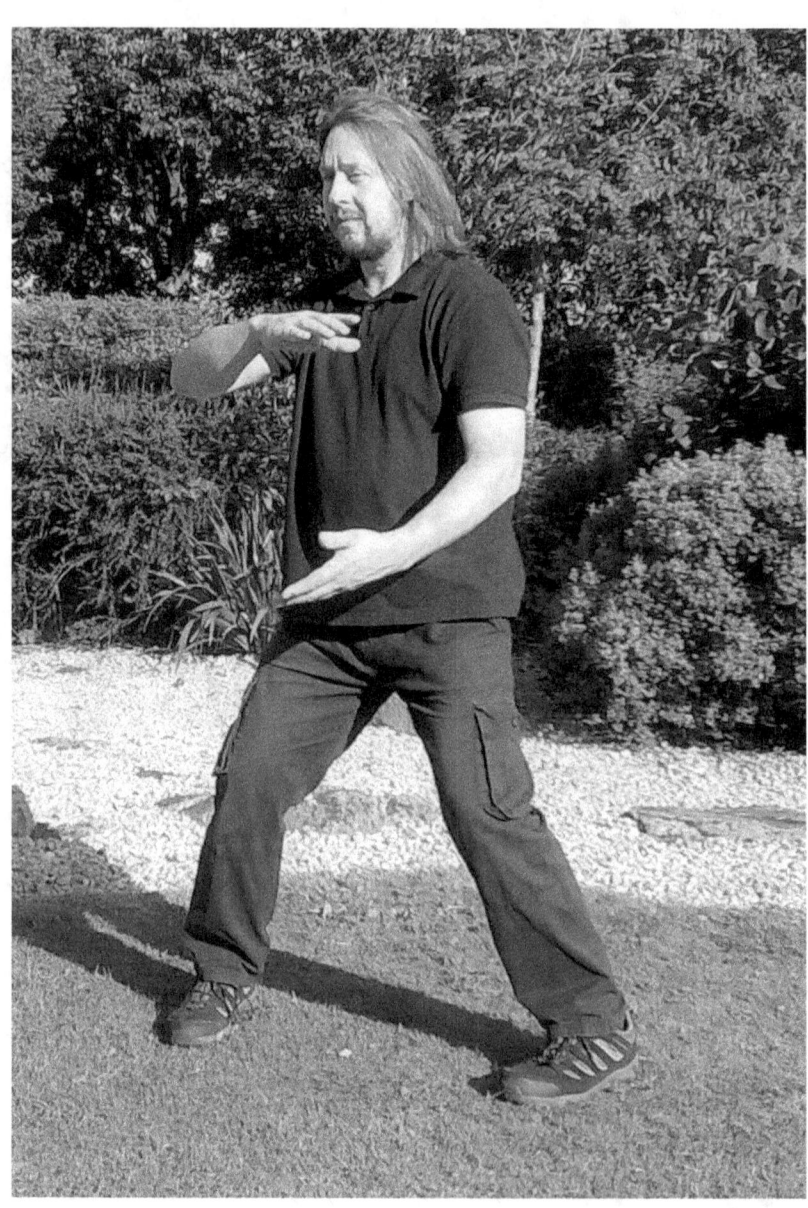

Push your right hand out in front of the right shoulder until the arm is straight, at the same time bend your right wrist until the thumb points downward, and place your fingertips around the tip of the thumb to make a beak.

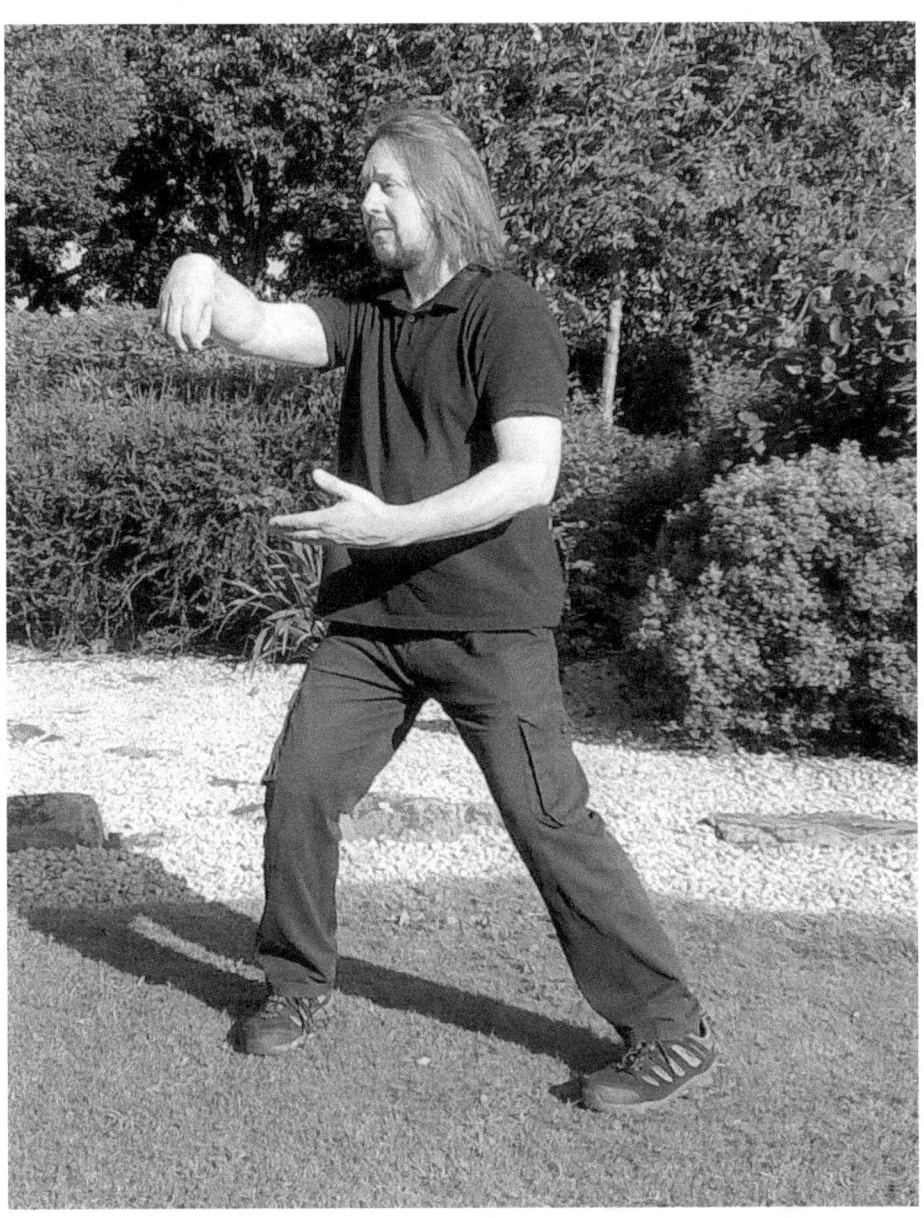

Turn back towards the left, your weight remains in the right leg. Lift up the heel of your left foot and pivot on the ball of the foot.

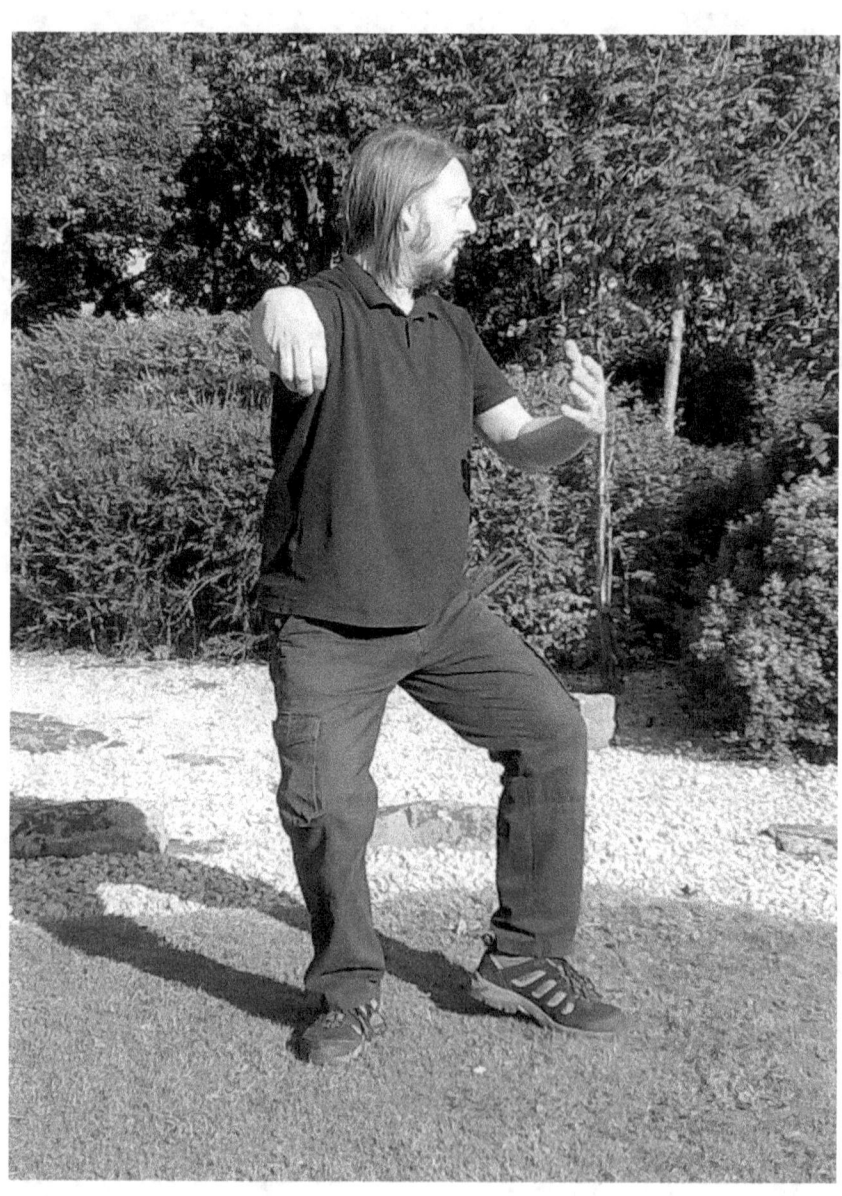

Step forwards and across to make a left footed Bow stance.

Bring your left hand up and across your body to your left side, rotate your palm until it faces out in front of your left shoulder.

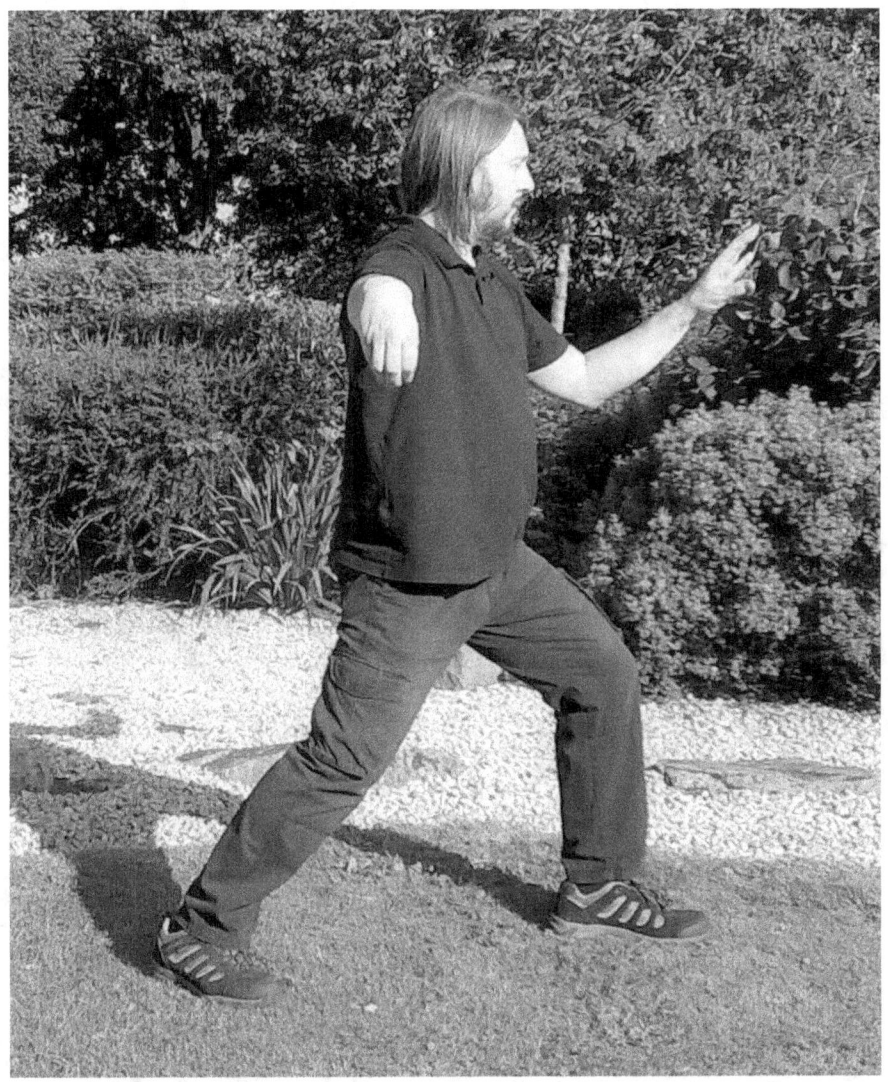

(Single Whip is different from the other Bow stances because your centreline turns to face your right corner, but you look forward)

5) Lift Hands

Shift your weight into your right foot; turn your body to your right side. Shift your weight into the right foot and step in with your left foot, raising the toes as you step into a Cat stance.

At the same time let go of the beak and bring your hands in towards each other.

Your arms should keep a rounded shape. Your body remains diagonal, and your right foot, face and hands are facing forward. The left hand is in front of your chest and your right hand is in front of the right shoulder.

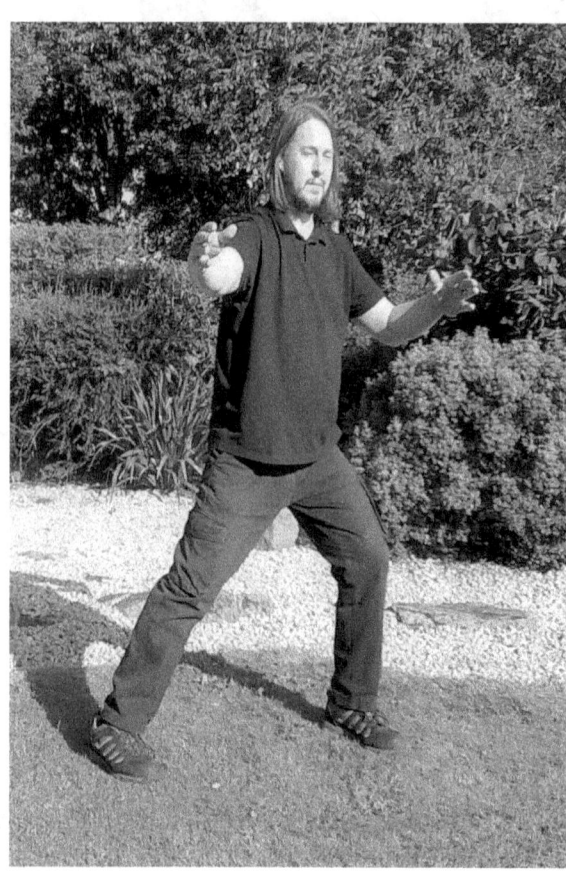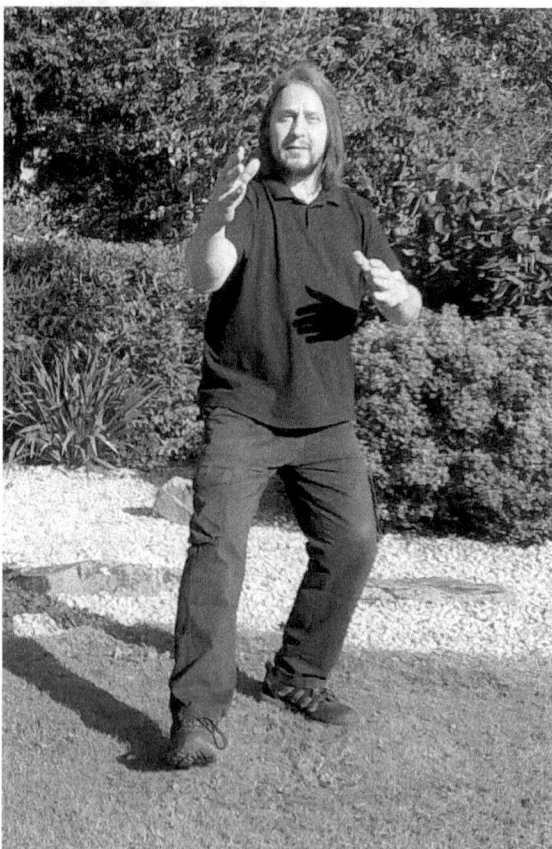

6) Pluck, Elbow, Shoulder Stroke

Bring your arms down towards your left side, the left hand in front of your left hip, the right hand in front of the Dantien.

As you lower the hands, step in with your right foot and place the toes where the heel was previously. Your body maintains a diagonal alignment. The right arm has a rounded Ward Off shape with a space between your arm and the lower abdomen.

Once you finish the plucking movement circle your left arm back, up and around, then bring the left hand up in front of your upper chest.

Step forward with your right foot into a seventy percent Bow stance. Keep the same shape to your arms throughout his movement. Your centreline is diagonal, but your eyes look forward.

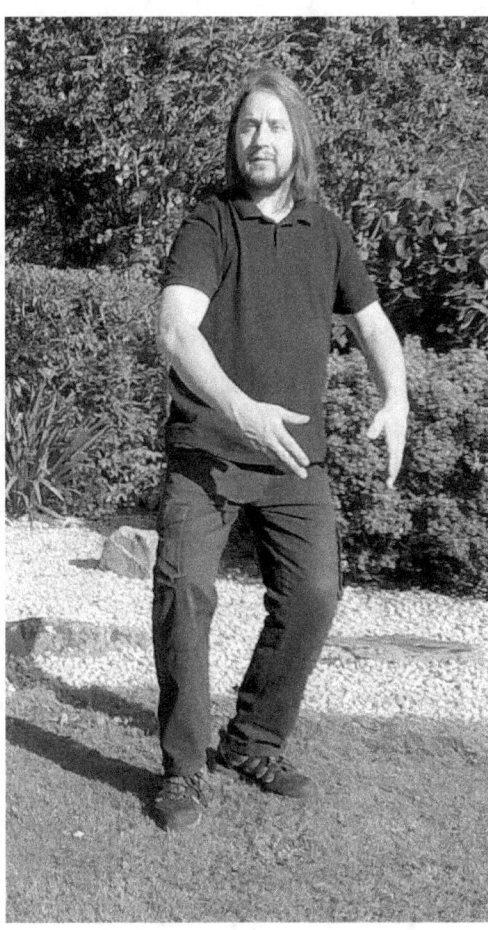
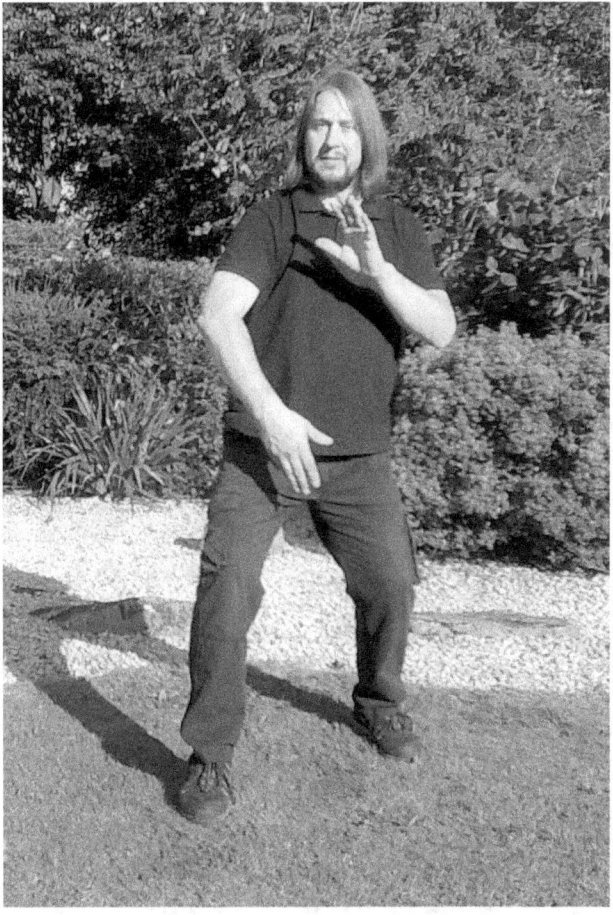

7) White Crane Spreads its Wings

Shift your weight gradually back into your left leg. Lift up your right toes and turn your body to the left, as you do this the right leg follows the movement of the body pivoting on the heel foot to your left side.

Shift your weight back into the right leg and sit fully on it, the weight remains in this leg throughout the rest of this movement.(This is a ninety to ten percent back weighted Cat stance)

Lift up your left heel and pivot on the ball of the foot until it faces forward.

Bring your left hand down and across your body in a sweeping motion. The left arms end position is at the outside of your left hip with the palm down. At the same time the right hand comes up and across the right side of your body, passing the chest to open out at the side of your right temple, the palm faces forward.

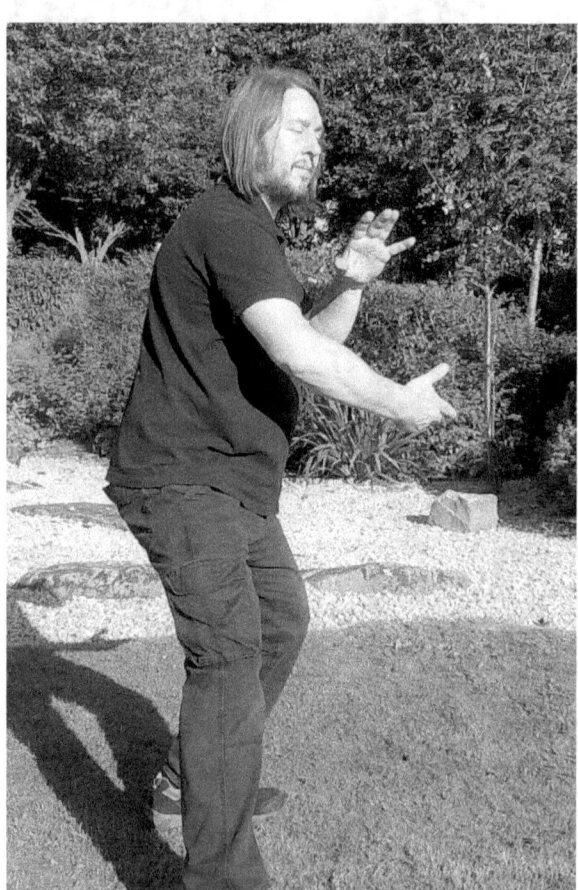
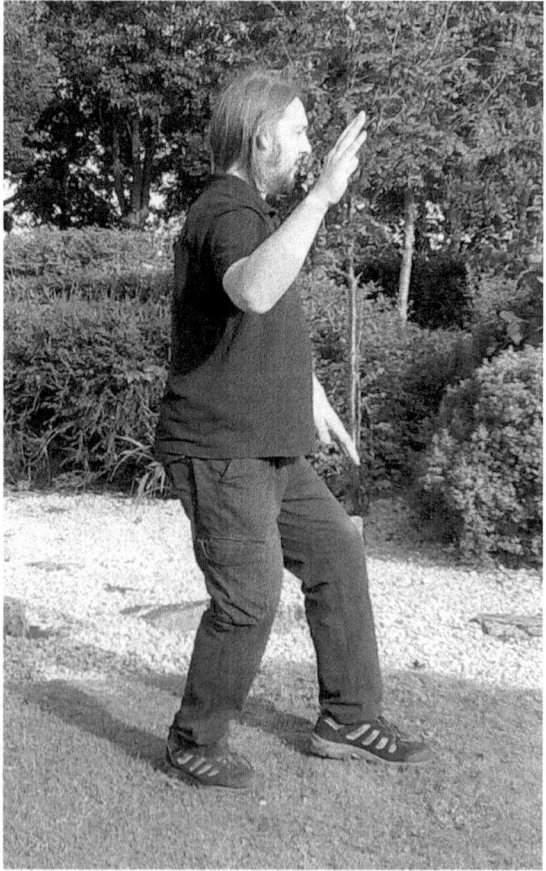

8) Brush Knee and Push

Turn your right hand until the little finger faces the floor and make a downward chopping movement and then circle it back behind you, it rises up and continues circling and around until it is near your right ear.

Synchronously bring your left hand up and across your body to the front of your right upper chest. Step forwards and diagonally, place your heel down first and slowly roll the foot into a left Bow stance.

As you step, your left hand sweeps down across your body to return to its starting position palm down. Your right arm sinks down two inches and then moves forward across the body to rest in front of your centre line. It makes a single hand push shape with the fingertips facing forward.

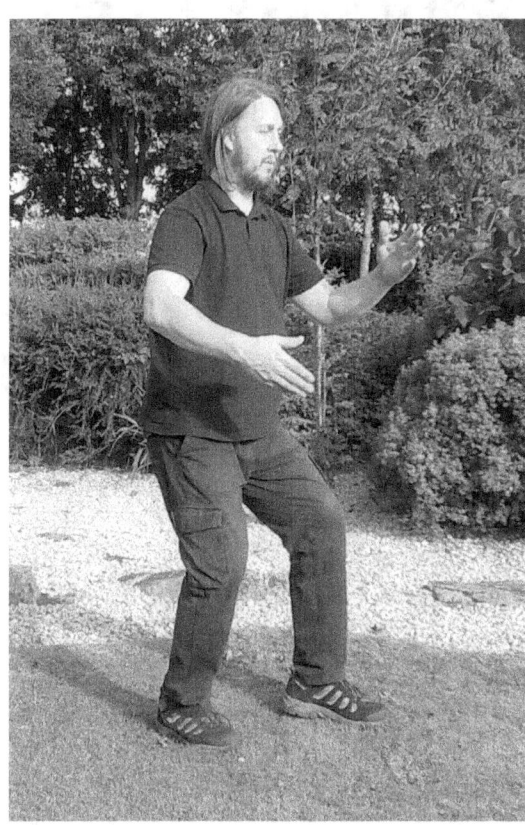 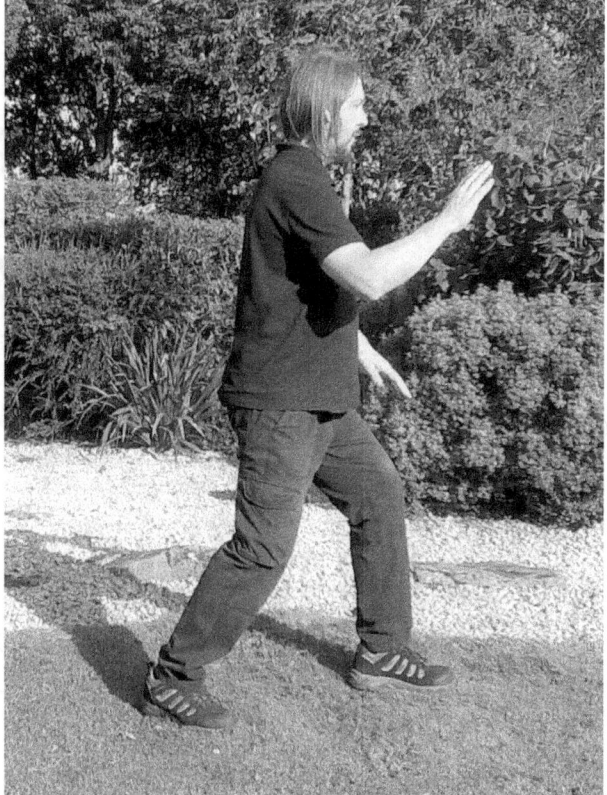

9) Play Guitar

Sit fully into your left leg. Step forwards with your right foot, the right foot remains at a forty-five degree angle.

Place your right foot carefully down, six inches behind the left foot and gradually shift your weight onto it and raise the toes of your left foot into a Cat stance.

As you do this, turn your right hand thumb side up and lower it downward two inches.

At the same time, turn diagonally so that the left shoulder is further forward than the right, lift up your left hand, and turn it so that the palm faces to your right side.

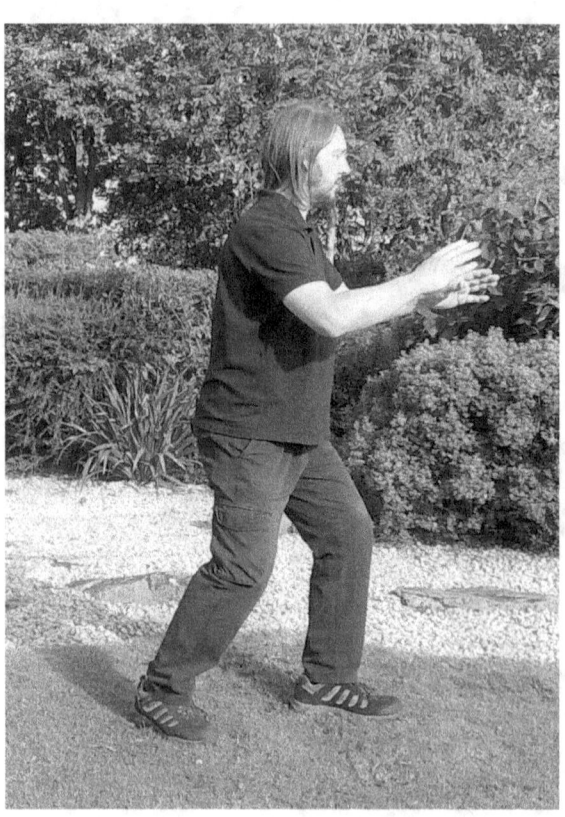 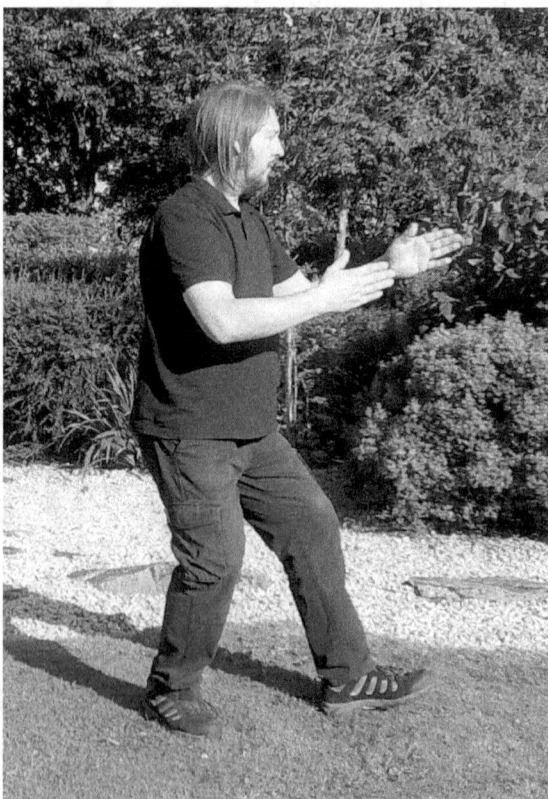

10) Brush Knee Push

Make a chopping movement with your right hand, it drops down and, circles back upwards and around until it comes up near your right ear.

Synchronously bring your left hand up and across your body in front of your right upper chest.

Step forwards and across into a left Bow stance. As you step, your left hand sweeps down across your body to return to its starting position. At the same time, your right arm sinks 2 inches and moves forward across the body to rest in front of your upper chest.

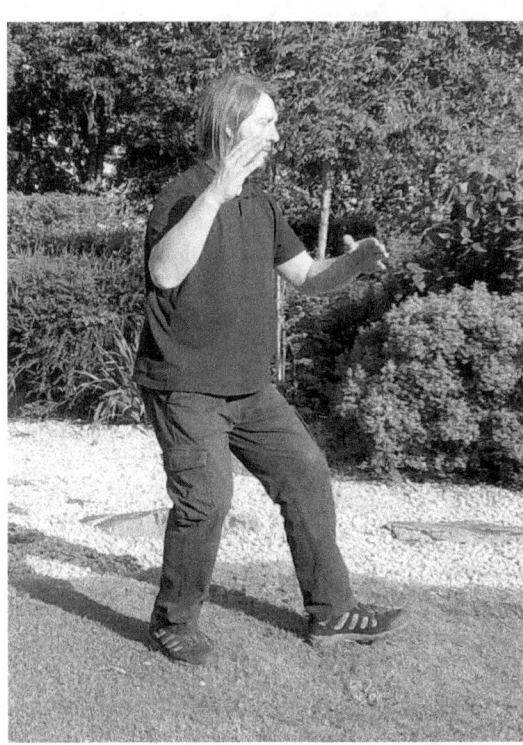 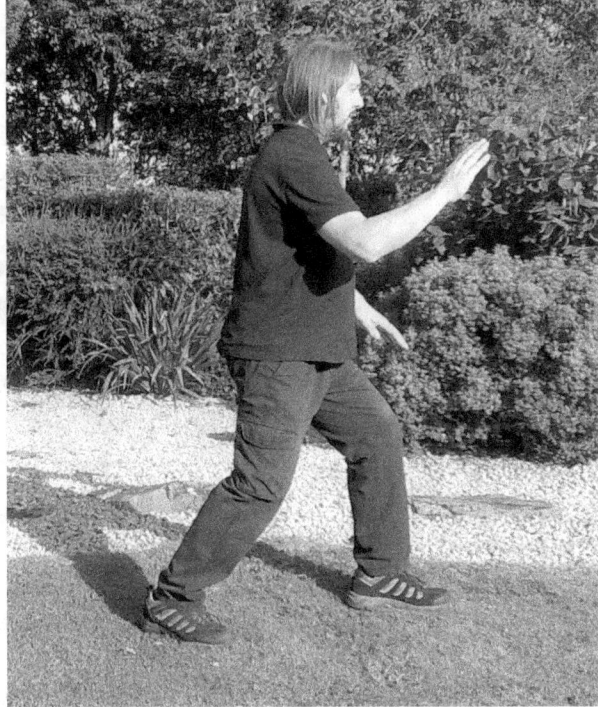

11) Parry and Punch

Shift your weight backward into your right leg and lift the left toes. Turn the left foot out to a forty-five degree angle pivoting on the heel, roll your foot down, and shift your weight fully onto the left foot.

Move both of your hands across by your left hip and make a relaxed fist with the right hand.

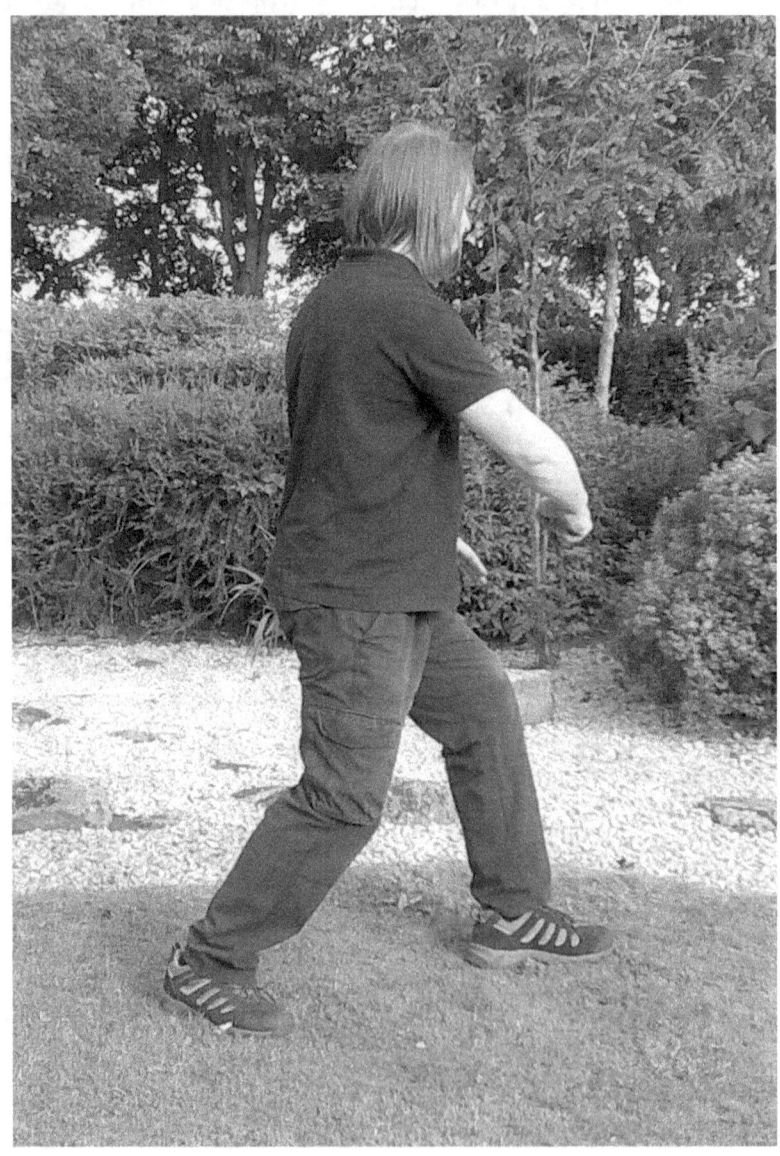

Once you complete this movement turn your body to your right corner; the hands and right leg follow the turning of the body.

The right fist travels in an arc across your body, rising in front of your chest and descending to the side of your right hip joint.

Your left hand follows the right hand until it is in front of your upper chest with the palm facing down, where it remains throughout the rest of the movement.

Now step out at a forty-five degree angle with your right leg and foot and shift your weight slowly onto it.

Step forward with the empty left leg into a left Bow stance.

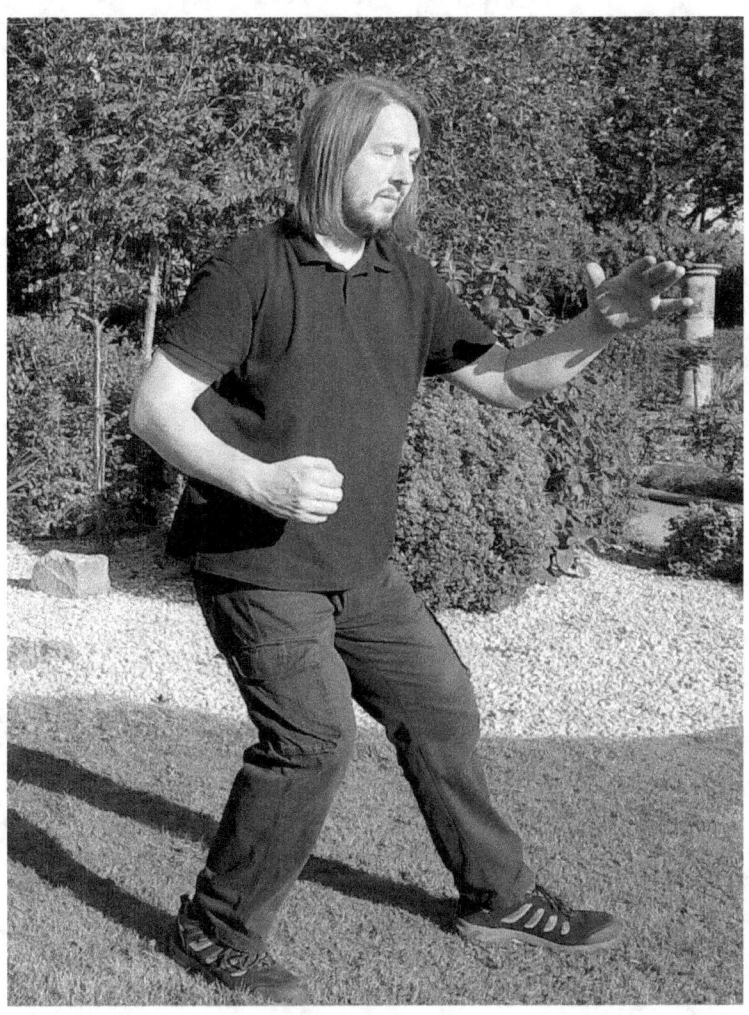

Punch the right hand forward and upward at a forty-five degree angle underneath your left palm.

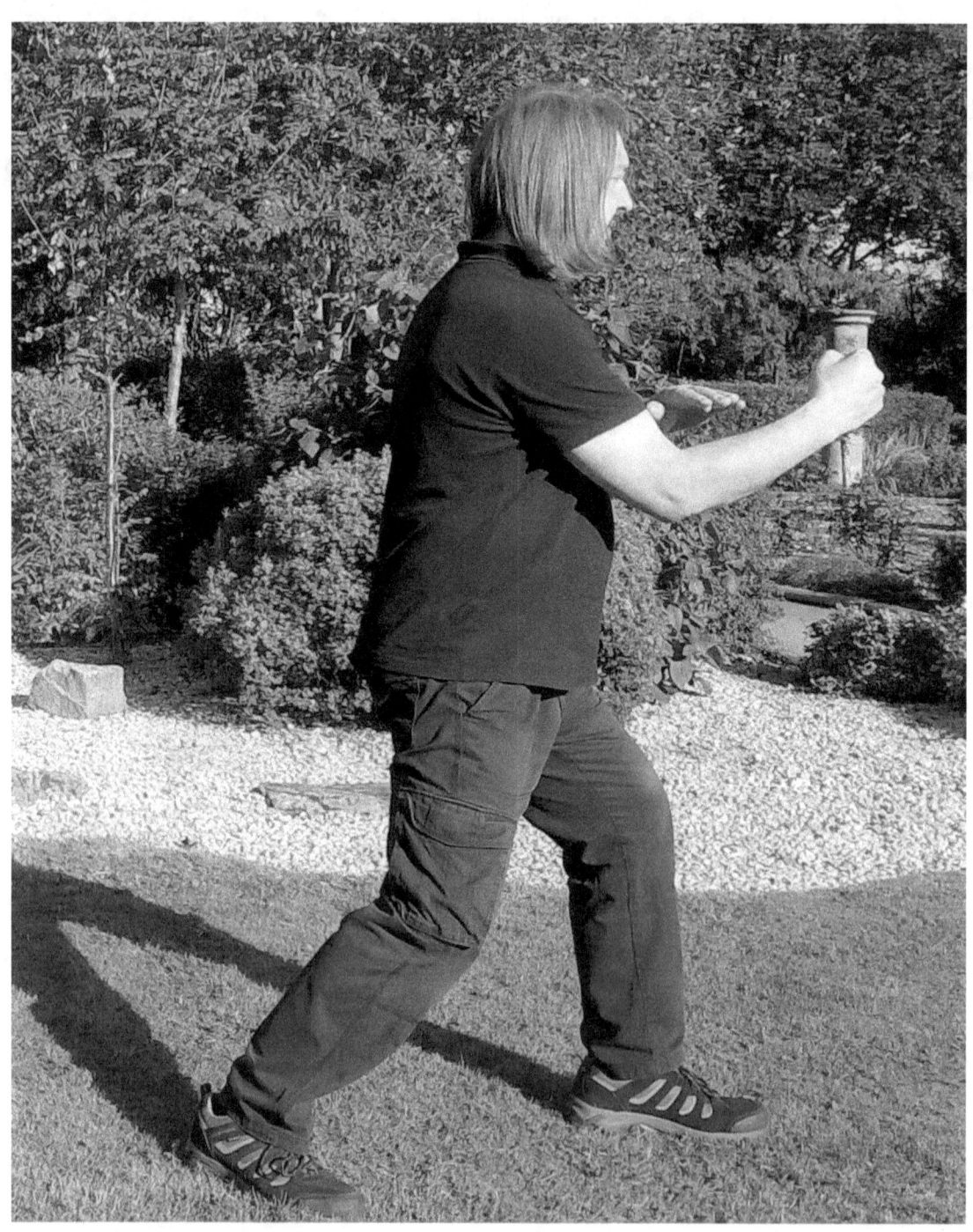

Apparent Close Up

Rotate your left hand palm upward and place it underneath the right elbow, shift your weight back into your right foot.

Bring the left hand forward and up so that both arms cross at the wrists, (the backs of your hands facing forwards) with the left hand on the outside.

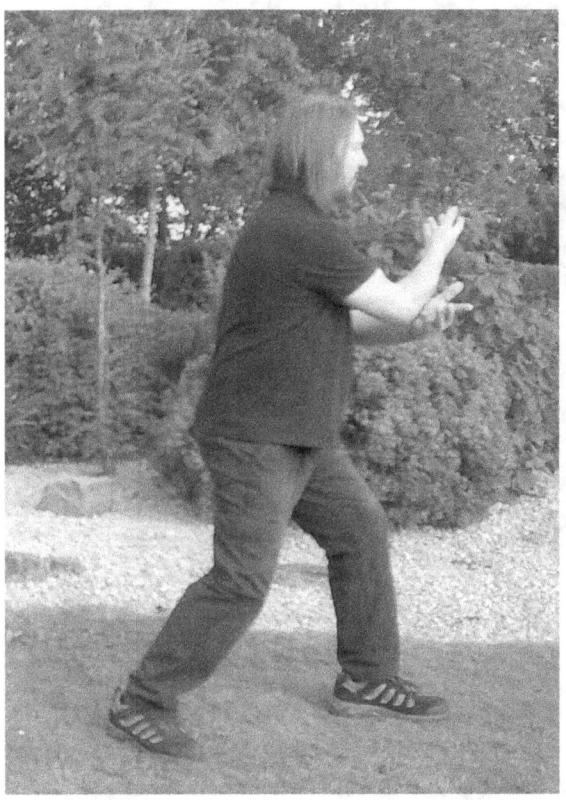 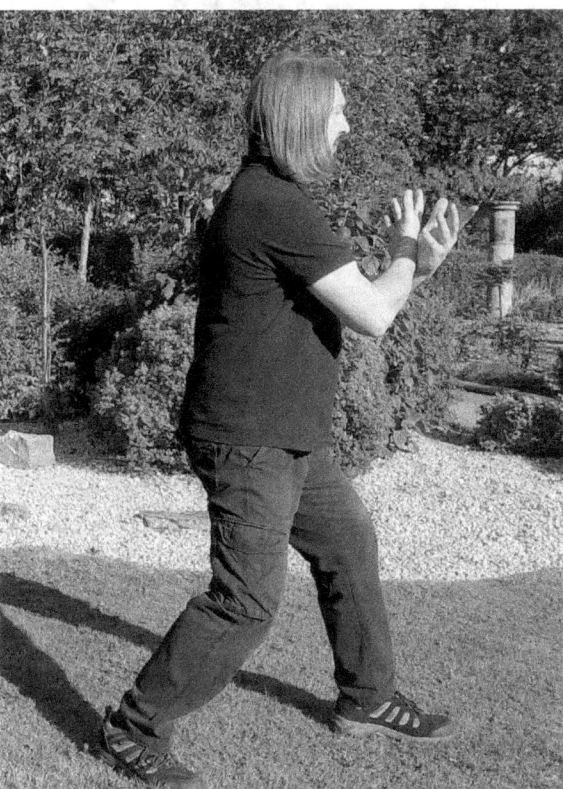

Push

Separate your hands to either side and rotate them until the palms face down at an angle. Move forward from your right leg into your left leg to make a Bow stance.

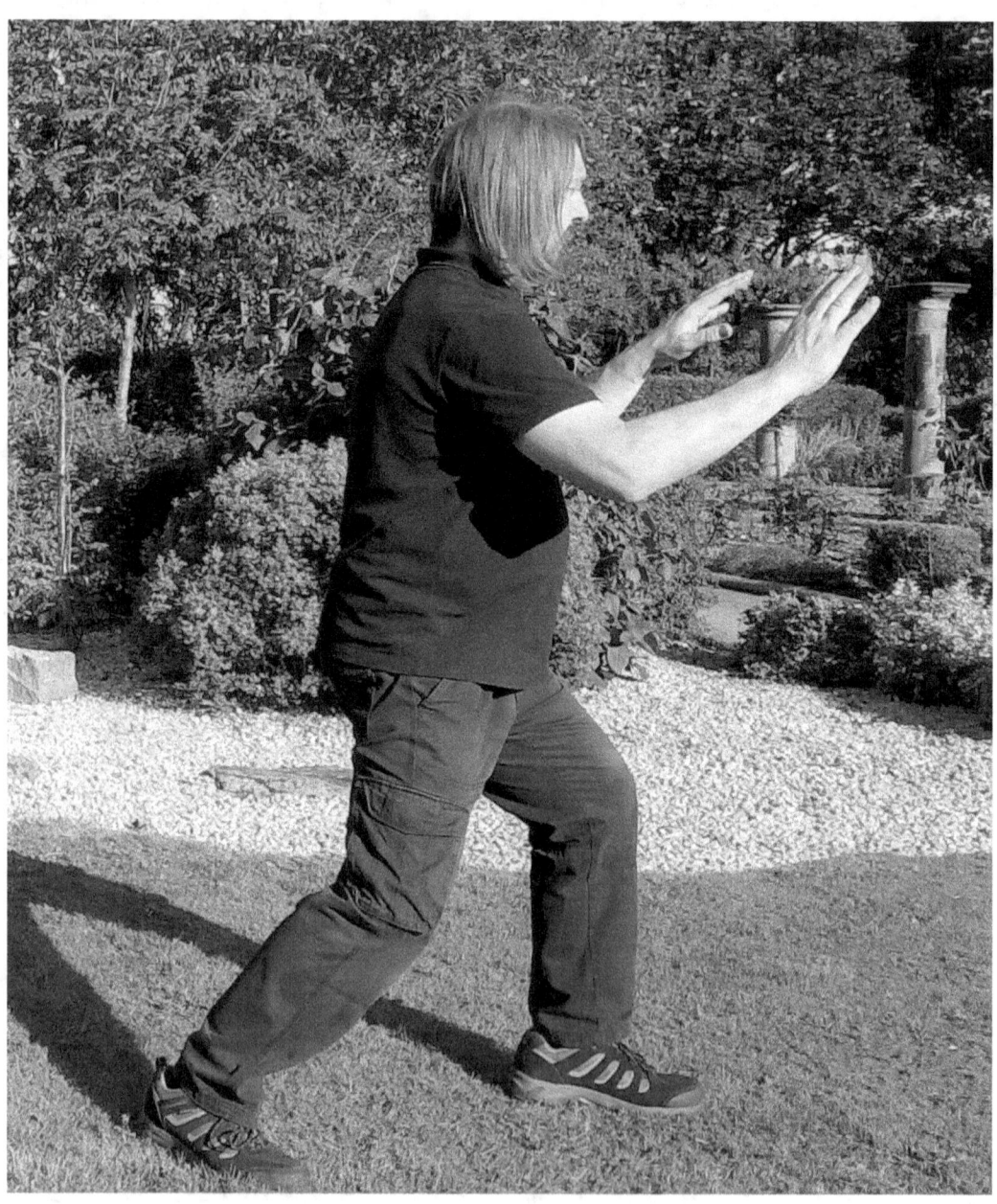

12) Seal the Knot

Shift backwards into the right foot, lift up your left toes, and turn to your right rear side, pivoting on the left heel.

Roll the left foot down, move all of your weight into your left leg, and step into a parallel stance with your right foot. Your feet are shoulder width apart and you now have equal weight in each leg.

At the same time, circle both arms out and downwards and then bring them up front of your chest, cross the wrists with your right wrist on the outside of your left.

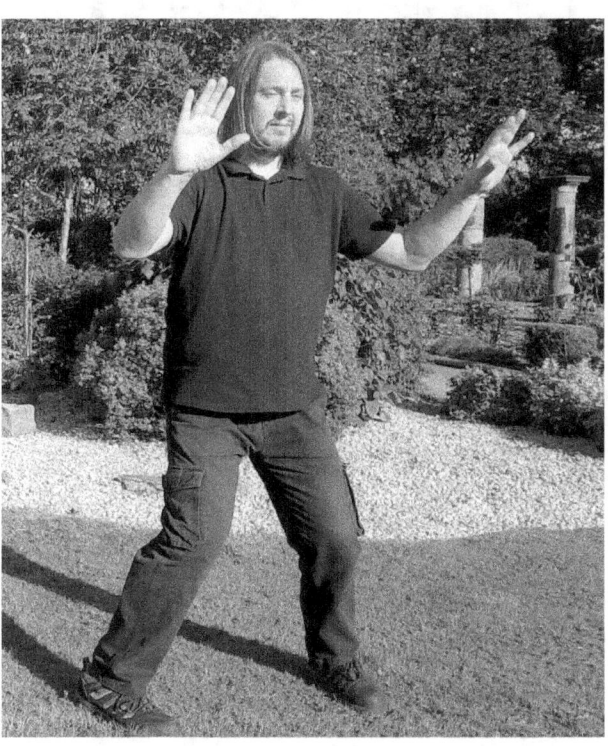 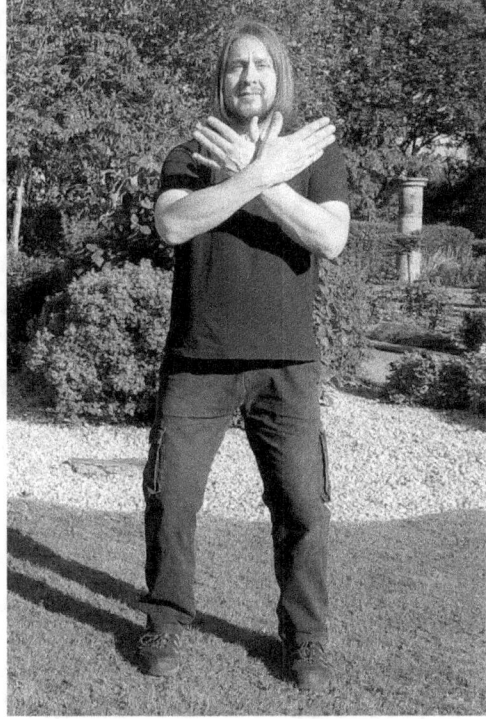

13) Carry Tiger Return to Mountain

Shift your weight fully onto the left leg and step out to your right rear corner with your right foot.

Place the foot down gently and move into a right foot forward Bow stance.

Circle the left hand down, back and round into a Push shape.

At the same time, sweep your right hand down and across into Brushing Knee posture.

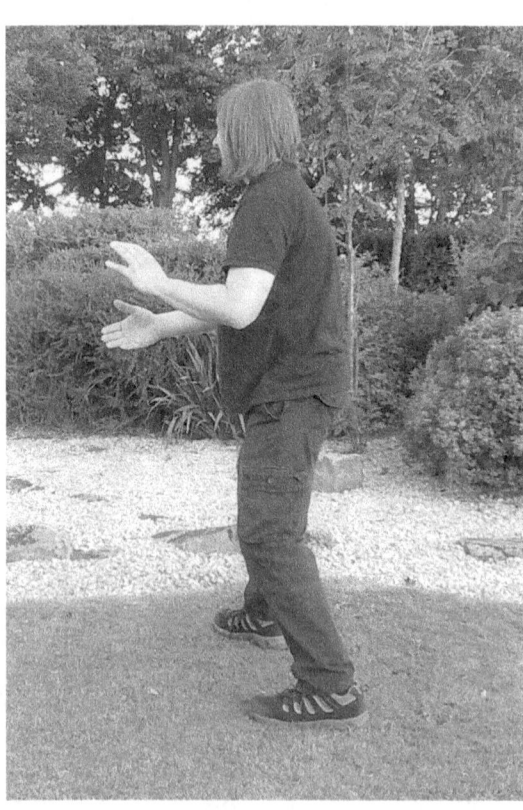 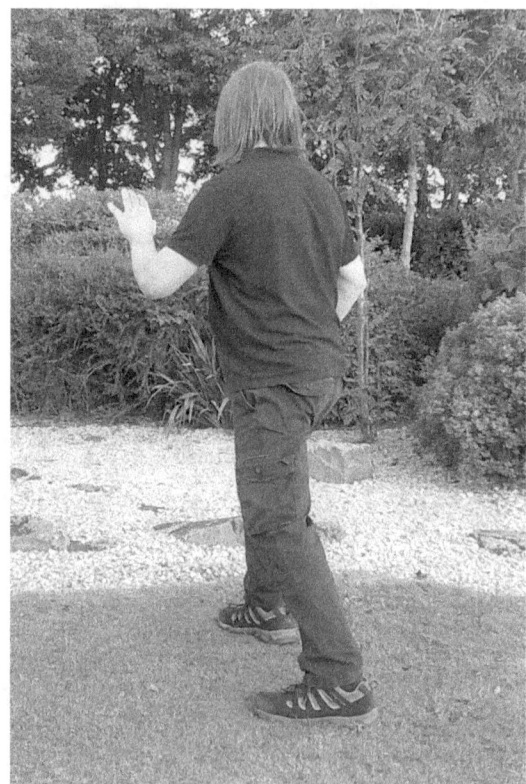

Ward Off Right

Leave the left hand in front of your chest and roll your right hand upwards in a curve to the 11 o'clock position in front of your right upper chest. The fingers of your left hand point to your right wrist and your elbows are heavy.

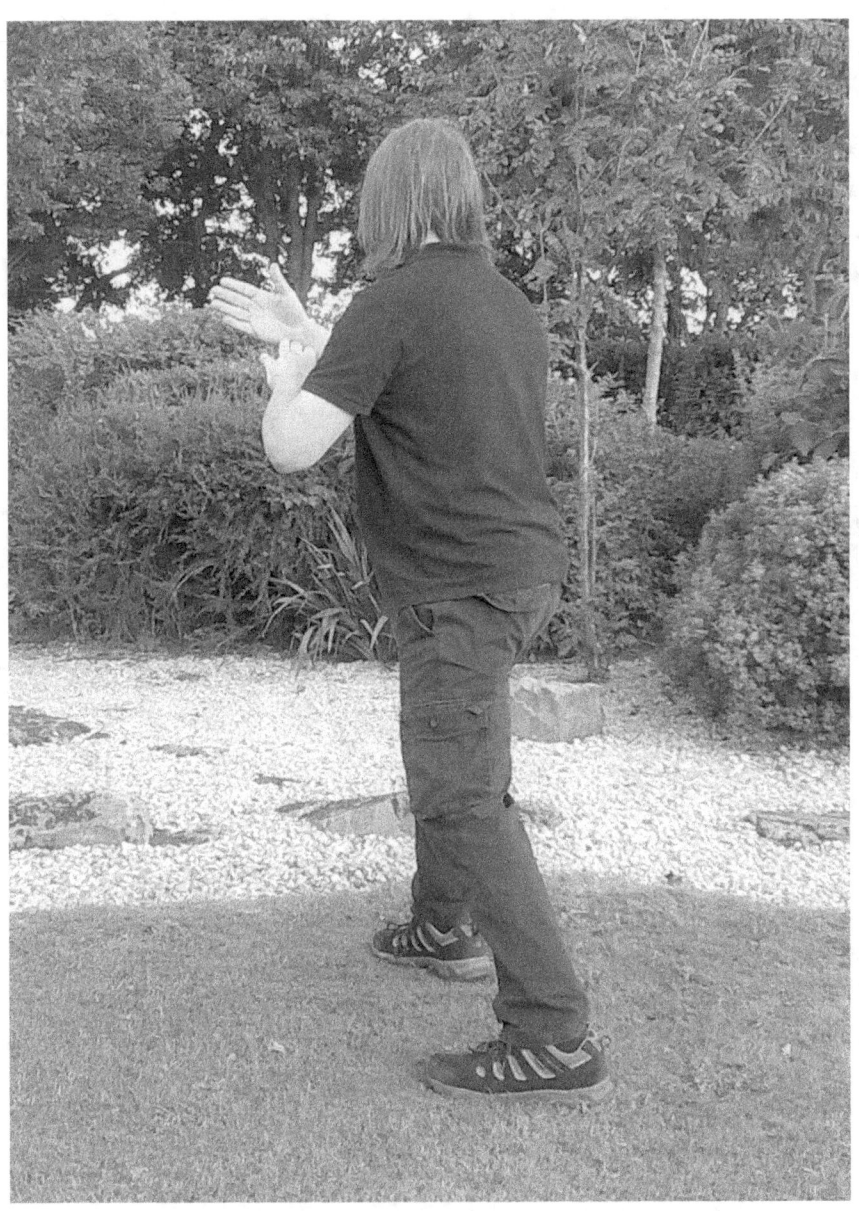

Rollback

Slowly lower your arms, keep a space between the arms and your body. At the same time move seventy percent of your weight into your left leg and turn your body towards your left corner. Keep your centreline alignment.

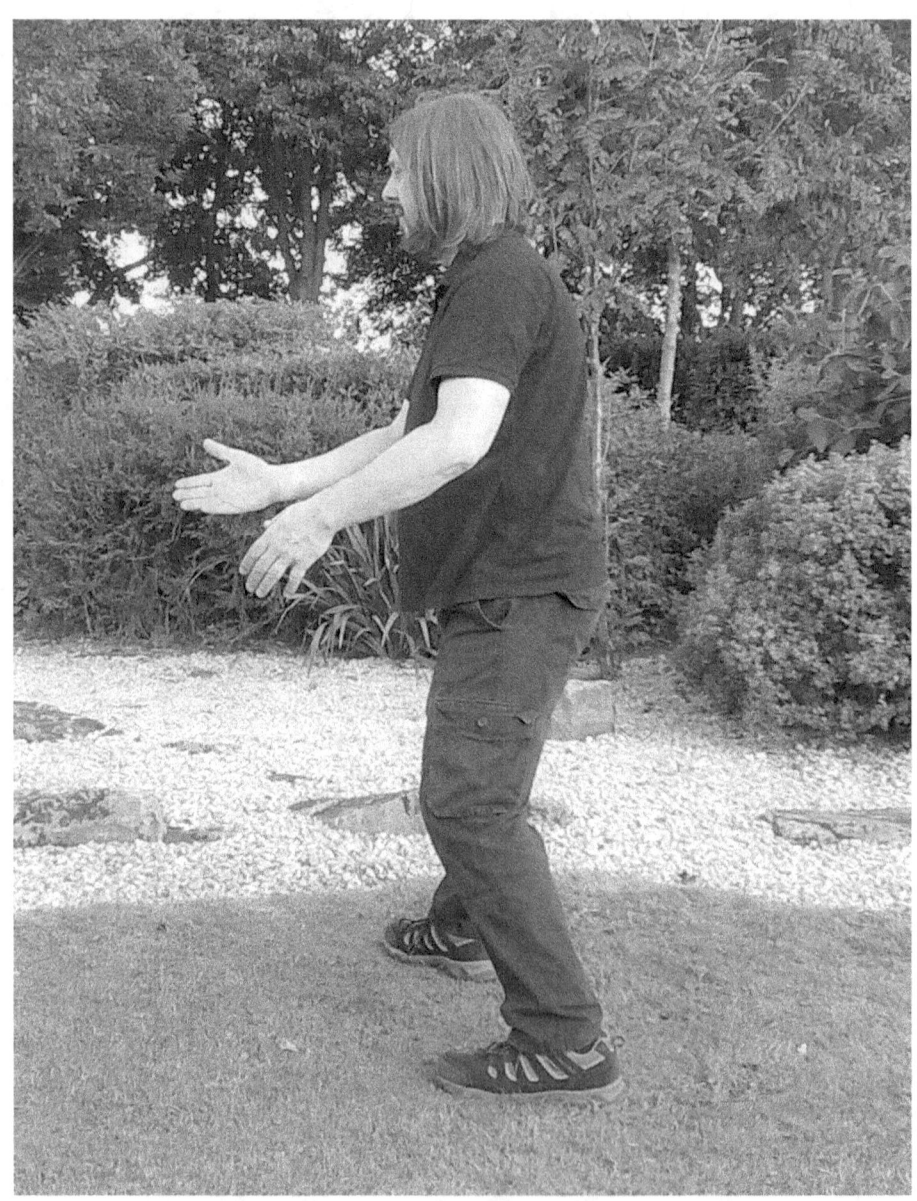

Press

Circle your left hand round and place your palm on your right inner wrist. Turn your body to square again and move your weight forward from the left leg into a seventy percent front weighted, right Bow stance.

At the same time, bring your connected hands up in front of your chest, and press them forward slightly. Your arms form a triangle shape.

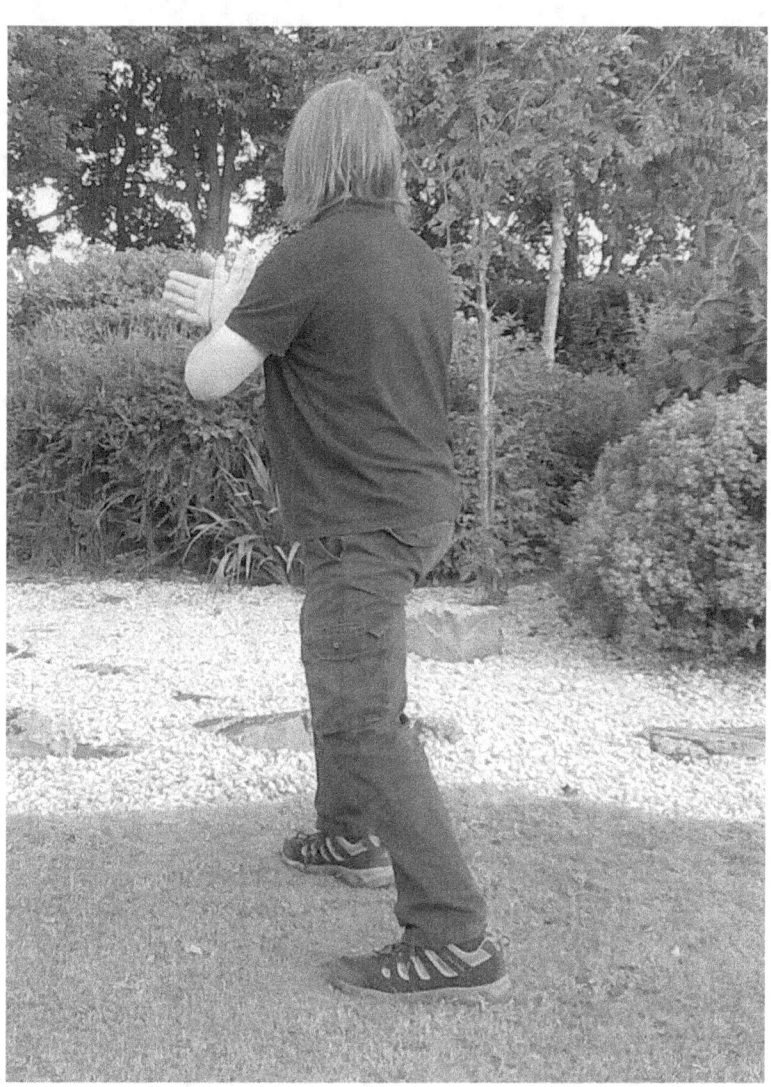

Separate Hands

Rotate your hands to palms down and at the same time cross your wrists, with the left hand on top. Immediately uncross wrists arms and separate your hands to shoulder width. At the same time, move backwards into your left leg.

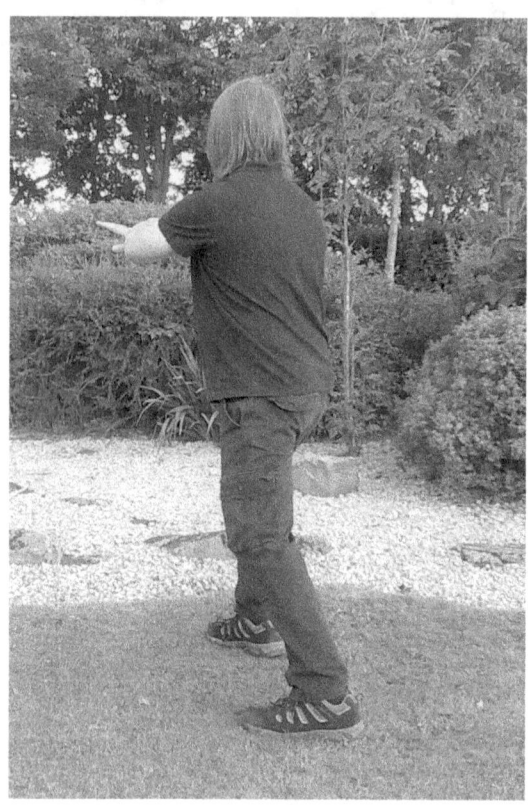
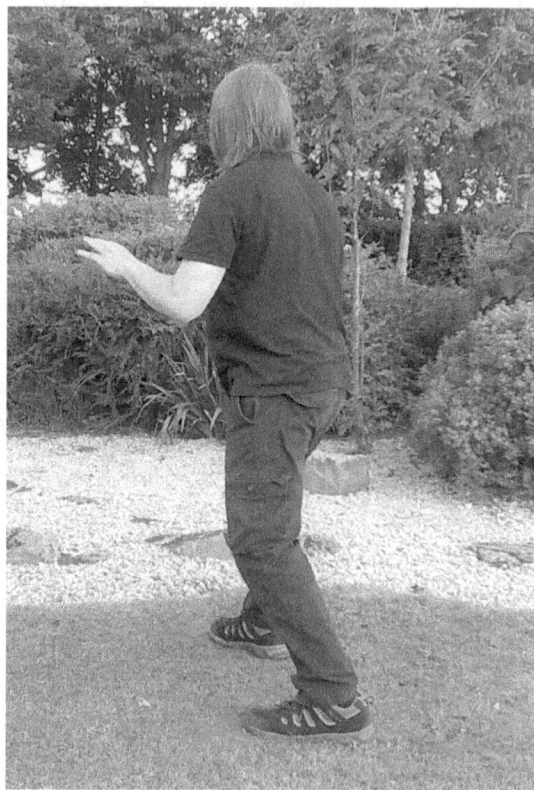

Push

Move forward onto your right leg, the hands follow the movement of your body. As you push forward both hands rise up at an angle in front of your shoulders, the movement ends with seventy per cent of your weight resting on the right leg.

.

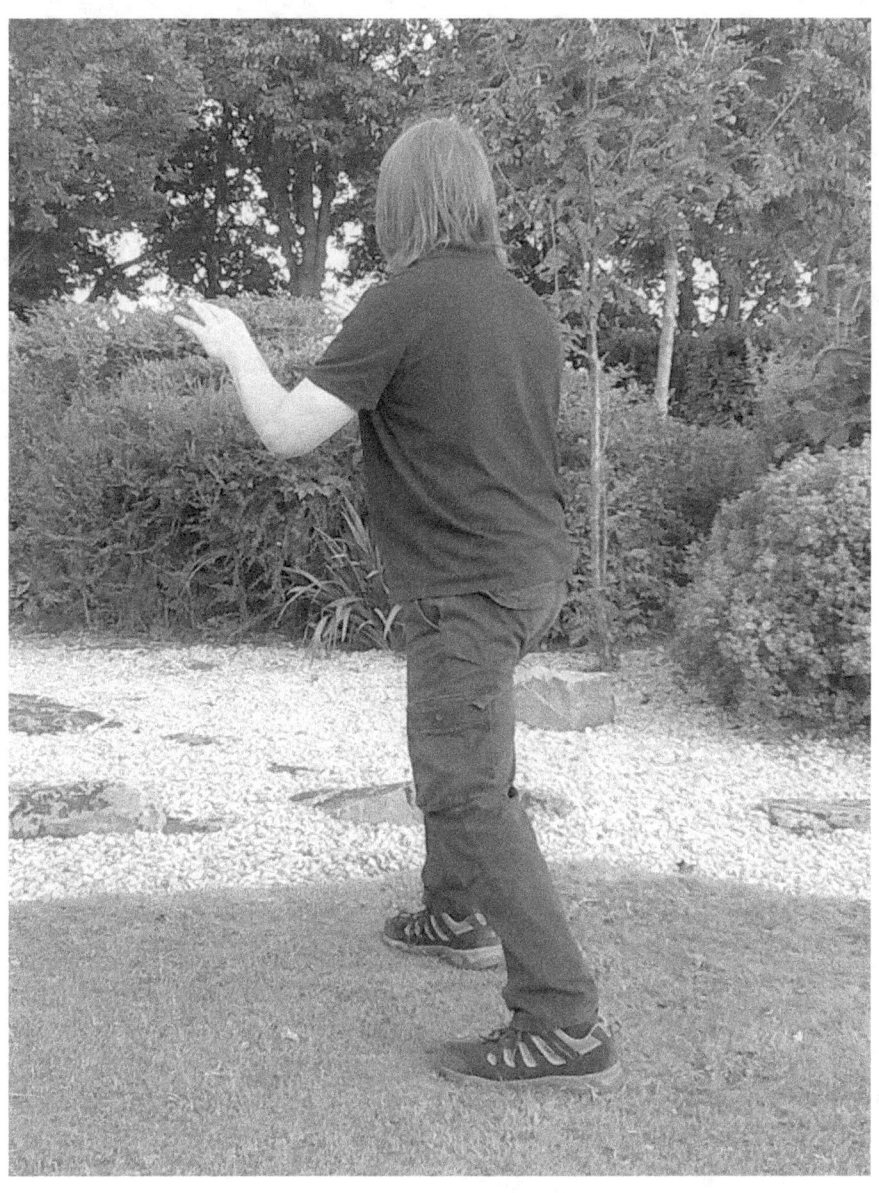

14) Diagonal Single Whip

Shift your weight back into your left foot.

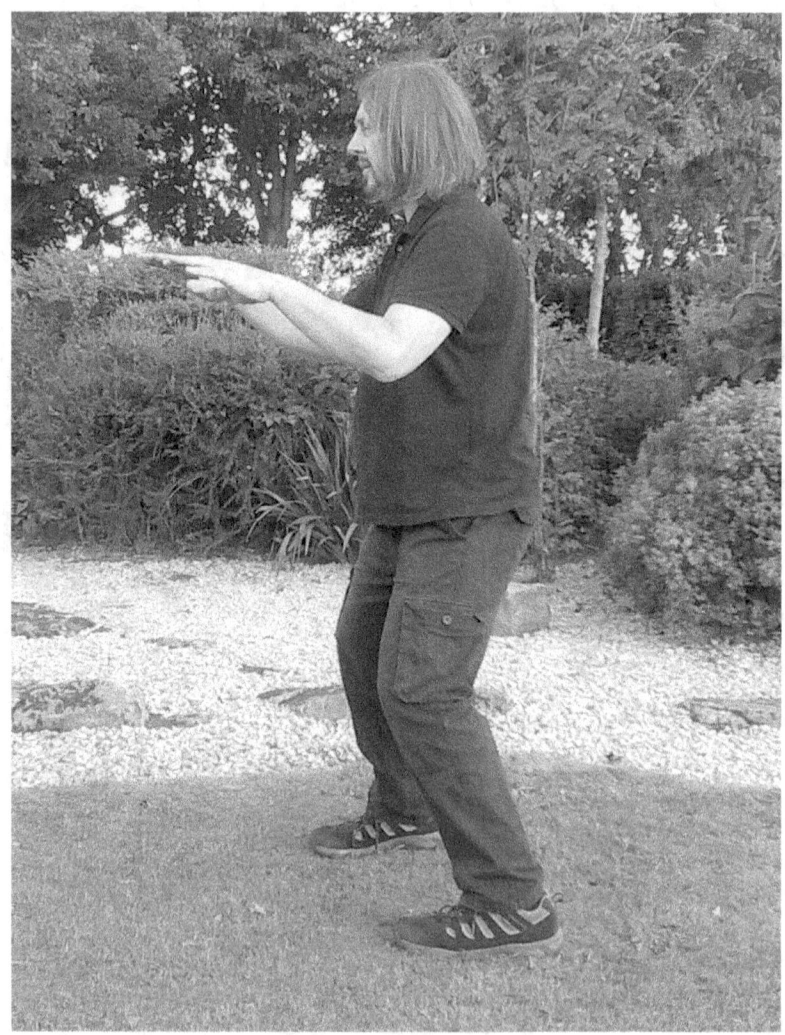

Lift the toes of your right foot. Turn to your back left corner; your hands remain in front of your shoulders.

Your right leg follows the bodies turning by pivoting on the right heel.

Hold a ball with the right hand on top and the left hand on the bottom.

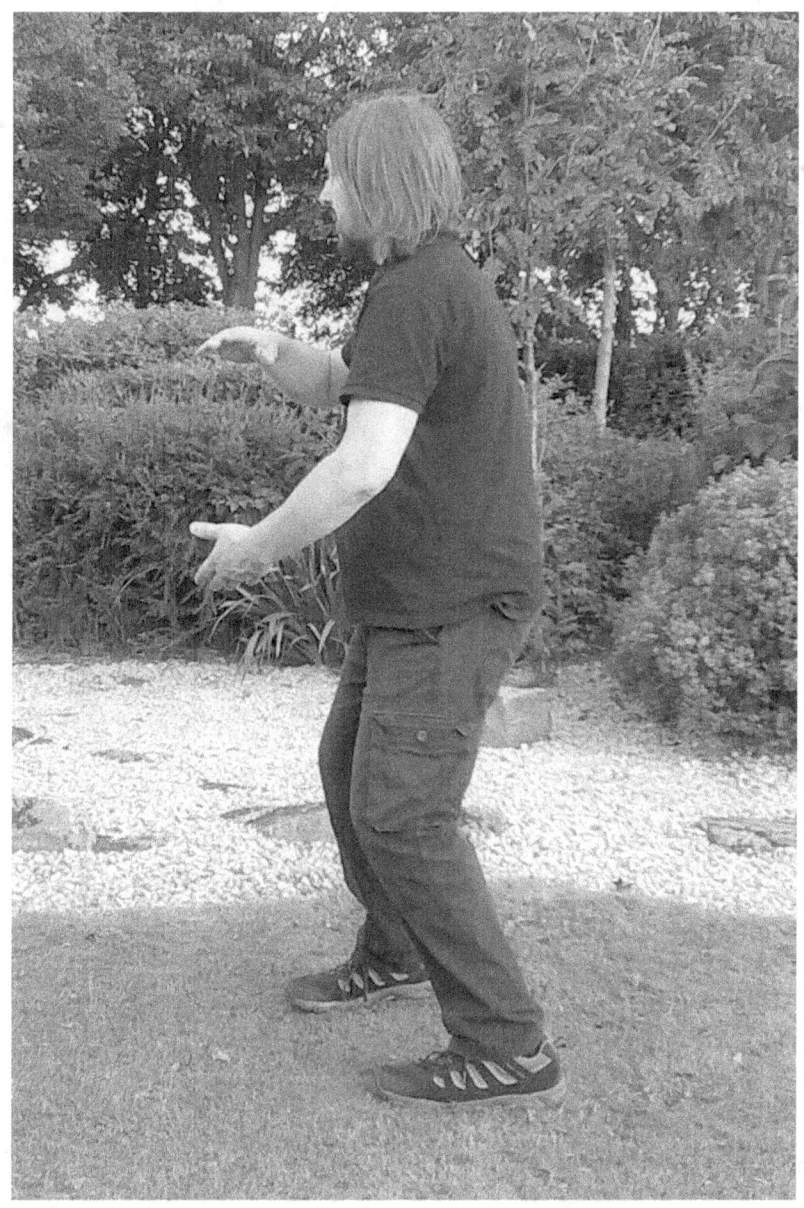

Push your right hand out until the arm is straight (but not locked out). At the same time bend your right wrist until the thumb points down and place your fingertips around the tip of the thumb to form a beak.

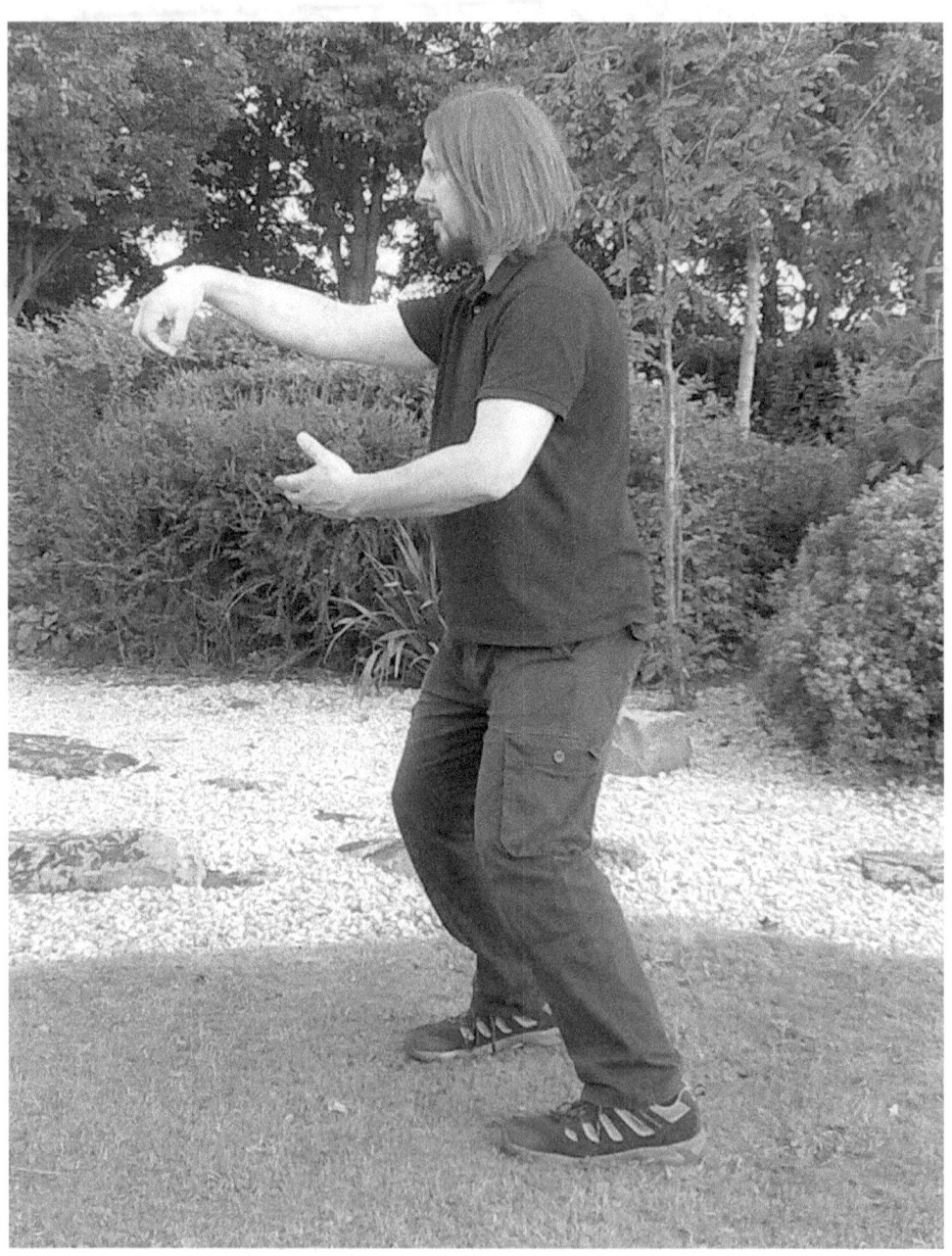

Turn back towards the left, your weight stays in the right leg. Lift up your left heel, pivot on the ball of the foot to the left and step forwards, place down your heel, and roll into a left footed Bow stance.

As you step your left hand rises in a Ward off shape, curving up and across your body to your left side, finally rotate your palm until it faces away from you in front of your left shoulder

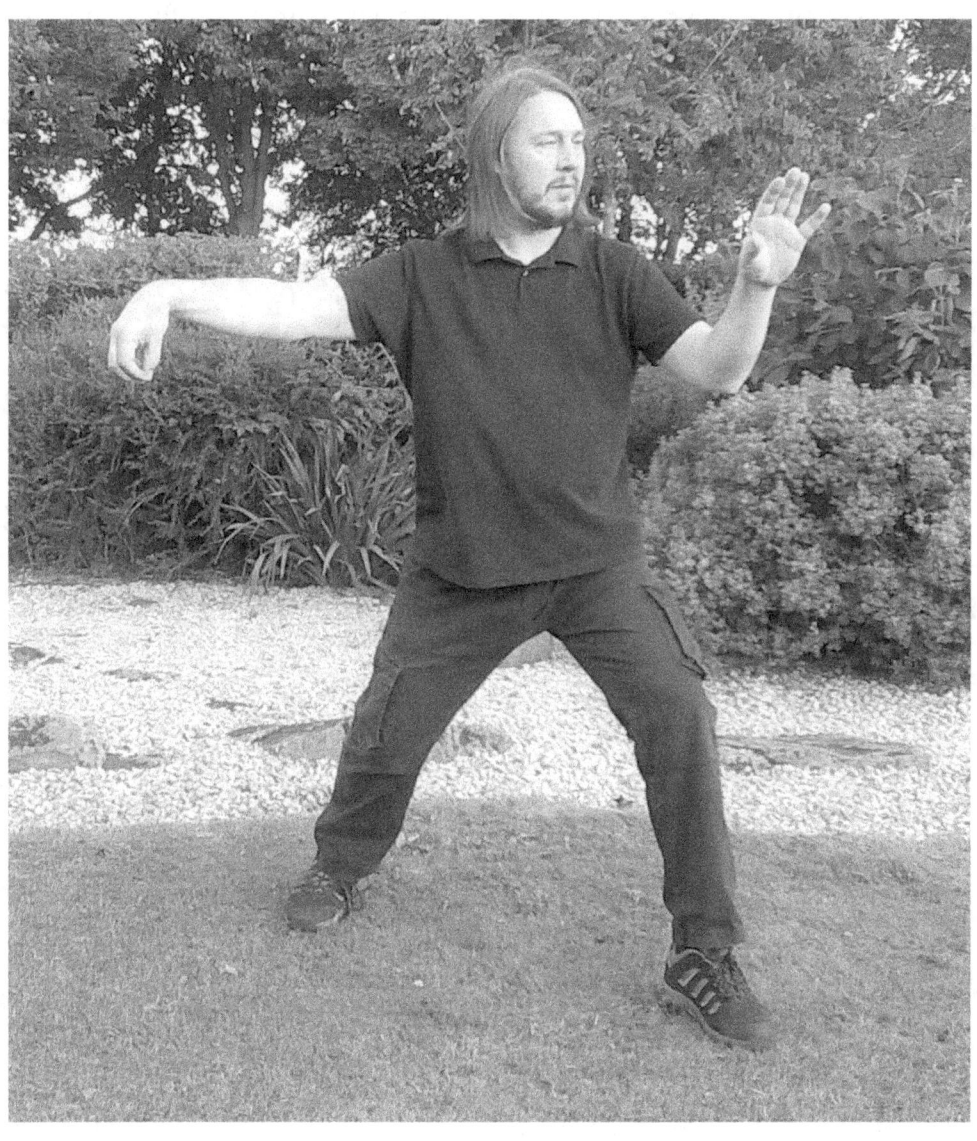

Step forward with your right foot, close the space between your feet, the left foot should be two inches further forward than your right foot, with the feet parallel.

Shift your weight across and sit fully into your right leg. Lift up your left heel. You will use the ball of the left foot to pivot on as you turn to your left, until your body is square to the front.

Once you have completed this movement, release the fingers of your right hand, and make an open hand with the palm facing in; your arms follow the turning of your body, the left hand making a sideways chopping movement, with the little finger side of the hand. The right hand makes a slapping movement.

The right hand finishes its movement with the fingertips facing straight forward at head height and with your left arm at an angle of twenty degrees out past your left shoulder.

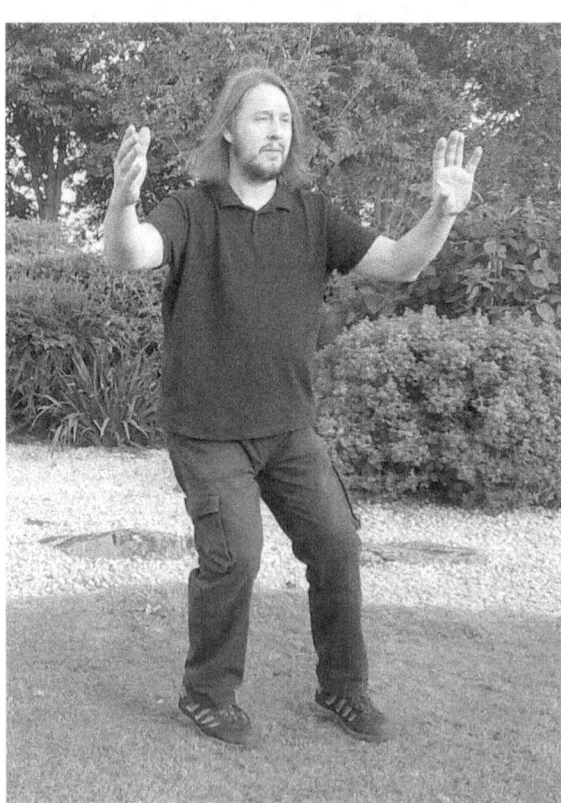 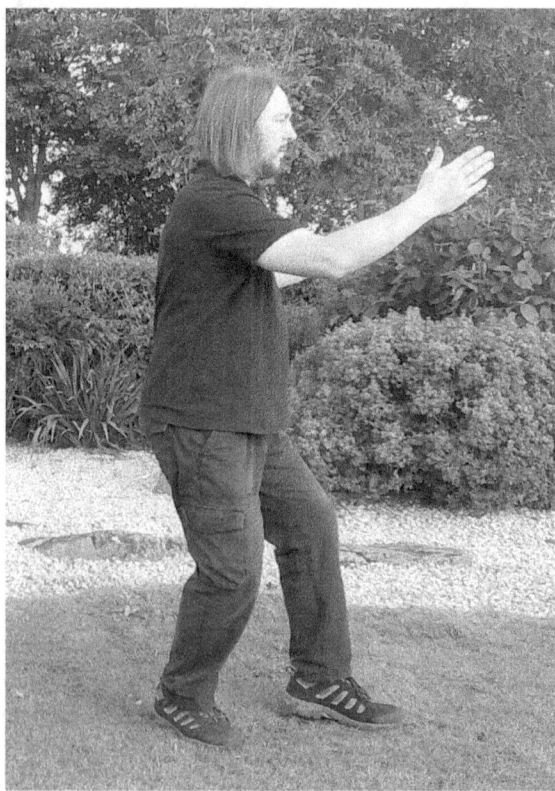

15) Fist Under Elbow

Your left hand chops downward and moves in a U shape, rising up in front of your left shoulder, the palm facing to the right side.

At the same time, your right hand descends in a curve down and to the left to make a fist with the thumb facing upwards, underneath your left elbow.

Lift up your left toes into a right rear foot, Cat stance.

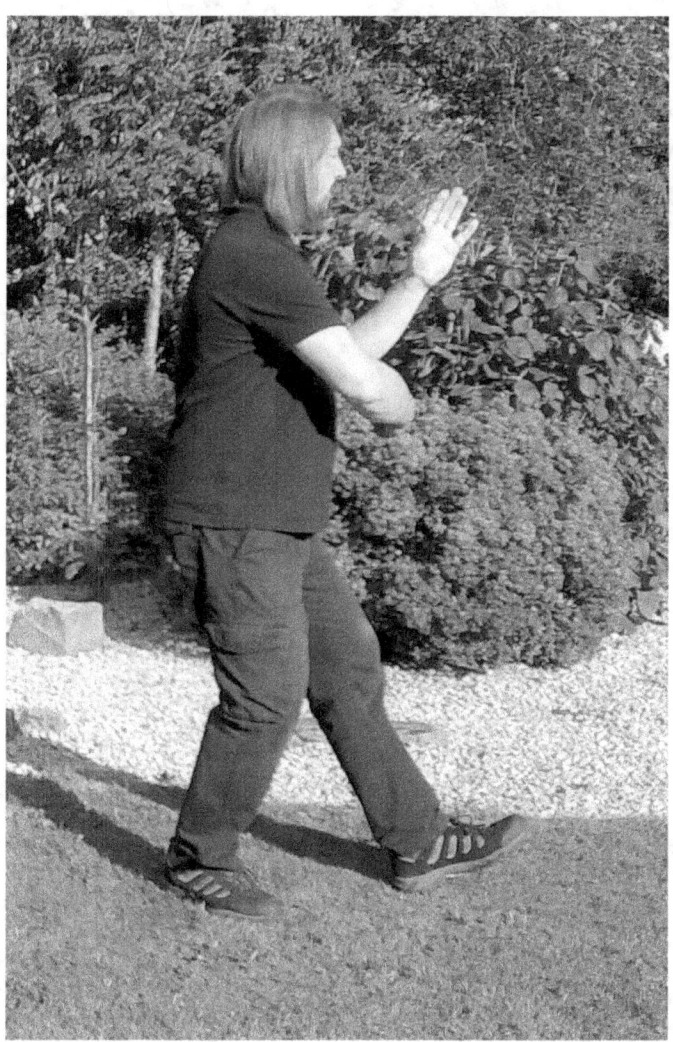

16) Repulse Monkeys

Release the fist and open your right hand. Turn the upper body to your right front corner. Bring your open right hand, palm up in a curve past the side of the right hip, bring it up and back behind your right shoulder.

At the same time turn your left hand palm up and bring it forward. (Both palms should now face upward.)

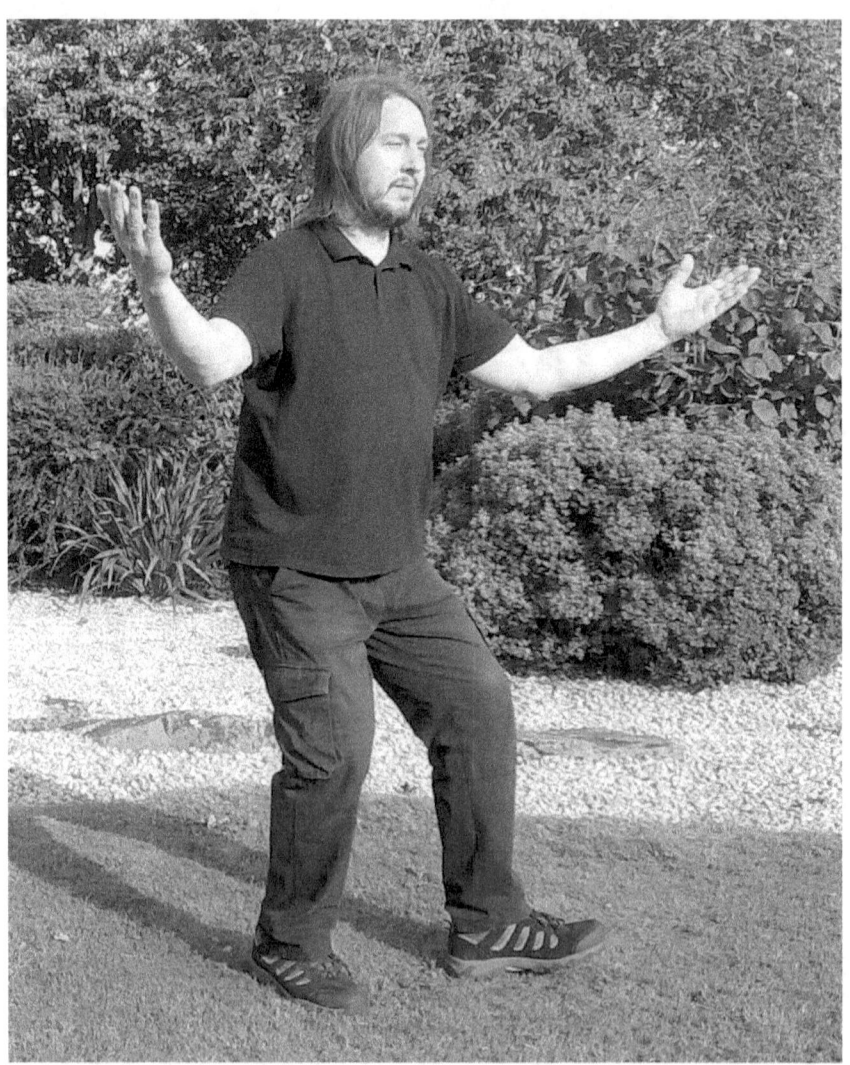

Step back and across with your left foot into a shoulder wide parallel bow stance. Place the toes down first and gradually roll your foot down onto the floor.

Slowly shift your weight into the left leg and then lift the heel of the right foot, pivot on the ball of the foot and place it flat on the ground. Both feet should be parallel in a shoulder width stance.

As you return to a forward facing posture, bring your right hand past your right ear, your fingertips face forward. The right hand moves forwards and the left hand back.

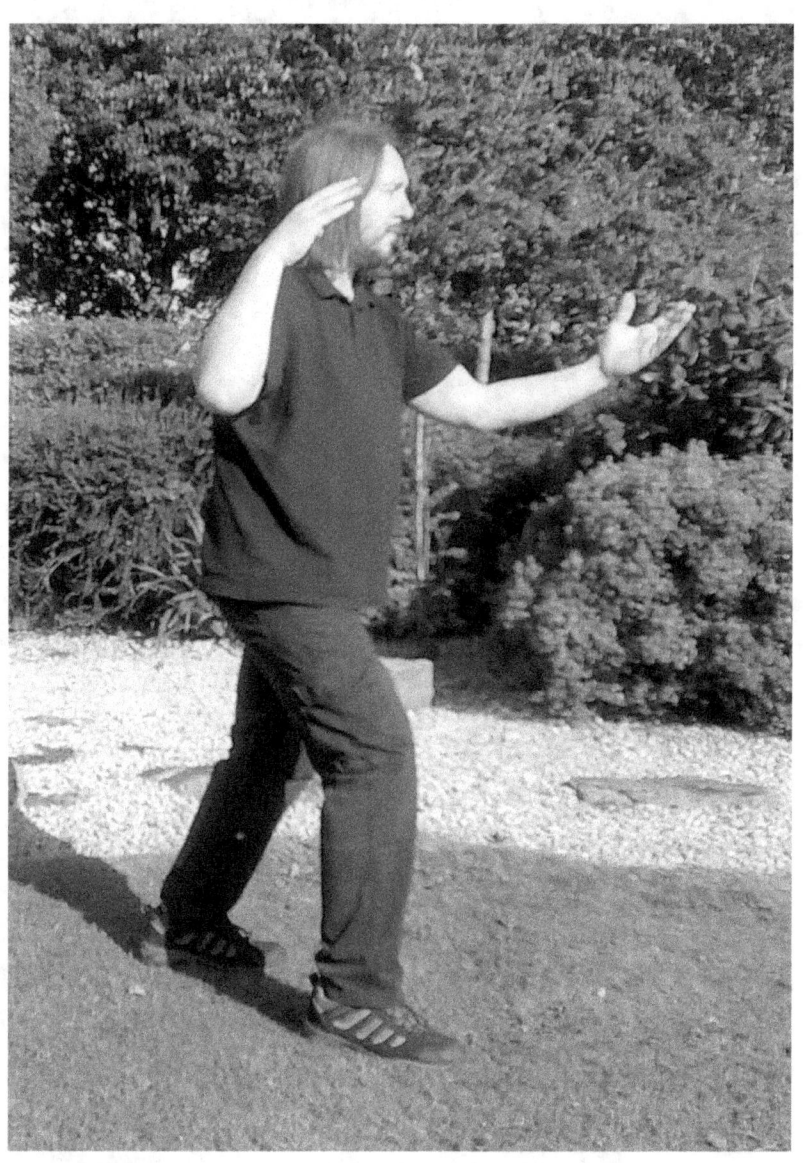

Roll the right hand over the left hand as if you are holding a ball in your left palm and the right hand rolls over it.

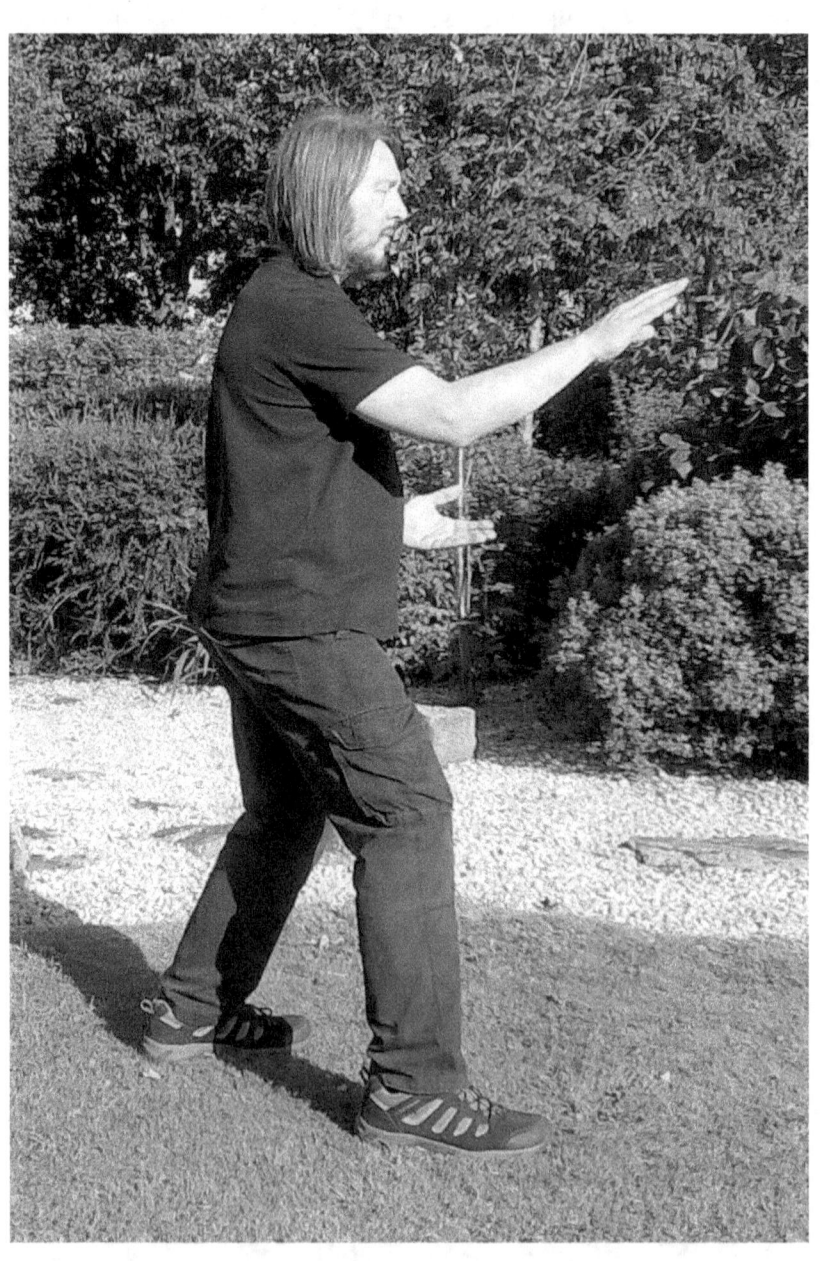

Turn your body to your left corner. Your right hand pushes forward and turns to face palm up.

At the same time bring your open left hand, palm up in a curve past the side of the left hip. The palm remains facing upward, as you raise your left arm to bring it up and back behind your left shoulder.

At the same time turn your right hand palm up and move it forward. Both hands are now facing palm upward. As this happens, turn your body to your left corner.

 Keep your centreline alignment (Nose, centre of chest and belly button) you should be able to see both of your hands with your peripheral vision.

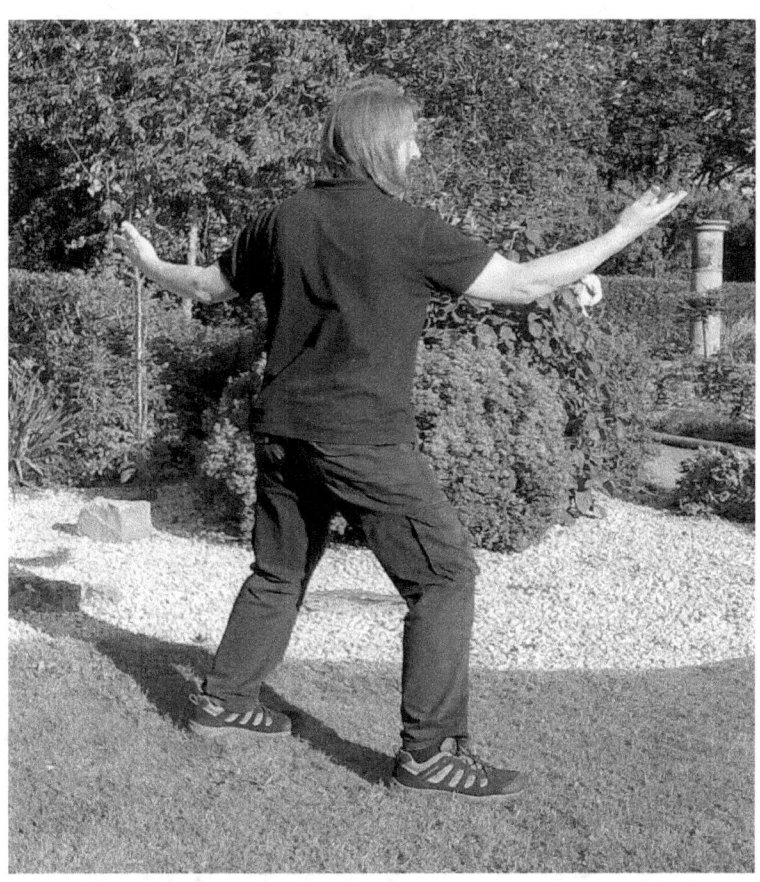

Step back with your right foot, put the toes down first, and roll the rest of your foot down until the whole foot is on the floor. Once you have planted the foot, shift your weight into the right leg.

As you return to a forward facing posture, bring your left hand past your right ear with the fingertips facing forward.

The left hand, palm facing down moves across in front of your centreline, as does your right hand with its palm facing upwards.

The left hand moves over the top of the right as if you are holding a ball in your right palm and the left hand rolls over the top of it.

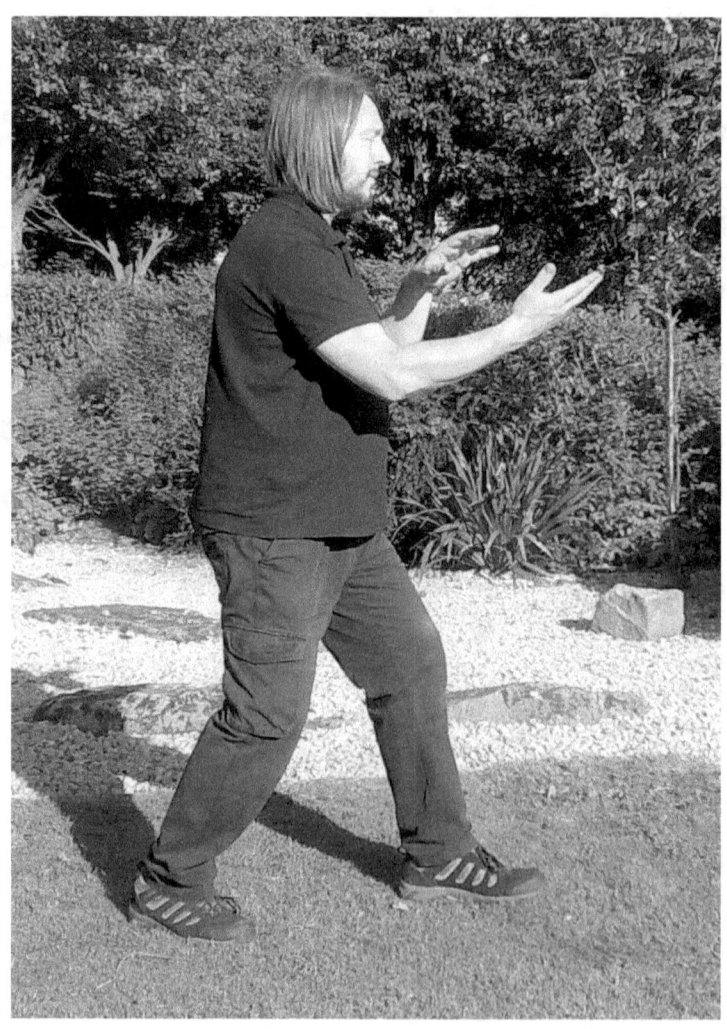

Turn to your right corner, with your arms following the turning of your body. Bring your open right hand, palm up in a curve past the side of the right hip. The palm remains facing upward as you raise your right arm to bring it up and back behind your right shoulder.

At the same time turn your leftt hand palm up and move it forward. Both hands are now palms upward, as this happens, turn your body to your right corner. Keep your centreline alignment you should be able to see both of your hands with your peripheral vision.

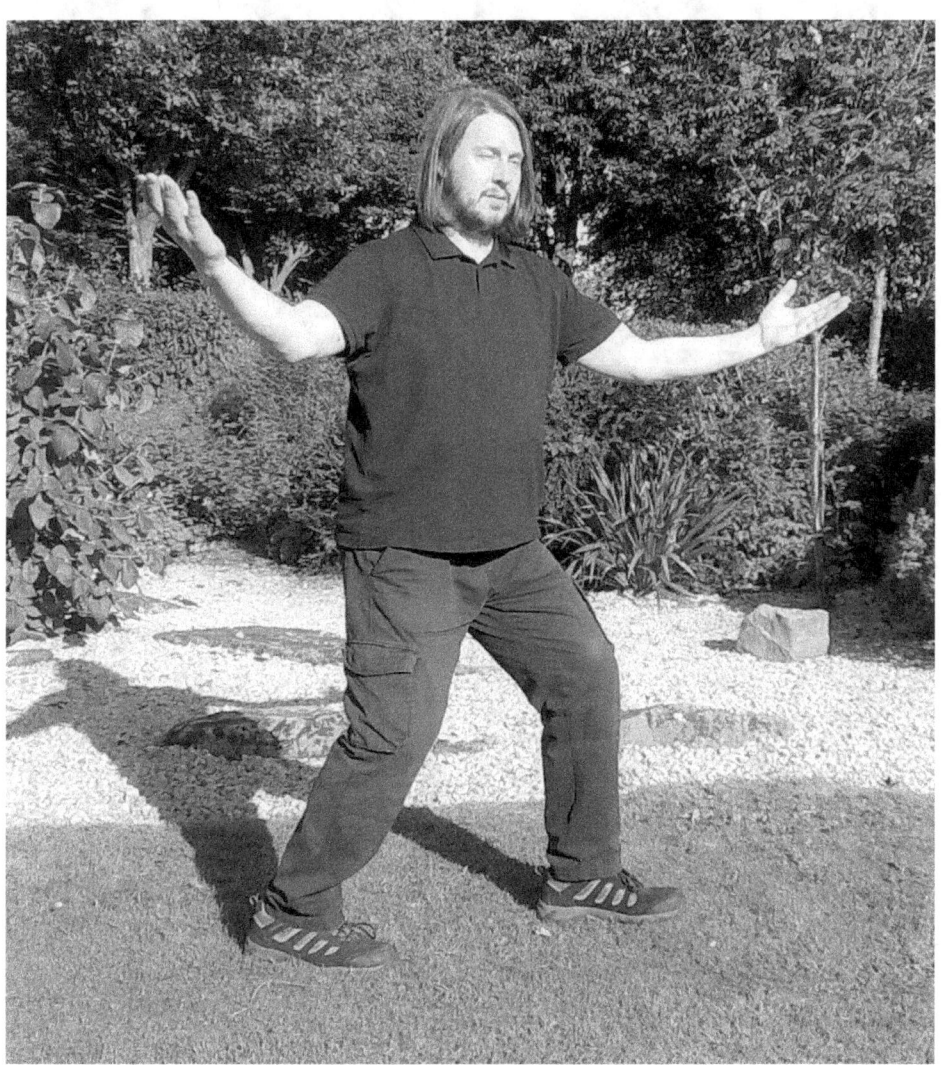

Step back with your left foot, roll the toes down first, and gradually roll the rest of your foot down until the whole foot is on the floor. Once you have planted the foot, shift your weight into that leg.

As you return to a forward facing posture, bring your right hand past your right ear with the fingertips pushing forwards.

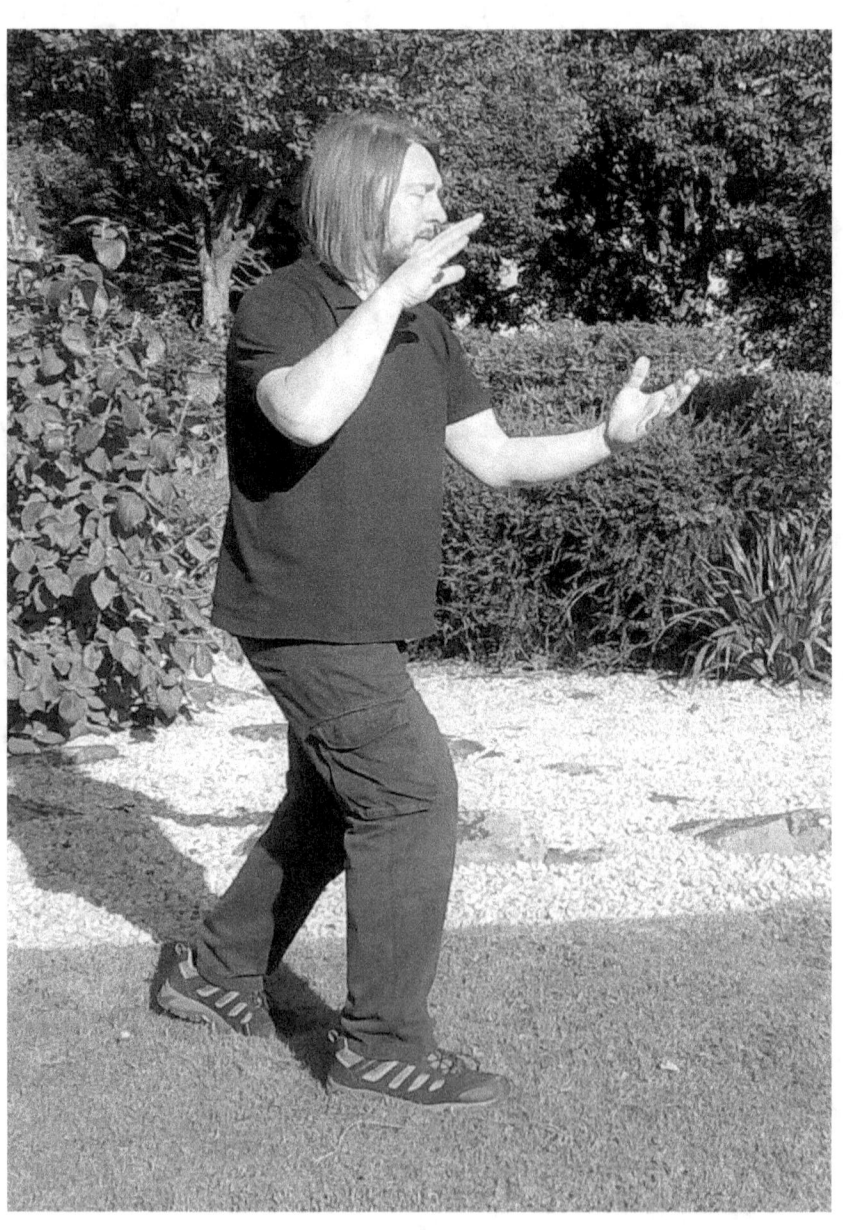

The right hand, palm facing down moves across in front of your centreline, as does your left hand palm facing upwards.

The right hand moves over the top of the left as if you are holding a ball in your left palm and the right hand rolls over the top of it pushing forwards with the fingertips.

Your left hand descends and moves in a curve to your left hip where it sits palm facing upward.

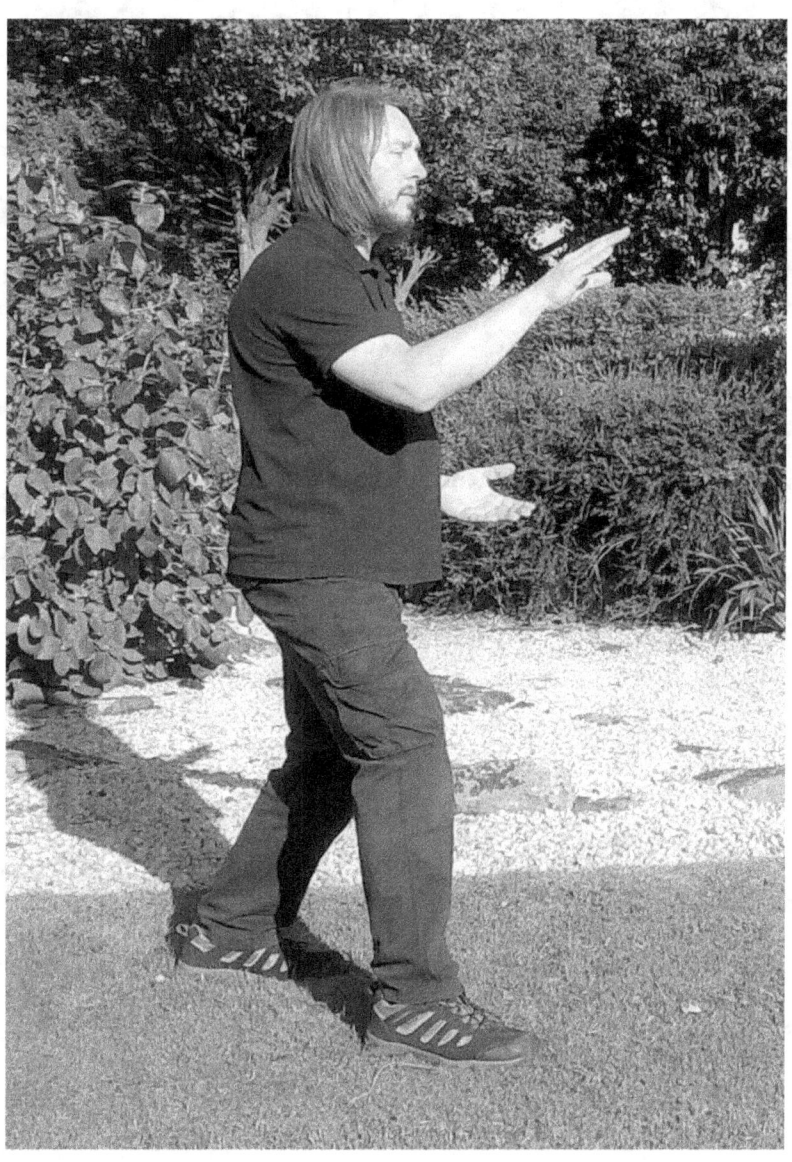

17) Diagonal Flying

Turn to the left rotating your hands to hold a ball with the left hand on top and right hand on the bottom.

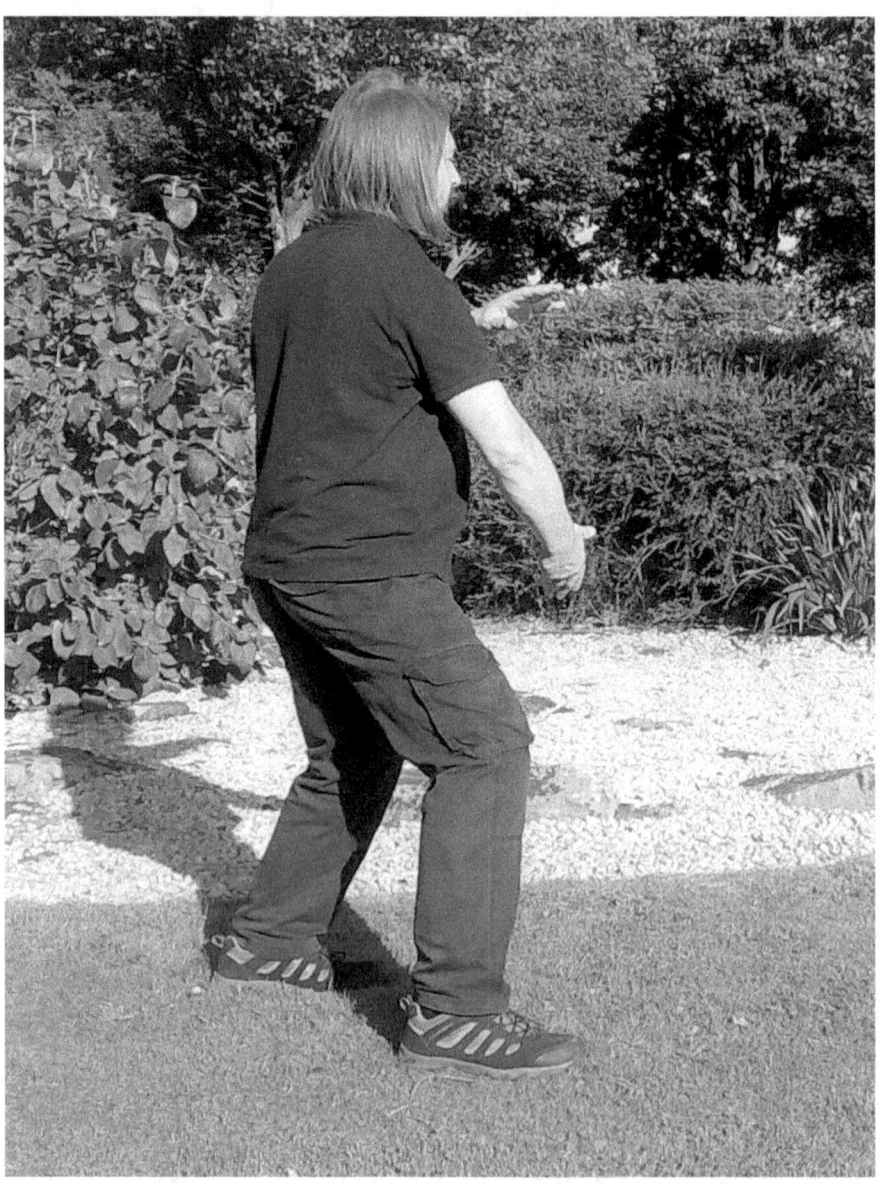

Take a large step to your right rear corner, moving into a right foot forward Bow stance.

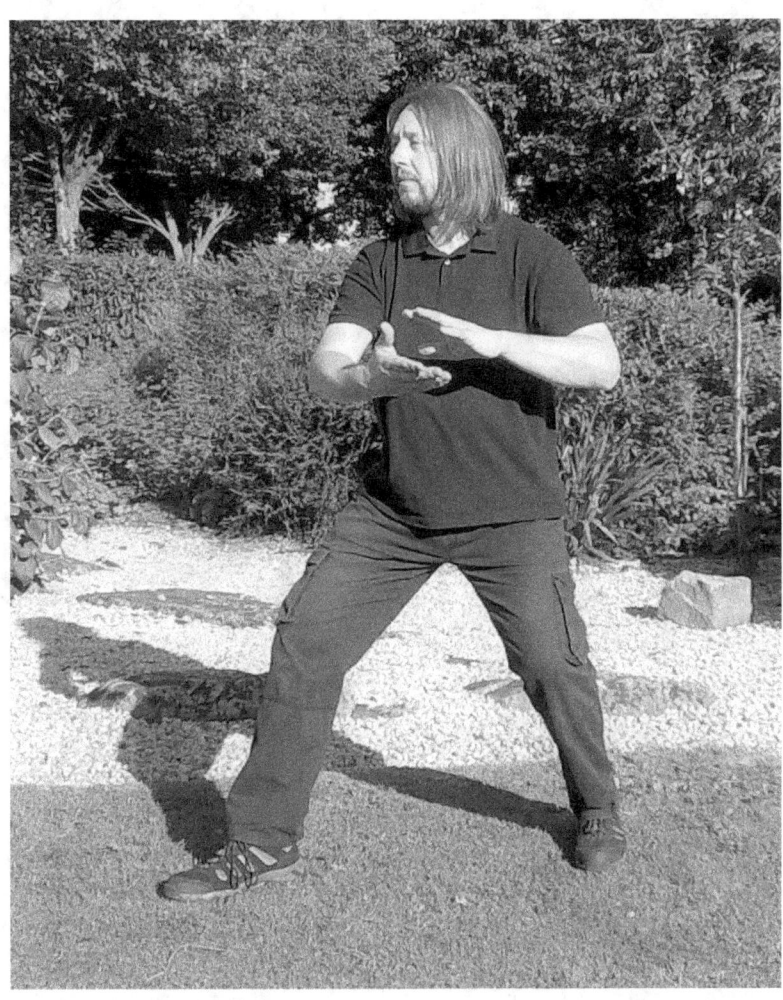

Bring your right hand, (palm facing upwards) up and across the right side of your body, its ending position is just past your right shoulder, at the same time as your left arm (palm facing down) descends to the outside of the left hip.

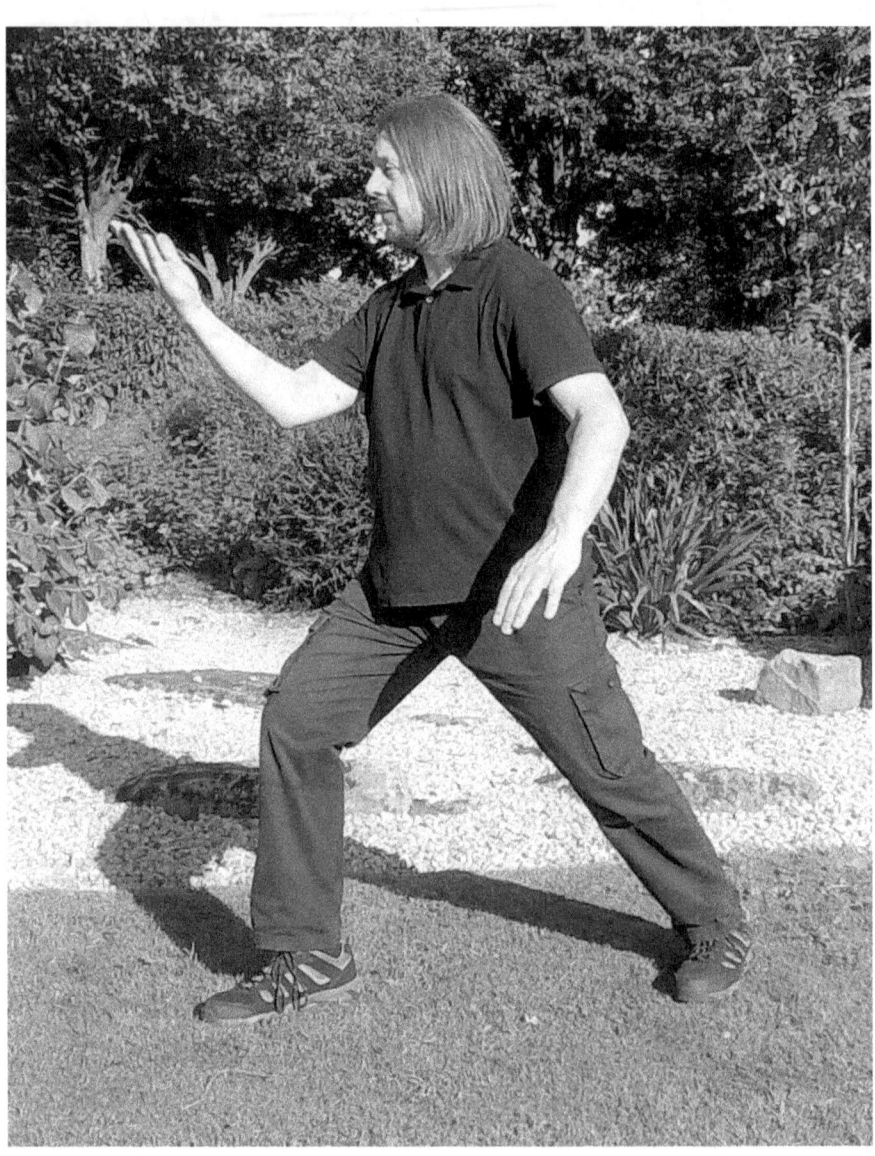

18) Wave Hands Like Clouds

Turn your body to face square and step forward with you right foot into a parallel stance. Slowly shift your weight to the left leg. Pivot on your right heel to square up the feet. Shift your weight fully onto the left foot.

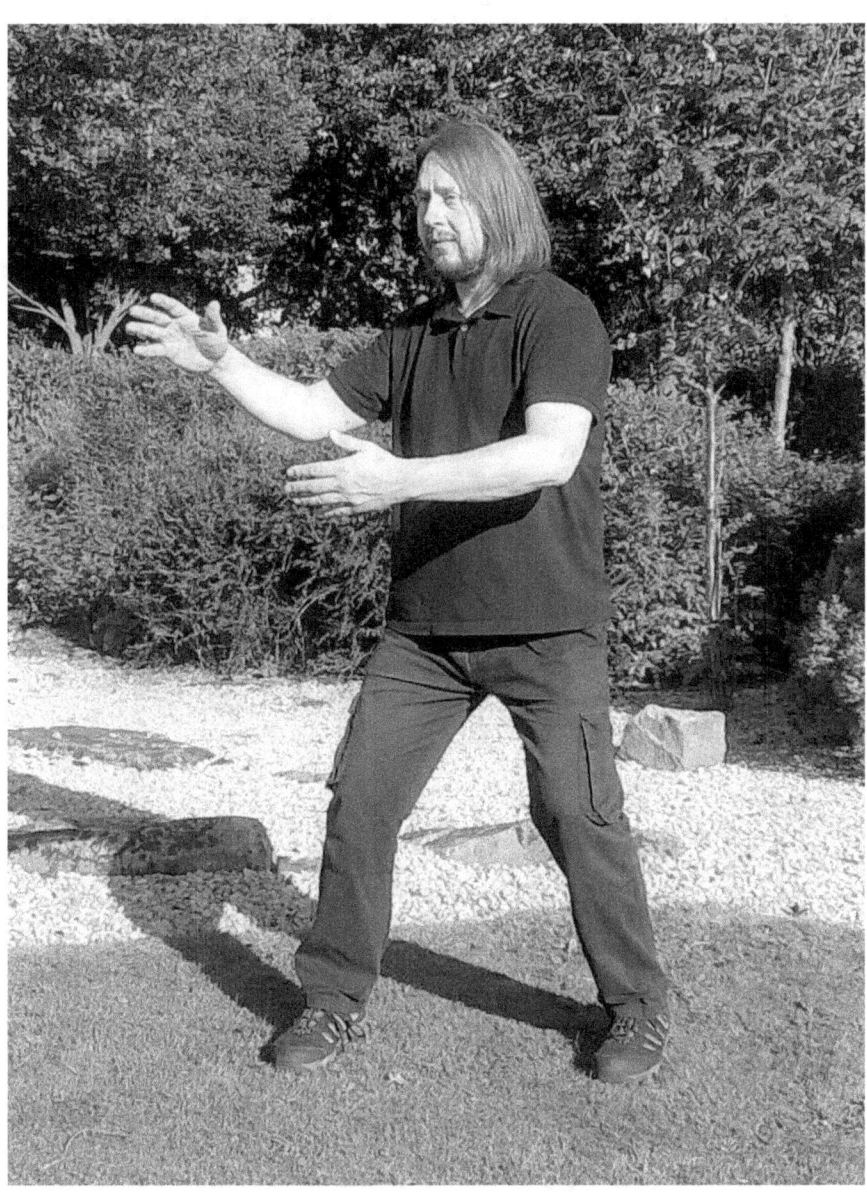

Your right hand turns palm in and sinks down to make a scooping shape at your right side. At the same time, turn your left hand to face to your right side and bring it in and up the centreline to make a left Ward Off shape.

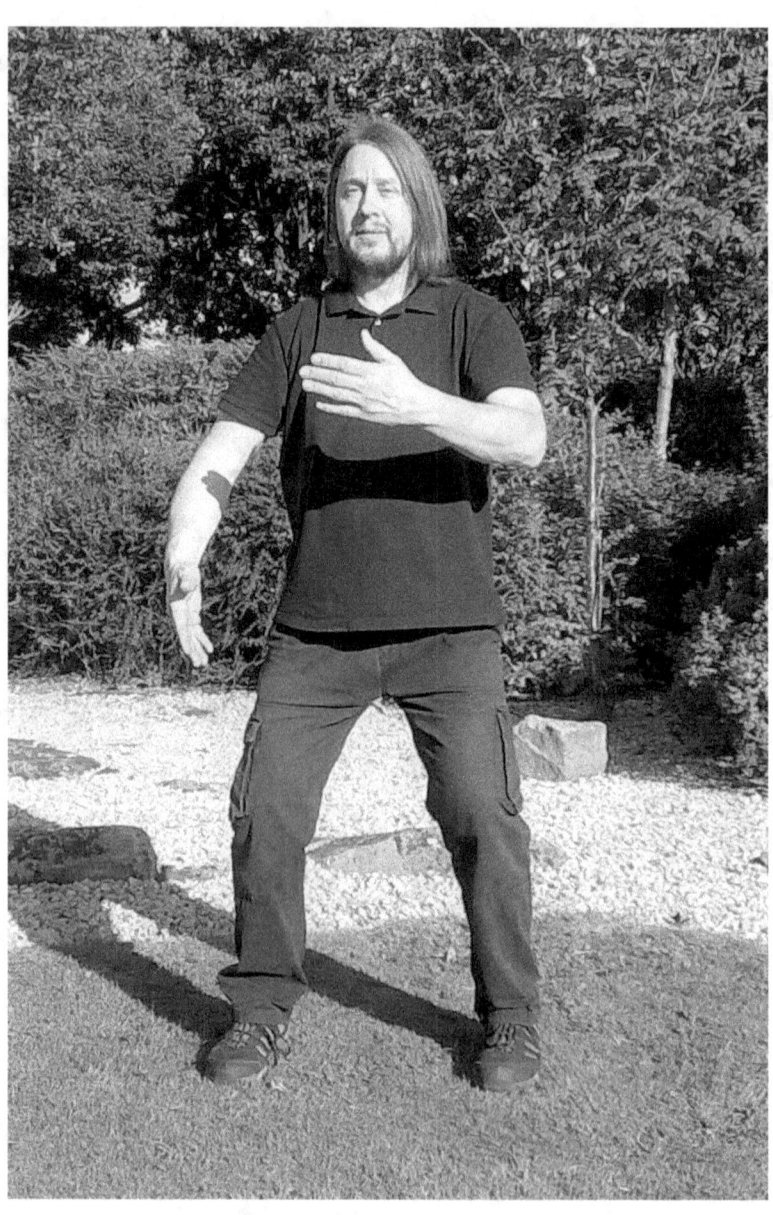

Turn your body to your left side, hold a ball, with the left hand on the top, and step in half a step with your right foot.

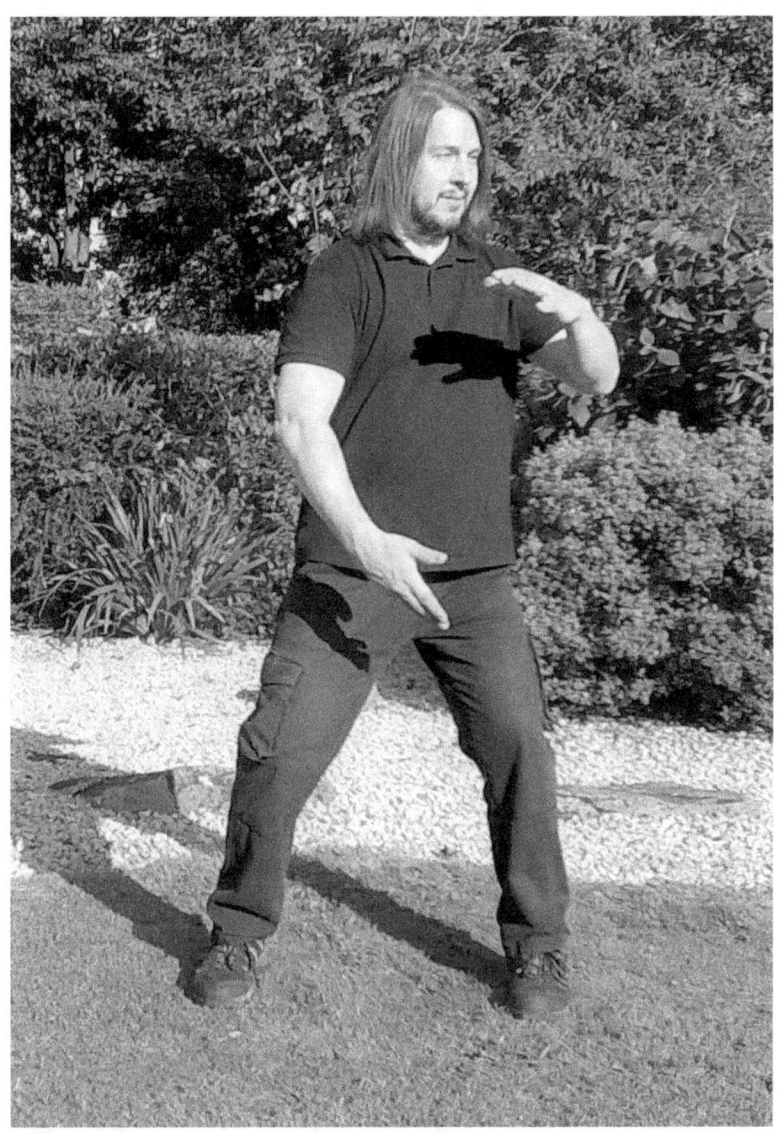

Turn to the forward position your right arm rises up, forming a Ward Off shape and the left arm sinks down to make a scooping shape at the left outside edge of your body.

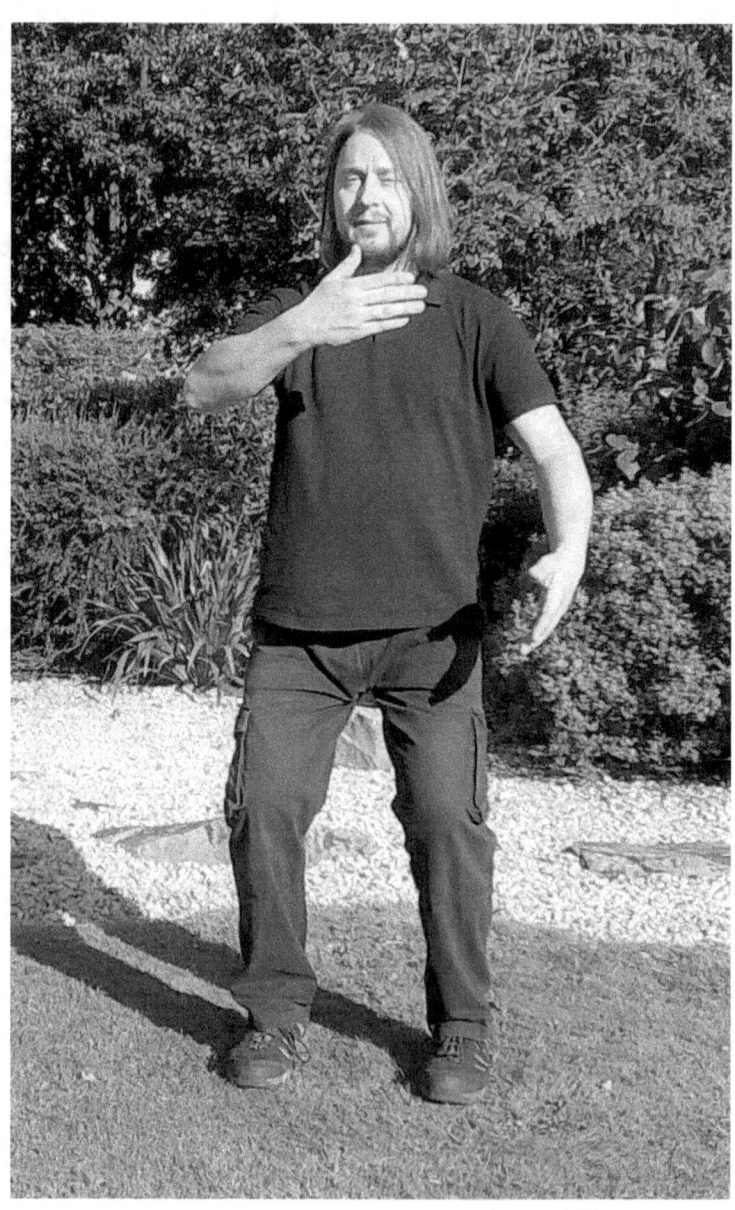

Turn to the right and hold a ball with the right hand on top as you do this, step out with your left leg, half a step.

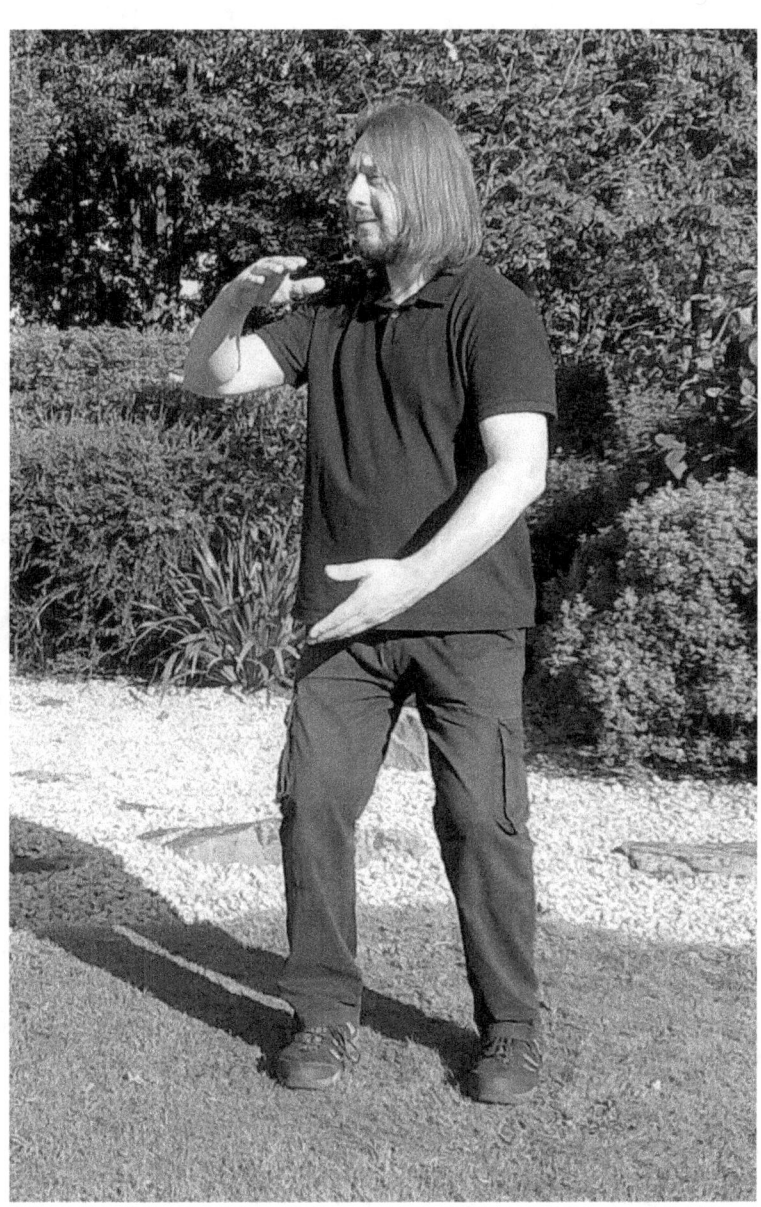

Turn to face square to the front and raise your left arm to Ward Off while the right arm scoops. Your weight begins moving into your left leg.

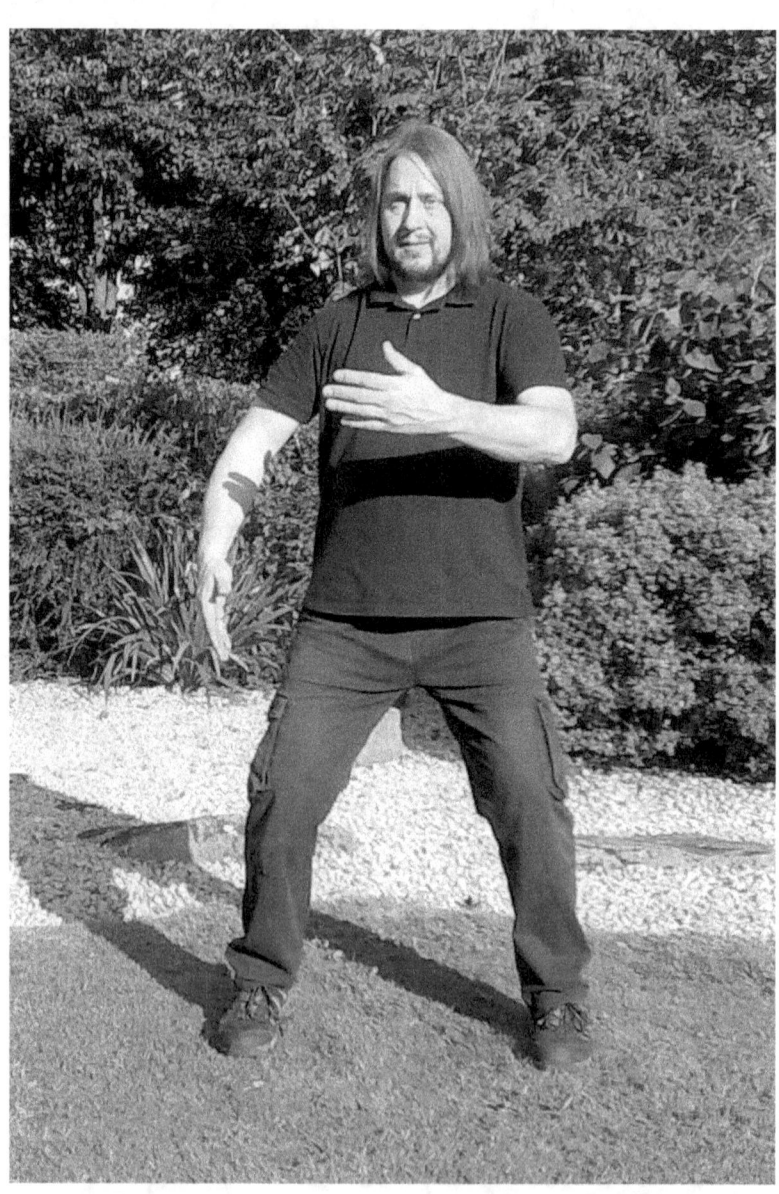

Make your last turn to the left, holding a ball, with your left hand on top and your right hand on the bottom, as you make this movement shift your weight fully into your left leg.

You step between a full shoulder width stance and a half stance each time, taking three steps to the left.

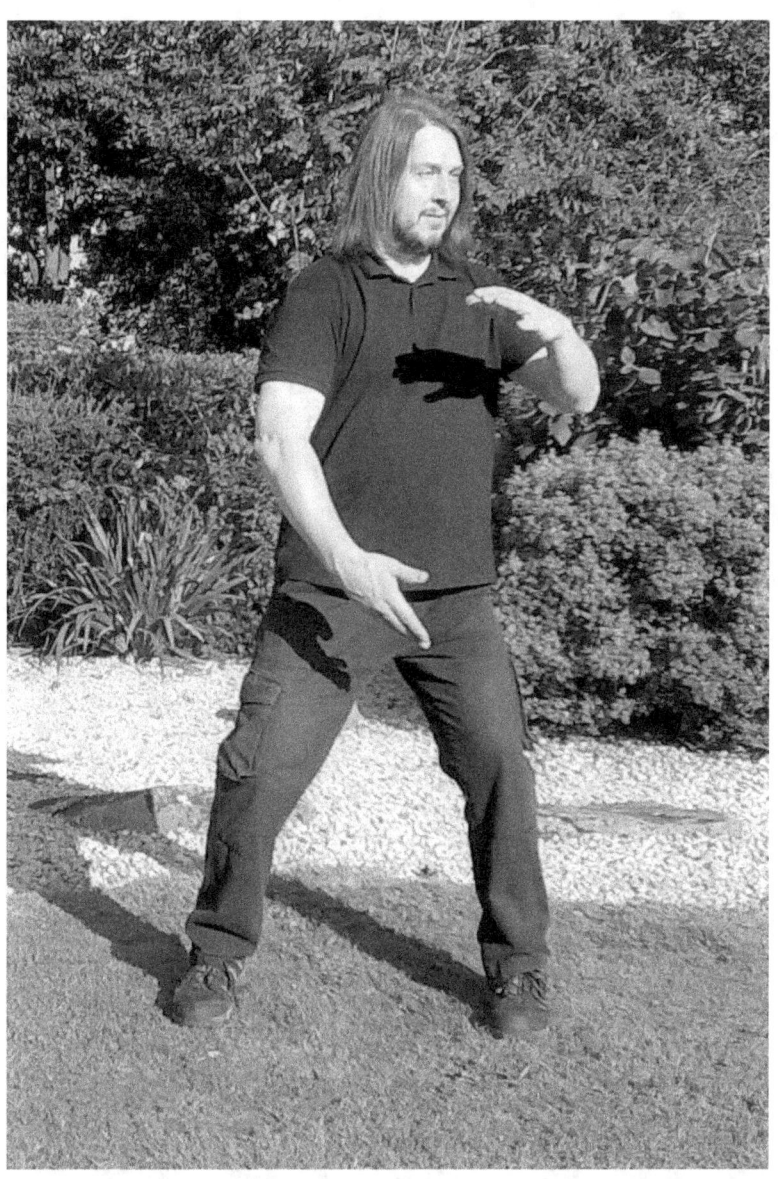

19) Snake Creeps Down

With your weight firmly on your left leg, step forward a short distance with your right foot, (keep a shoulder width stance) and gradually transfer your weight fully onto it. At the same time, roll your right arm straight out in front of your right shoulder and form a beak shape. (The Thumb tip is dropped towards the floor with the fingertips touching it)

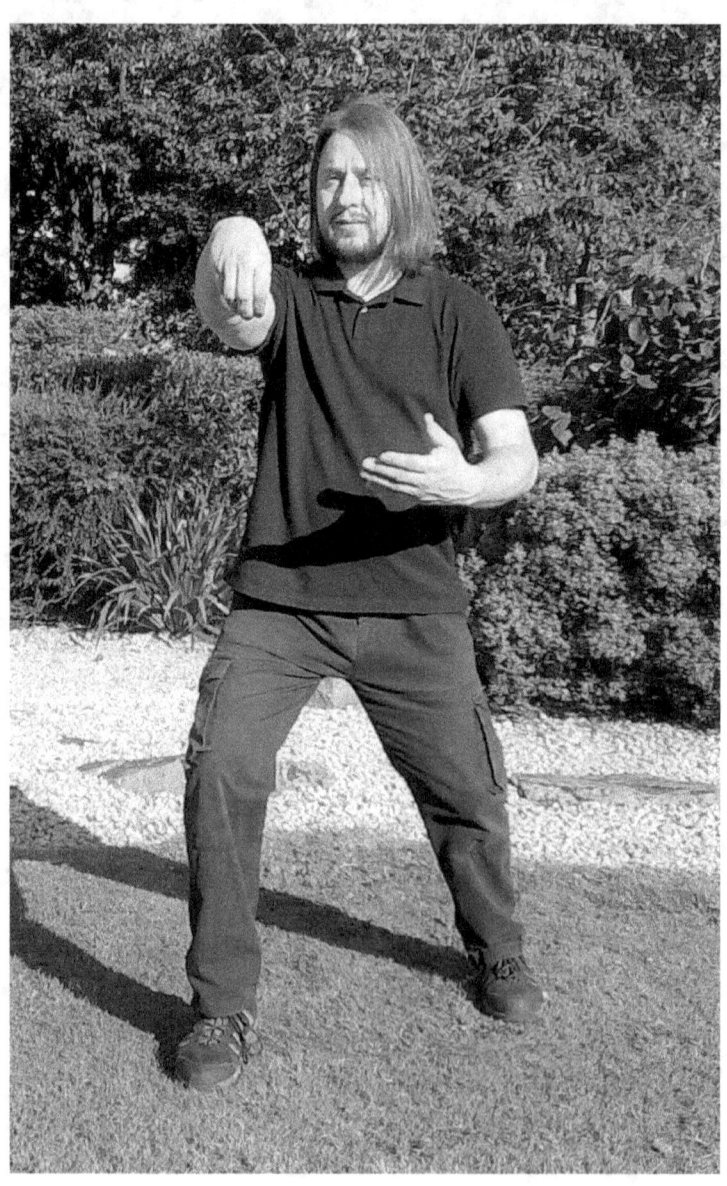

Lift up your left heel and pivot on the ball of the foot, turning to your left, and step into a front Bow stance. At the same time, bring your left hand up and across your body to make the posture, Single Whip.

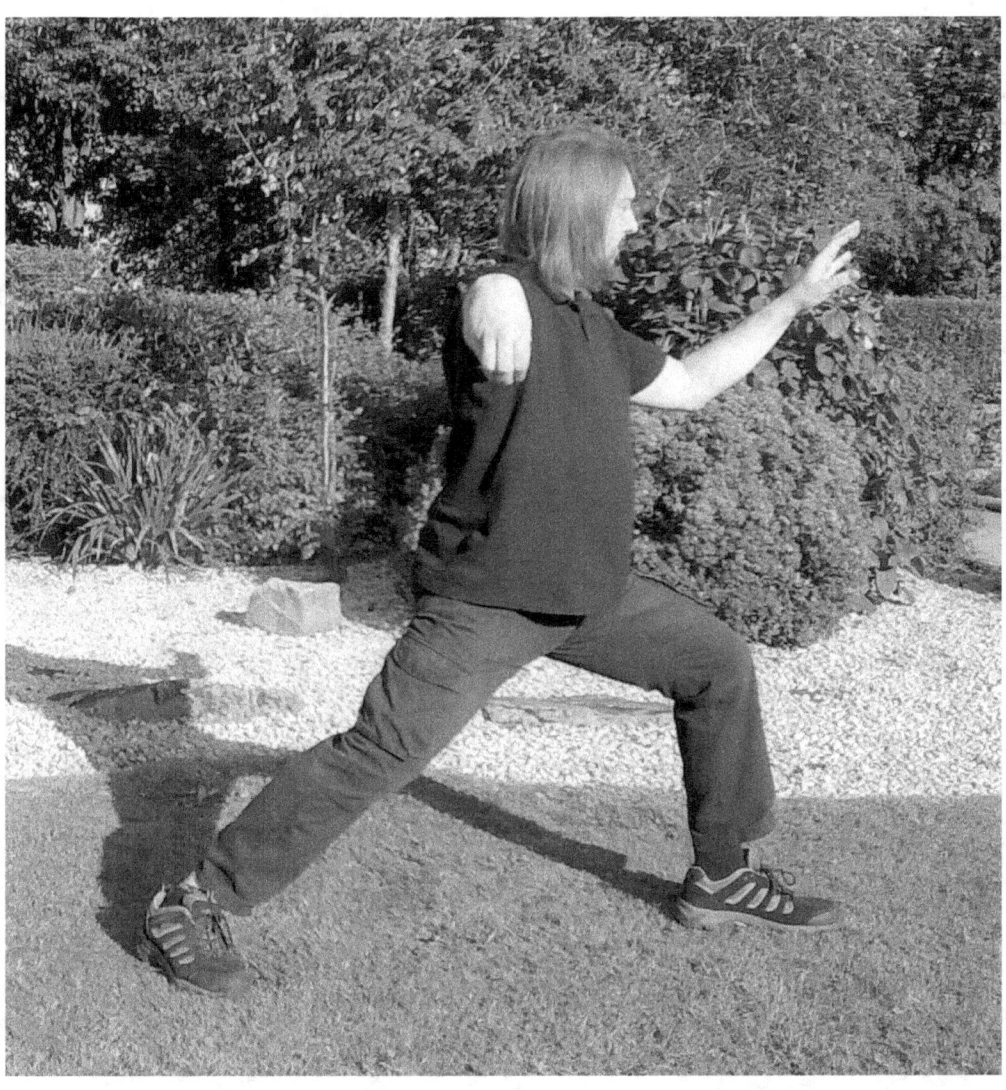

Move your weight back into your right foot and turn your body to your right. Sit down deeply on the right leg. Pivot on your left heel so that your toes turn to your right. Bring your left hand across to point to your right wrist.

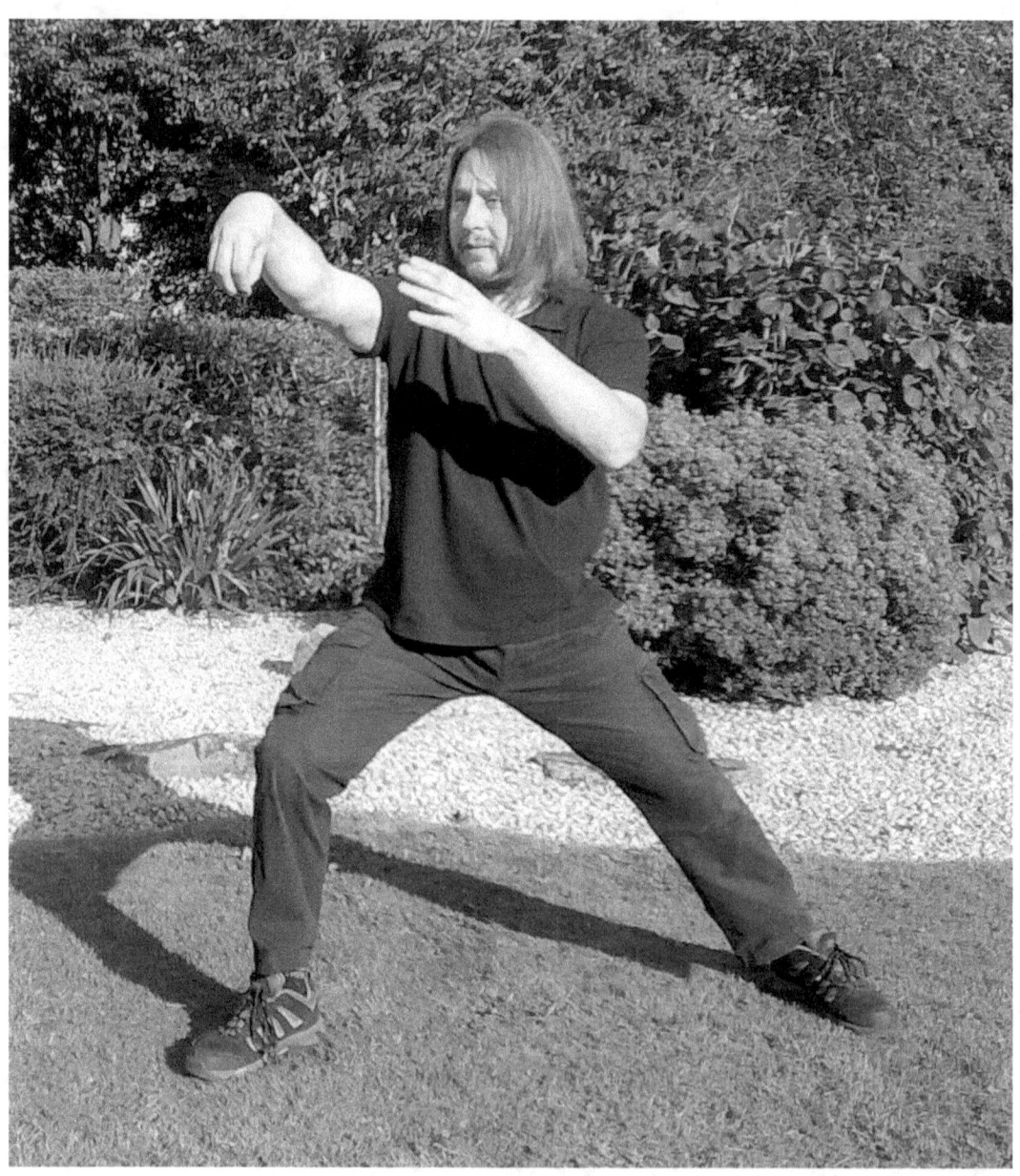

Turn the toes of your left foot back towards it's starting position and at the same time move your left hand down and forward to the inside of the left leg.

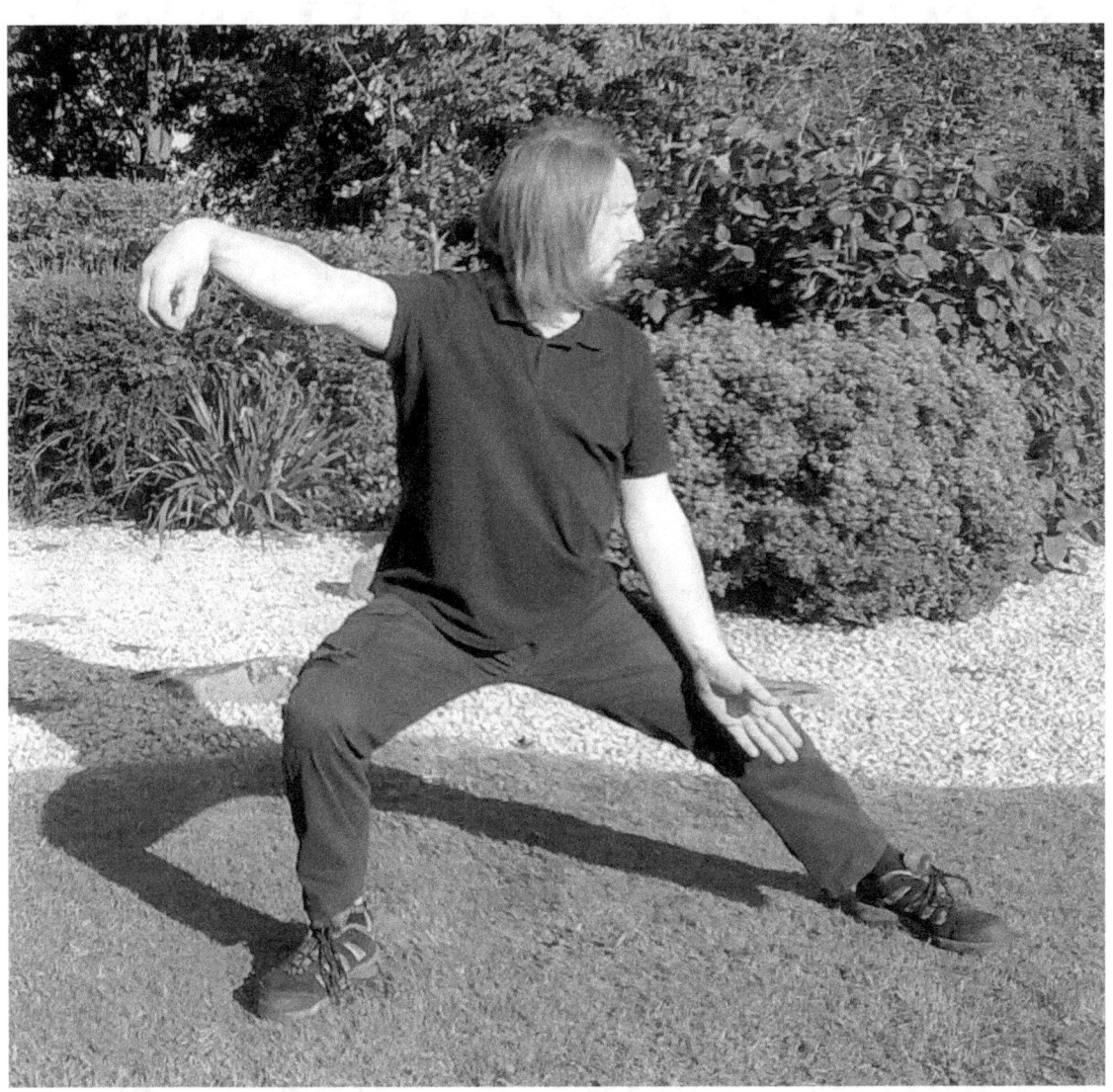

Move into the left leg, as you do this the fingers of the left hand point forwards.

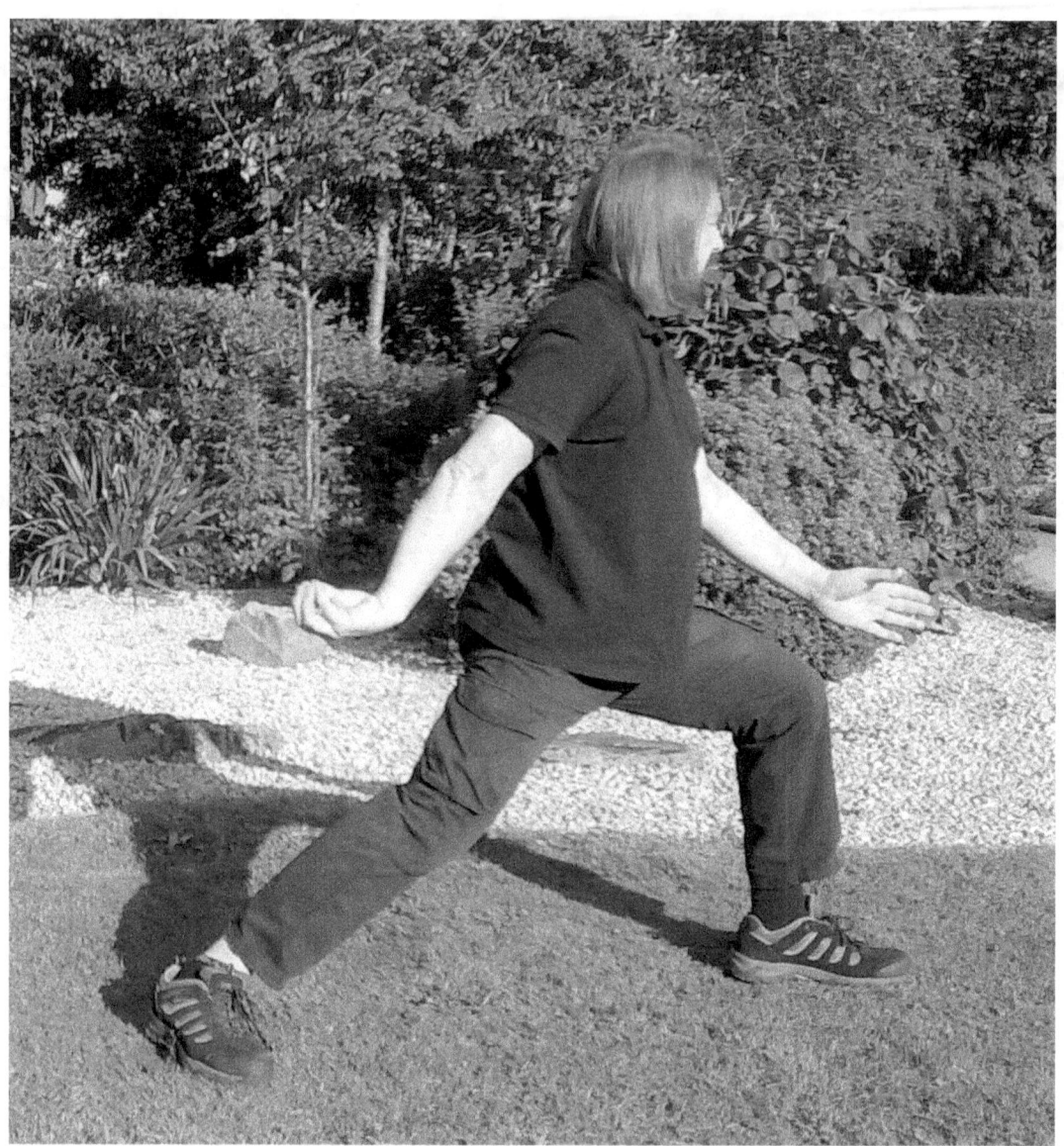

Return your right toes to their starting position and turn your left toes out to forty-five degrees. The fingers of the left hand should now be pointing upward. Turn your right hand over until the beak faces backward behind your body.

Shift one hundred percent of your weight into your left leg.

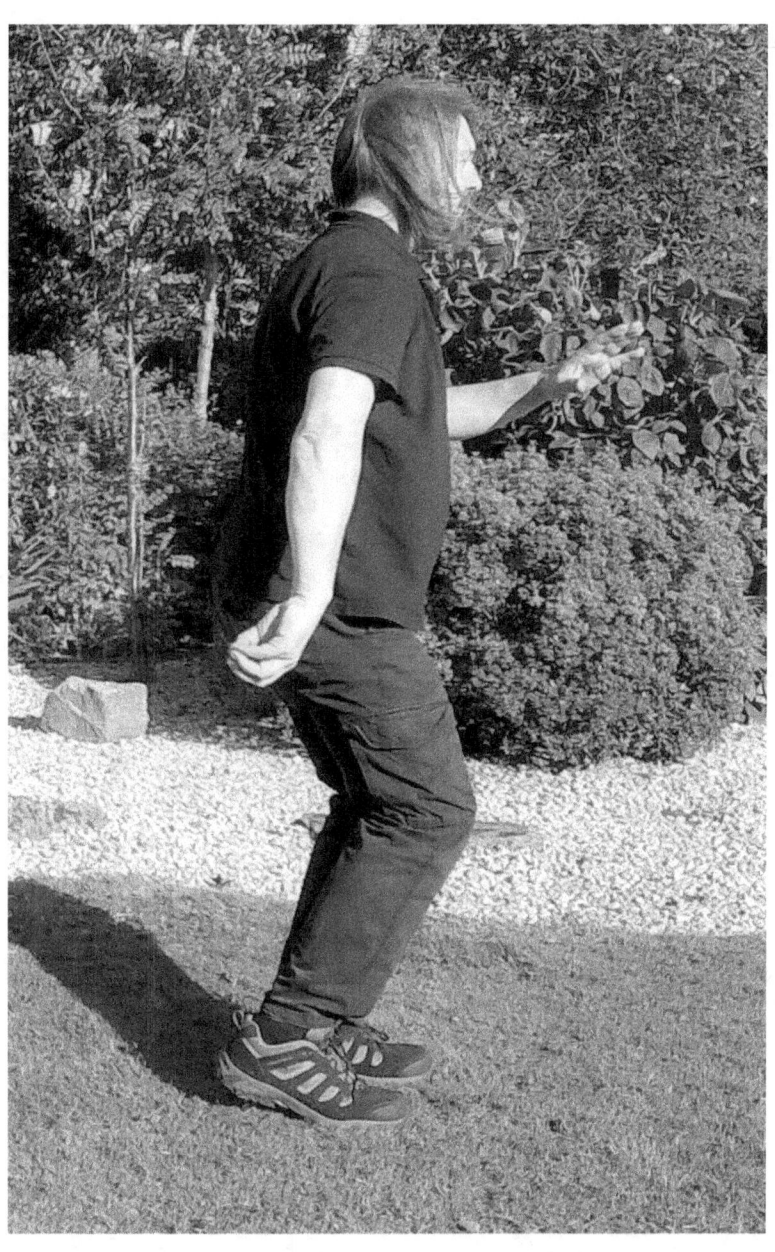

20) Golden Phoenix Stands on the Left and Right Legs

Golden Phoenix Stands on the Left Leg

As the right hand travels past your right hip, release the beak.

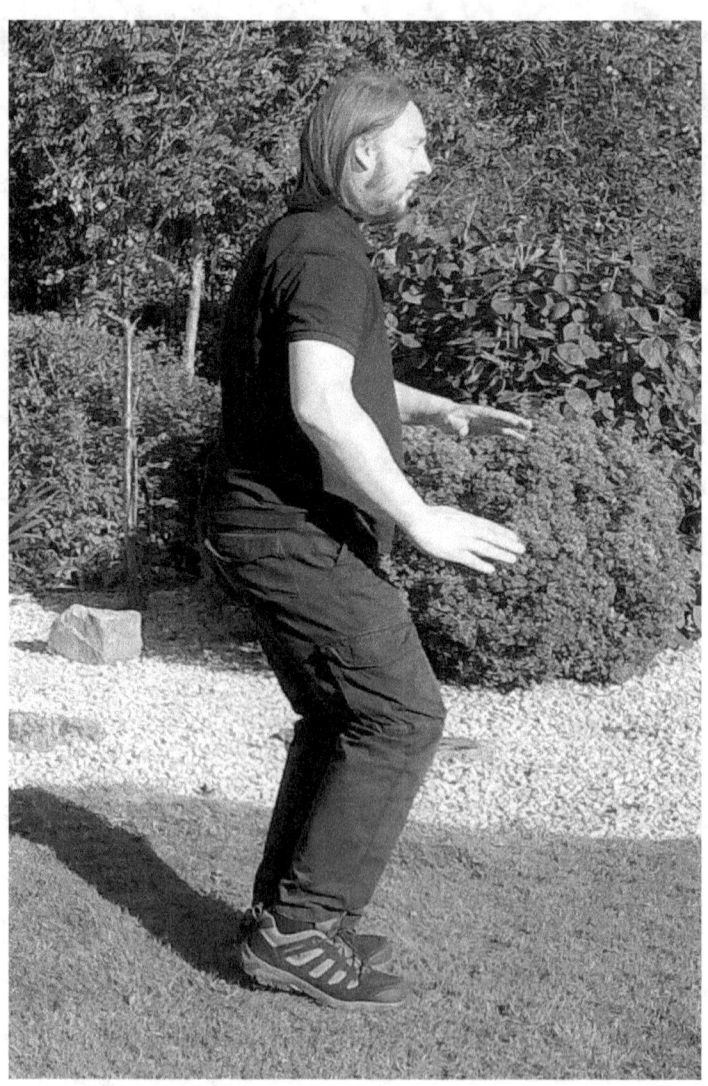

Point your fingers upwards and bring them up in front of your upper right chest.

The left hand settles down to your left side. At the same time, bring your right knee up until it is parallel with the floor.

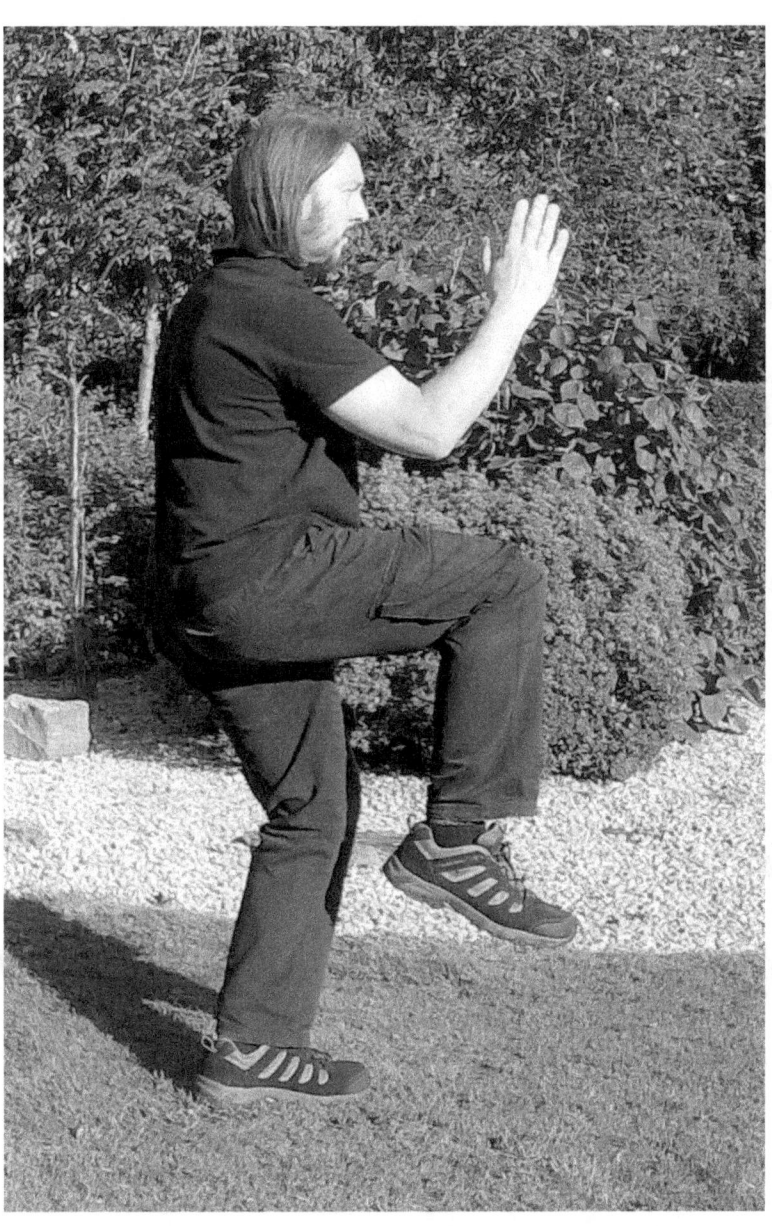

Golden Phoenix Stands on the Right Leg

Place your right foot down, (heel down first) at a forty-five degree angle and then shift your weight fully onto the right foot. Bring your left hand up in front of the left side of your upper chest.

The right hand settles down to your right side. At the same time, bring your left knee upwards until it is parallel with the floor.

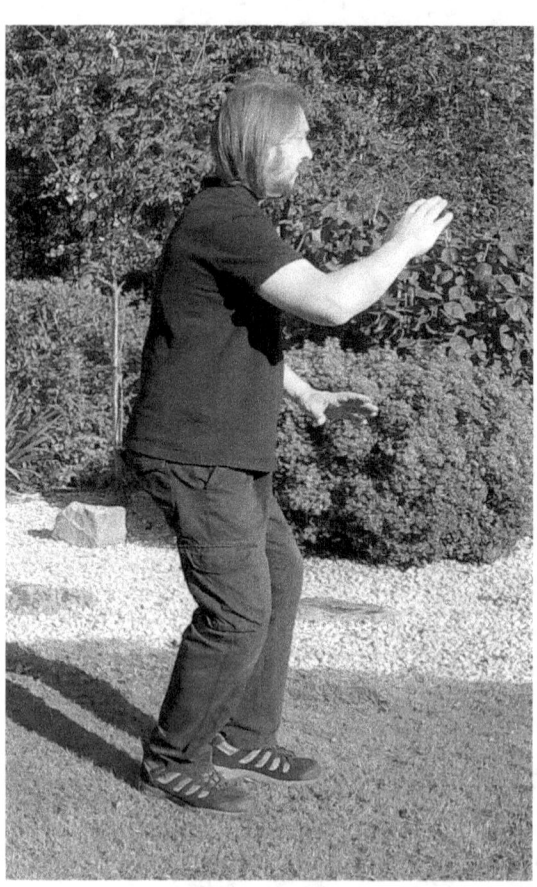
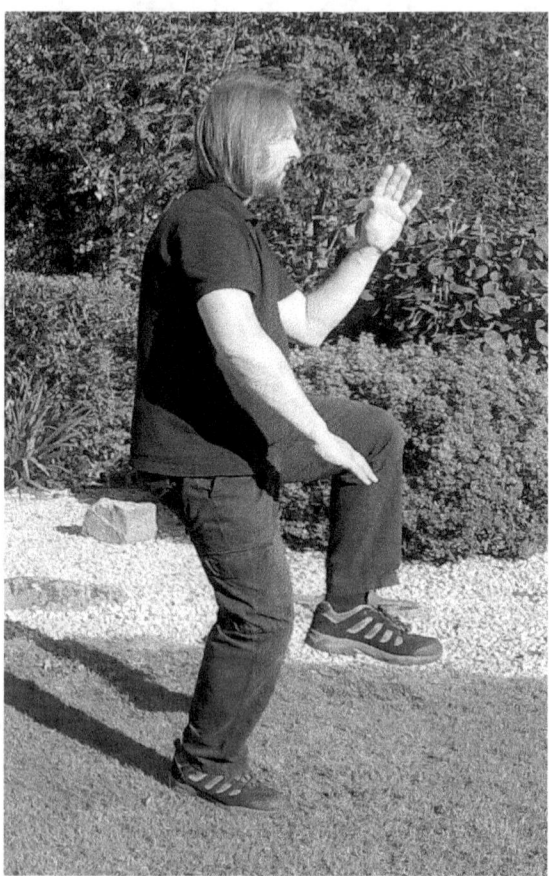

21) Separate and Kick with Right and Left Foot

Separate and Kick with the Right Foot

Place the left foot on the floor and shift one hundred percent of your weight across onto it. Turn your head to face your right corner, lower the left hand in front of your chest, and lift your right hand up to form a Play guitar shape to your right corner.

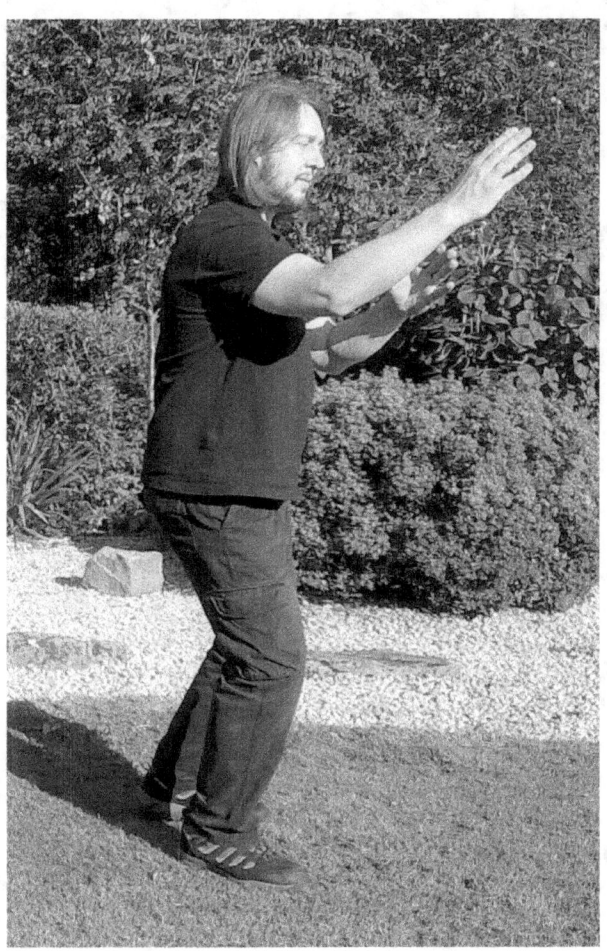

Lower both hands downwards, in a small plucking movement and at the same time raise the right heel.

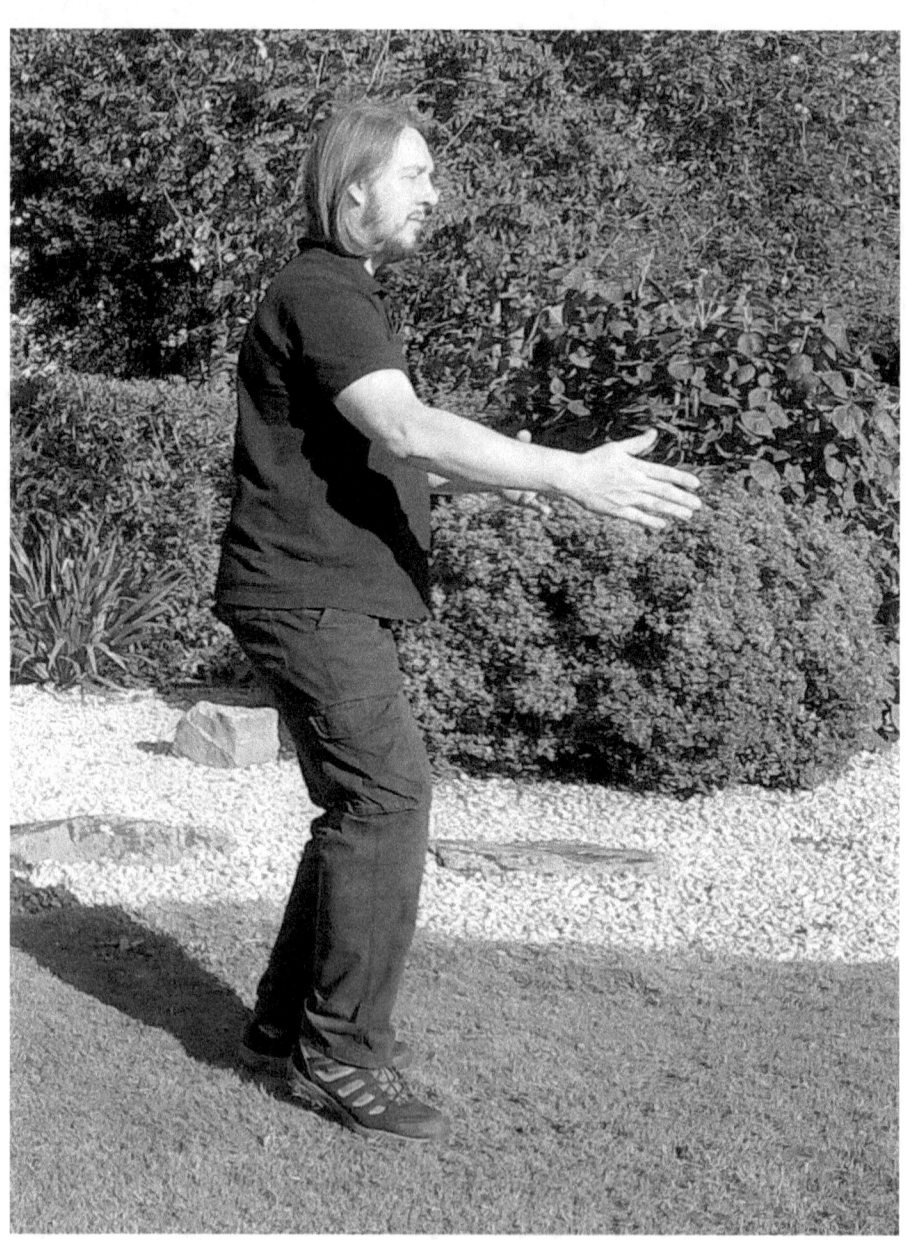

Bring your hands up in front of your chest, with the arms crossed at the wrists and the right hand on the outside.

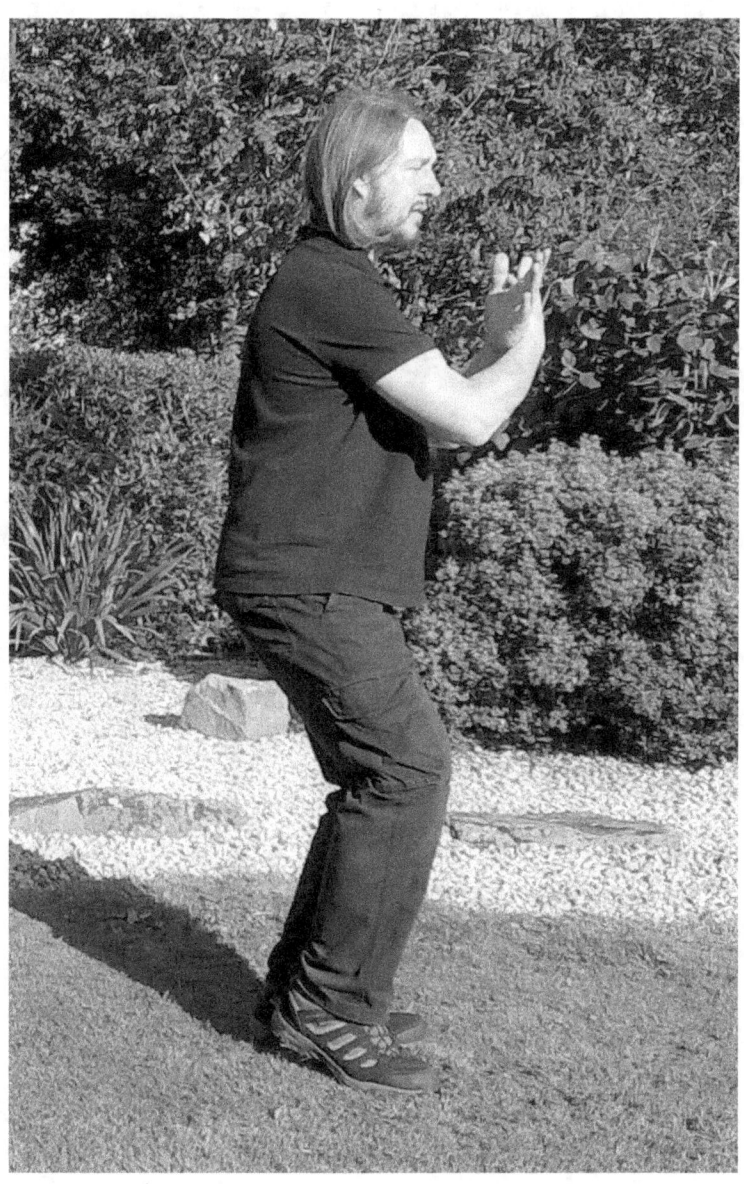

Uncross and separate your arms, the right arm moves forward and the left hand backwards. As you open out your arms, lift up your right knee and kick upwards with the toes of your right foot.

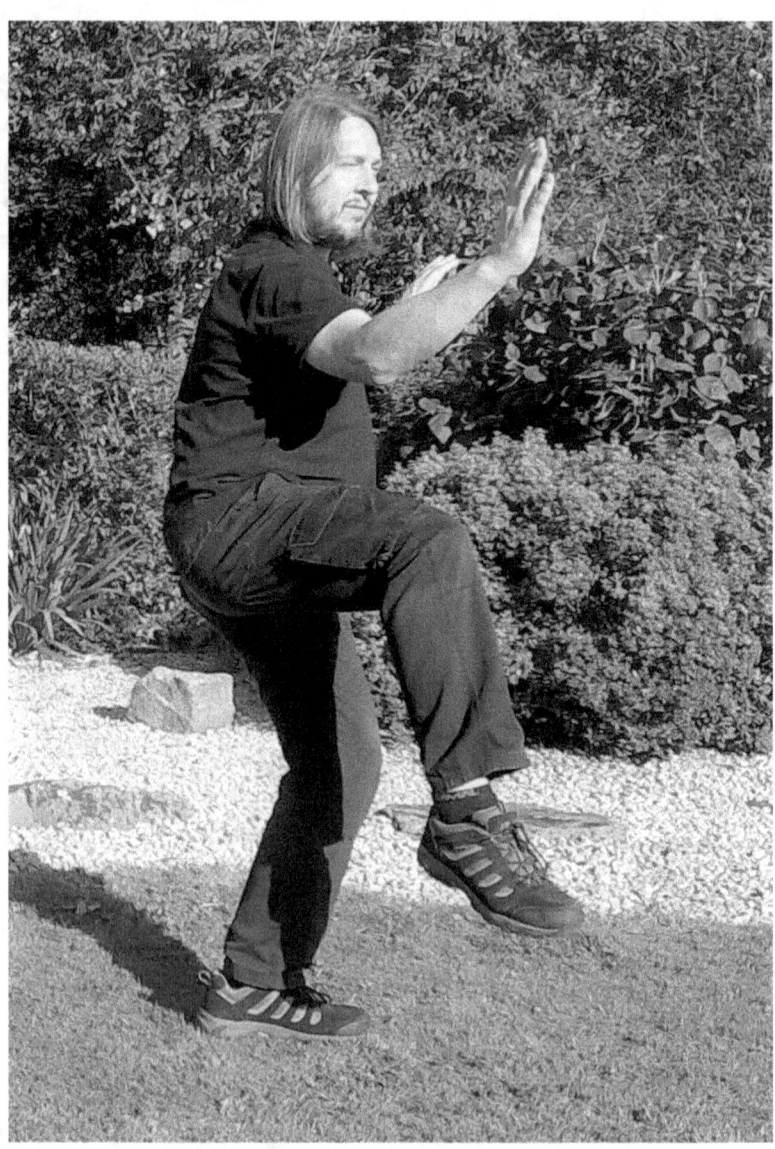

Seperate and Kick with Left Foot

Place the left foot on floor and shift your weight across and fully into it. Turn your head to face to your right corner, place the left hand in front of your chest, and lift your right hand to form Play Guitar to right corner.

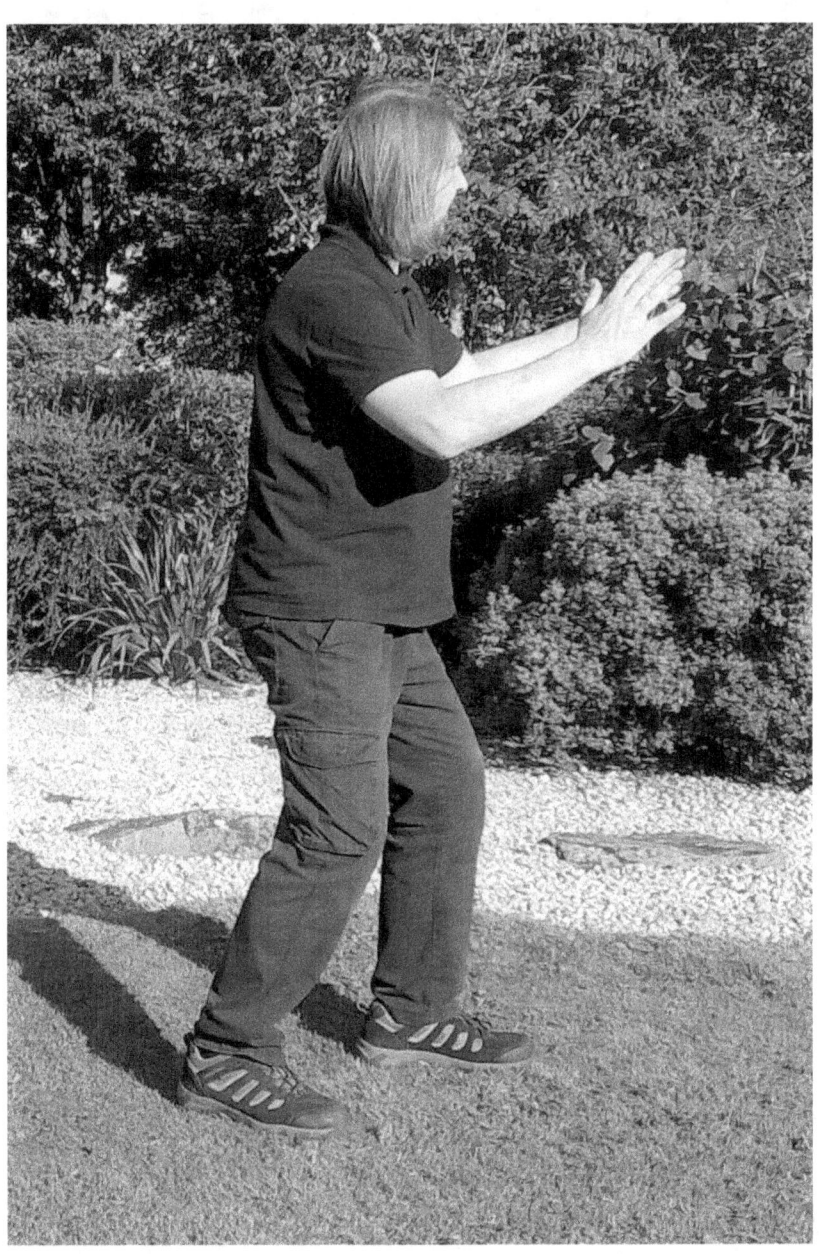

Lower both hands downwards, in a small plucking movement and raise the left heel.

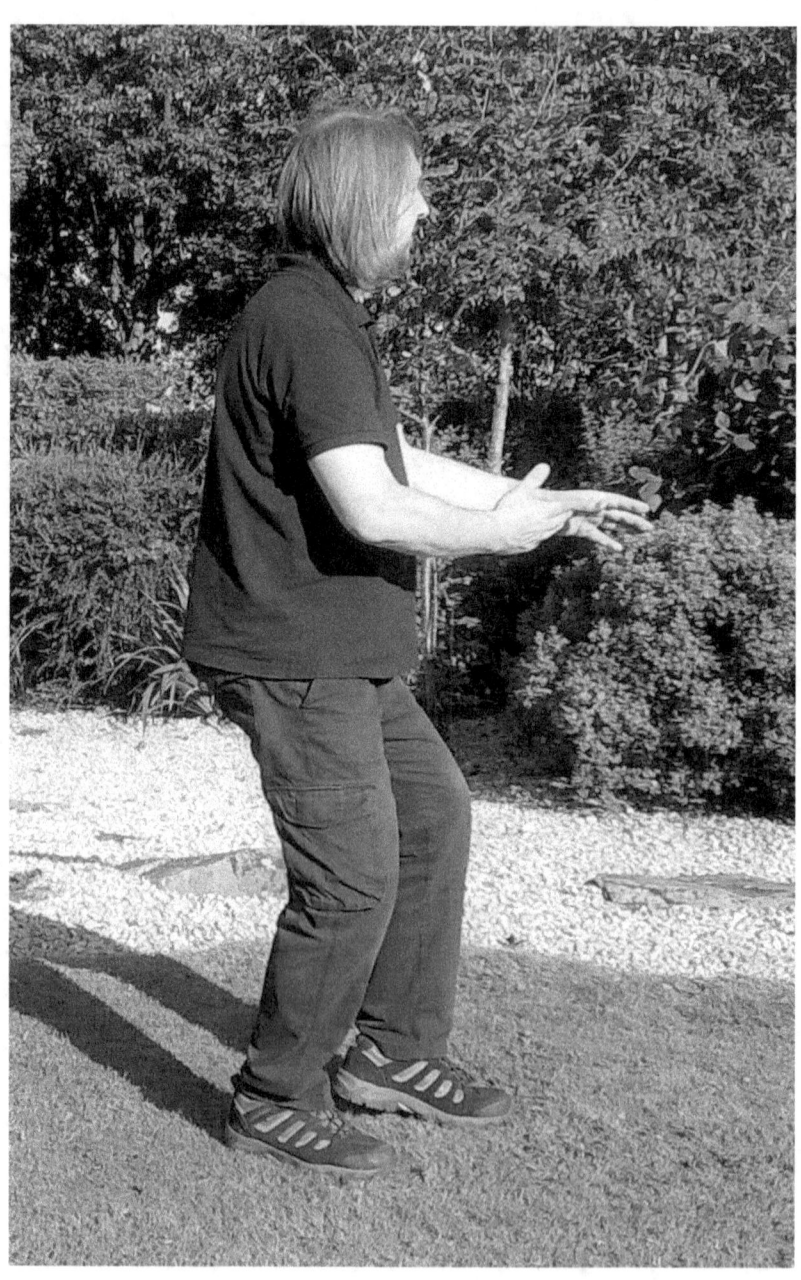

Bring your hands up in front of your chest, with the wrists crossed and the left hand on the outside.

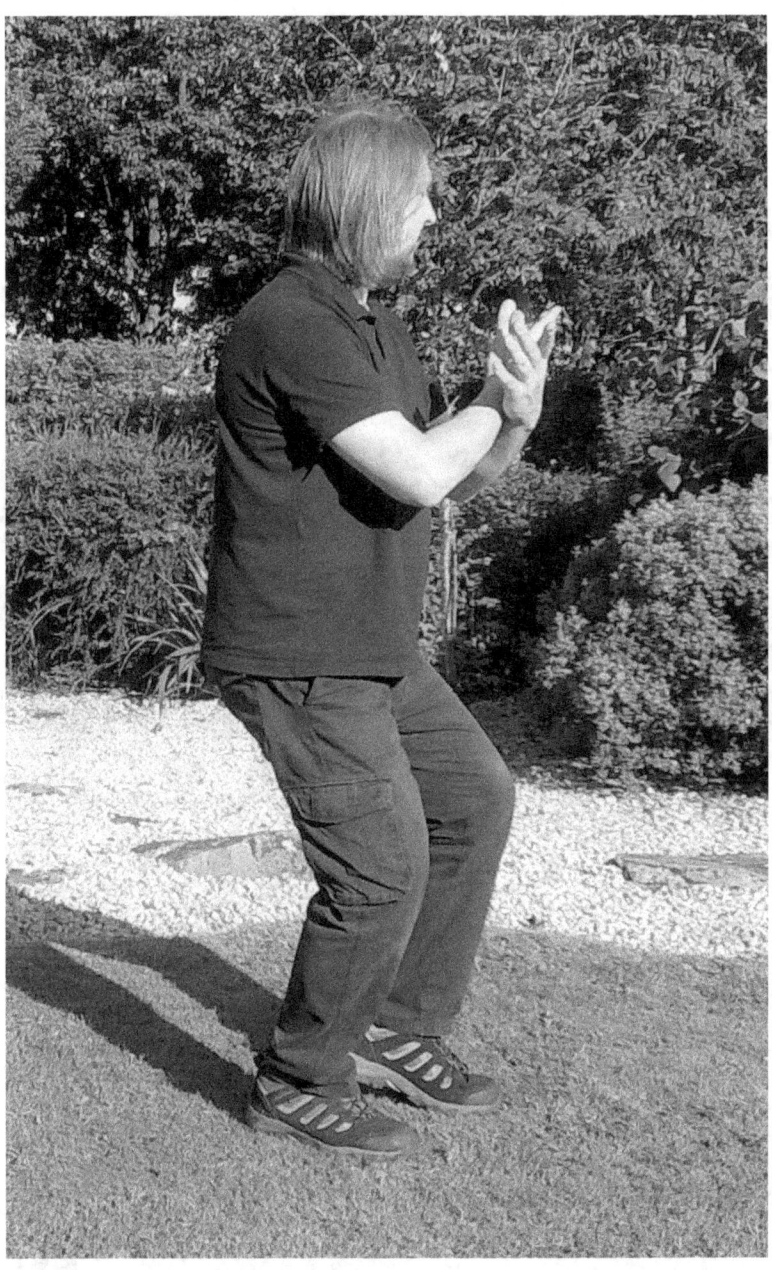

Uncross and open your hands out and across your body, the left hand goes forward and the right hand backwards. At the same time that you open out your arms, lift up your left knee and kick upwards with the toes of your left foot.

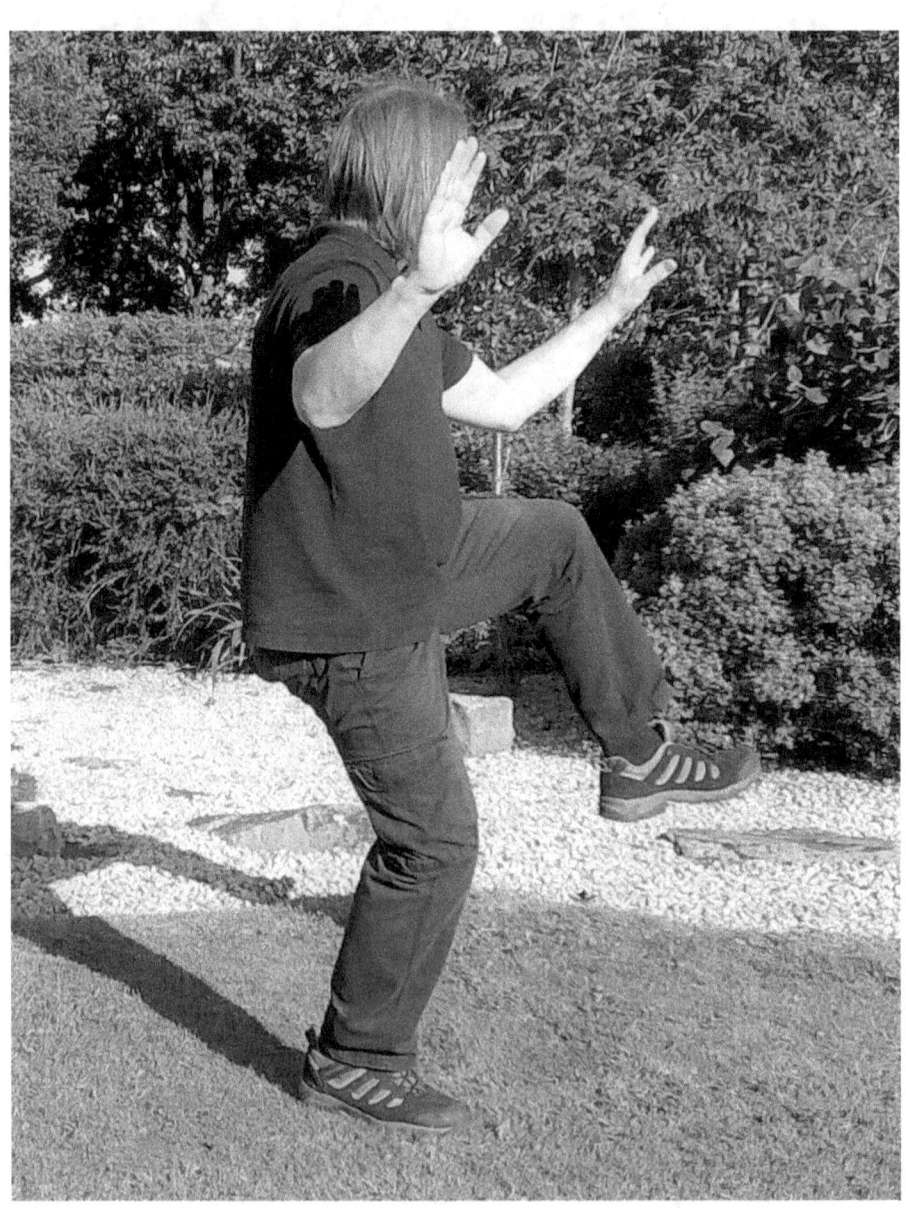

22) Turn and kick with Heel

Place the ball of your left foot behind the heel of your right foot, with about eight inches between them.

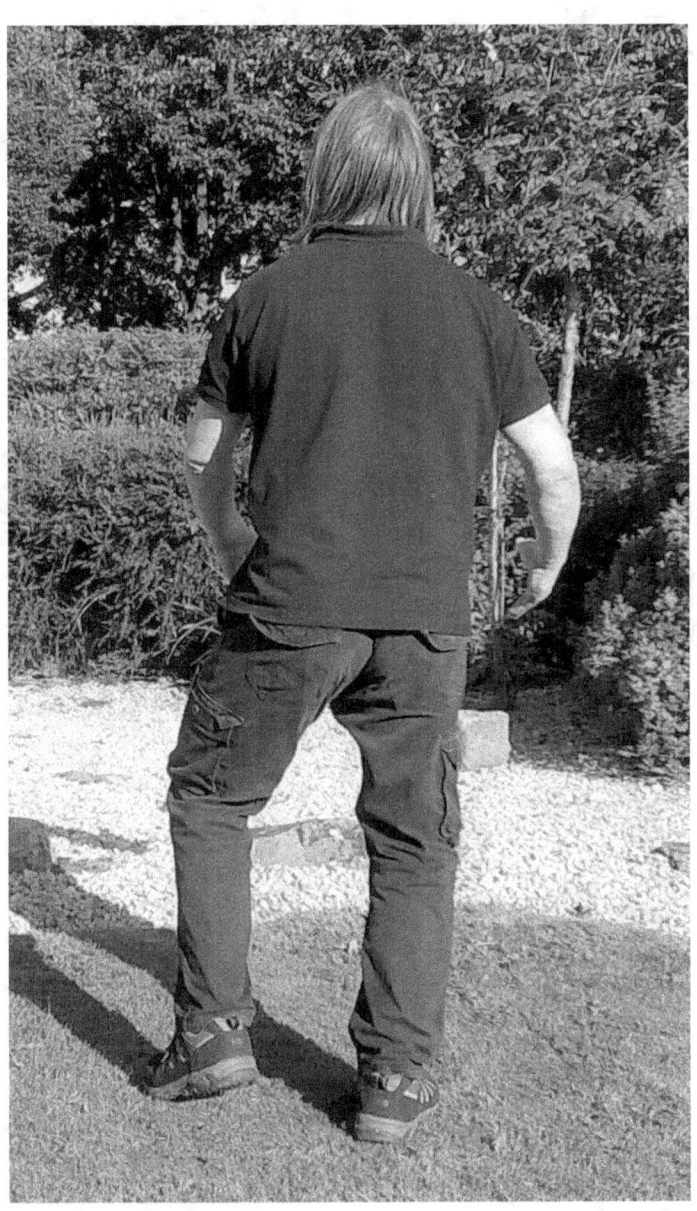

Pivot on your right heel to your left until you have spun one hundred and sixty degrees. Sit fully into the right leg and form a cat stance with the left heel up.

Gather your hands up as you turn, move them up in front of your chest, cross the hands at the wrists with your left hand on the outside.

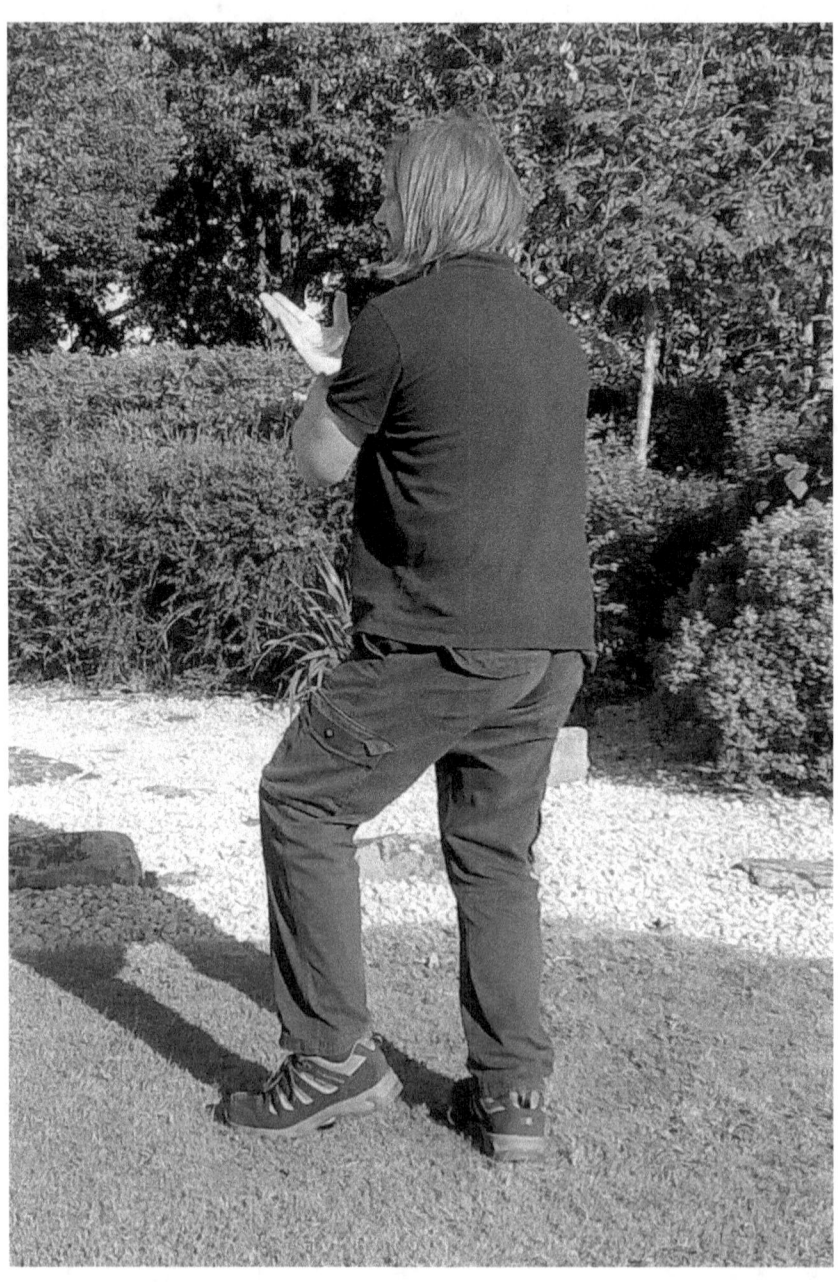

You look forward, but your body is diagonal. Separate your hands, the left going forward and the right hand back, and at the same time lift the left knee and kick out with the left heel to stomach height.

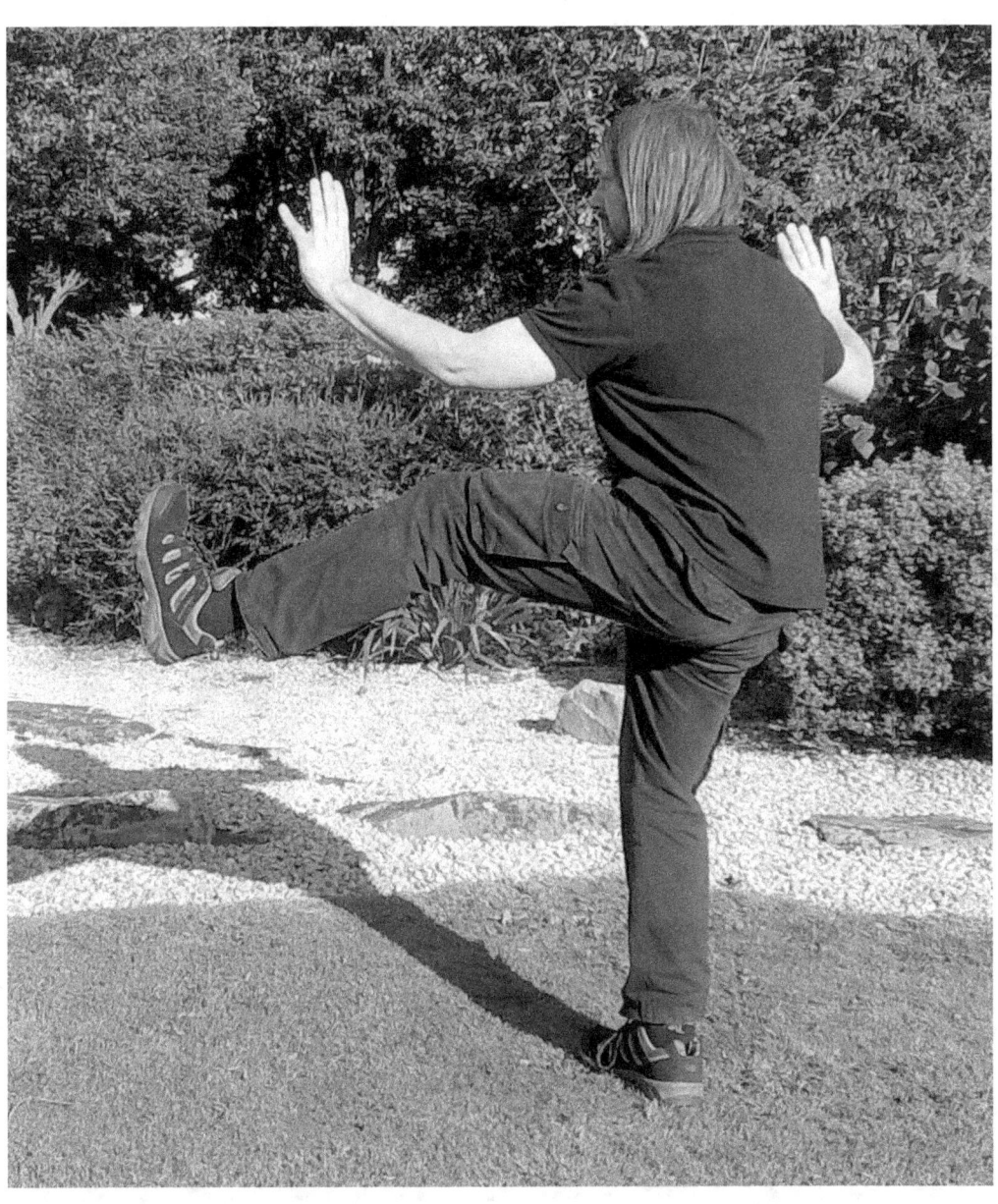

23) Brush Knee and Push Right and Left

As you finish the heel kick, step forwards with your left foot into a Bow stance. Turn your body from diagonal to square on to the front.

Your left hand sweeps down and across in an arc to rest by the outside edge of your left thigh.

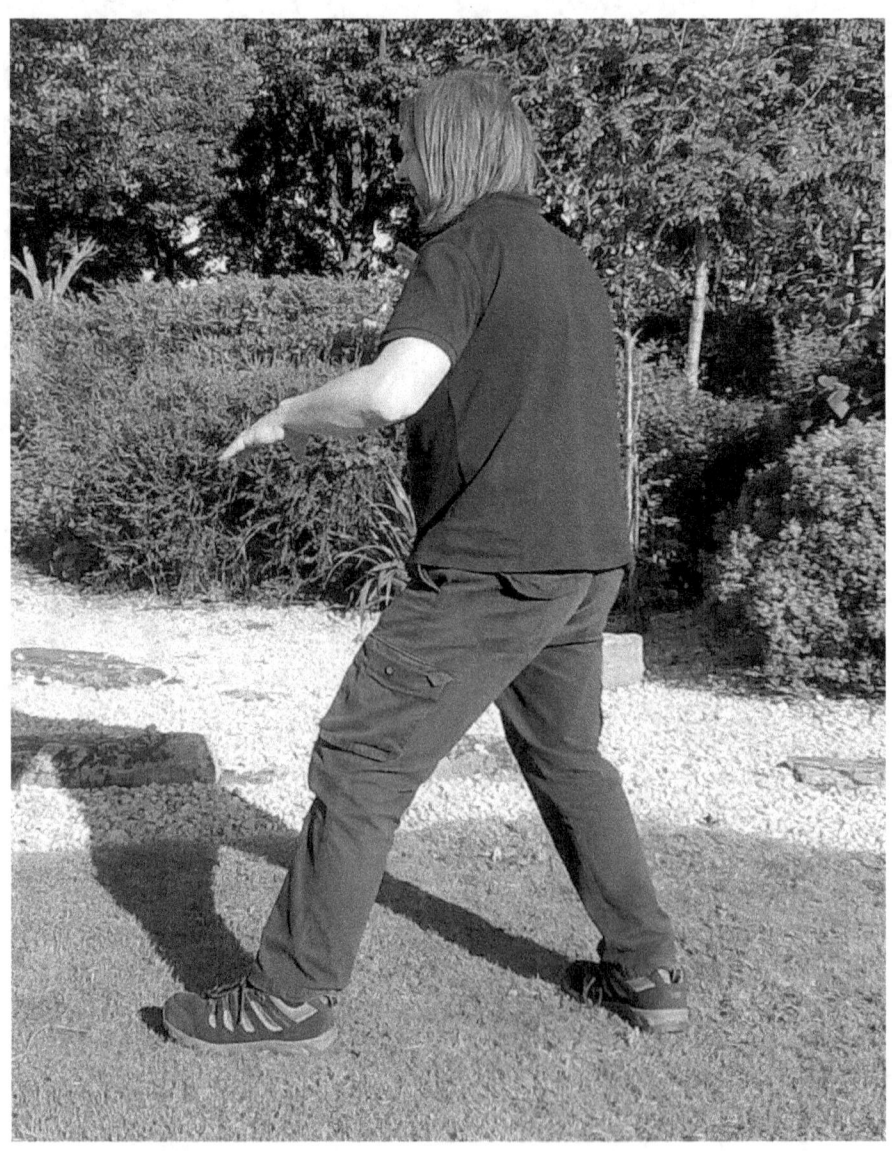

Bring your right hand forward in front of the upper chest in a push.

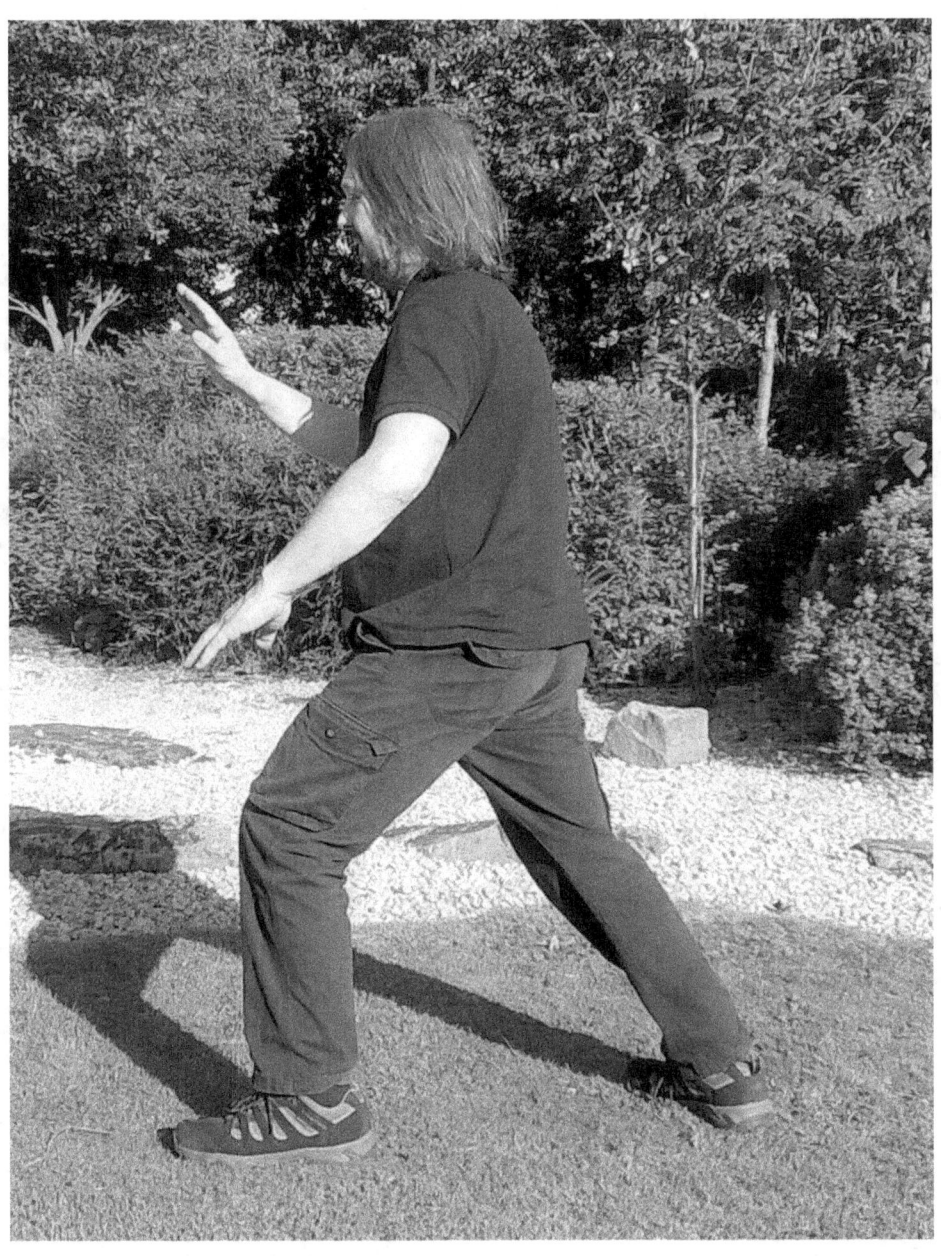

Brush knee Push Right

Move slowly backward into the right leg; lift the toes of the left foot, turn on the foot out to a forty-five degree angle.

Move forward into the left leg, circle your left arm back, around, and up to come up by your left ear, bring your left hand forward and across in front of the upper chest in a push.

Move your right hand across your body to the left in a beckoning motion, then sweep it back down and across in an arc to sit by the outside edge of your right leg.

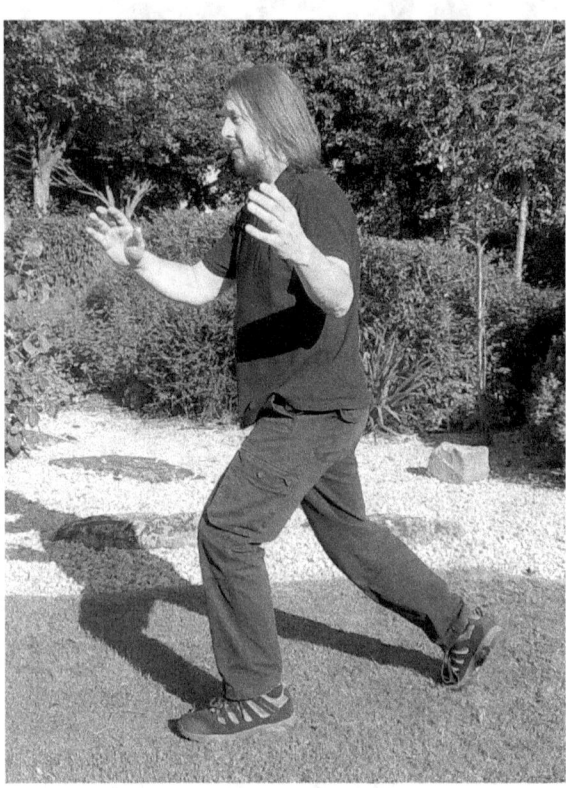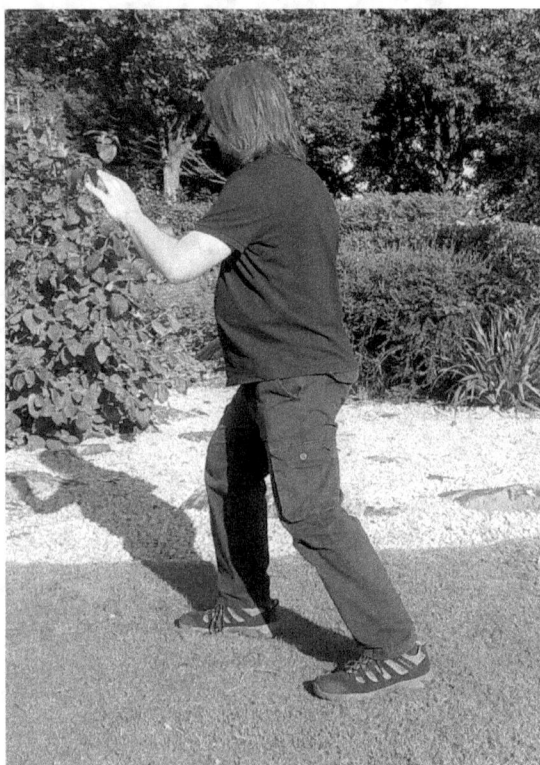

24) Brush Knee, Punch to Groin

From the preceding posture, shift your weight back and turn your body and right leg (by pivoting on the heel) to your right side.

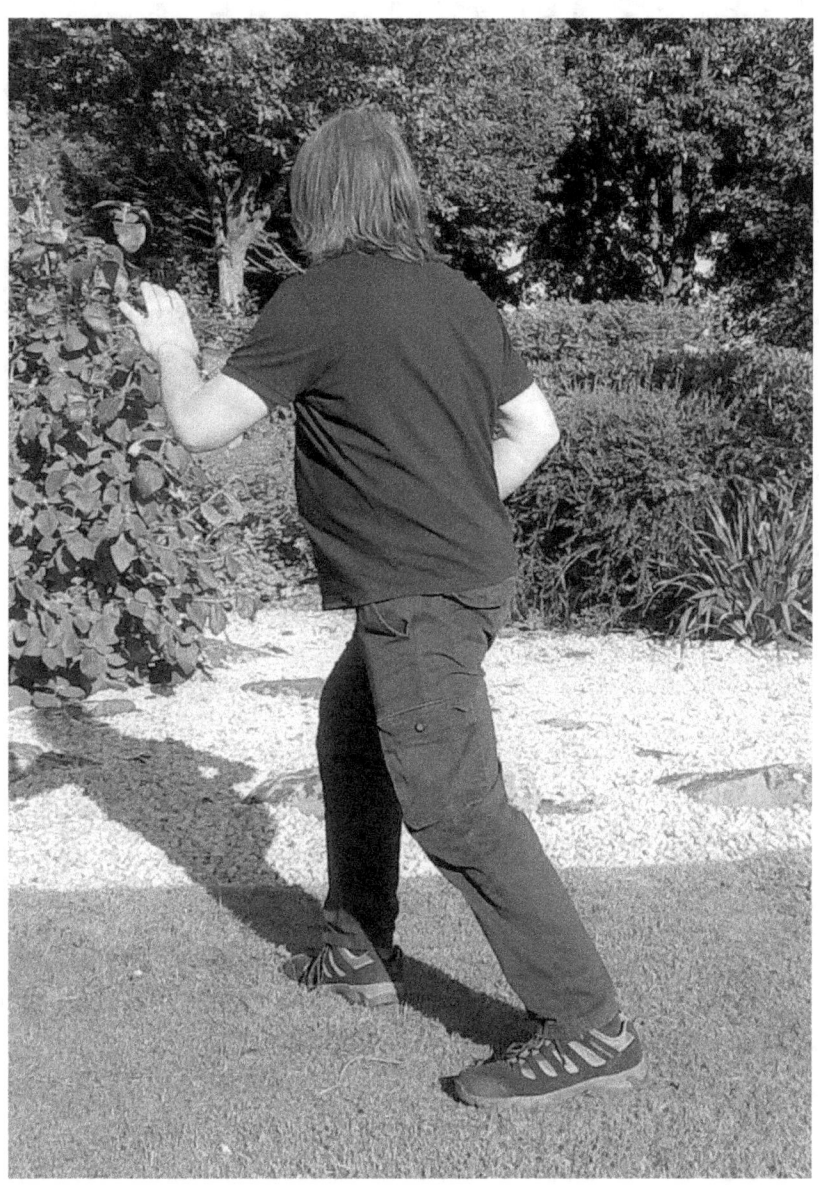

Make a fist and bring your right hand to the side of your right hip. Step forward with the left foot into a Bow stance. Brush across to your left side with your left hand and punch in front of the Dantien with your right hand.

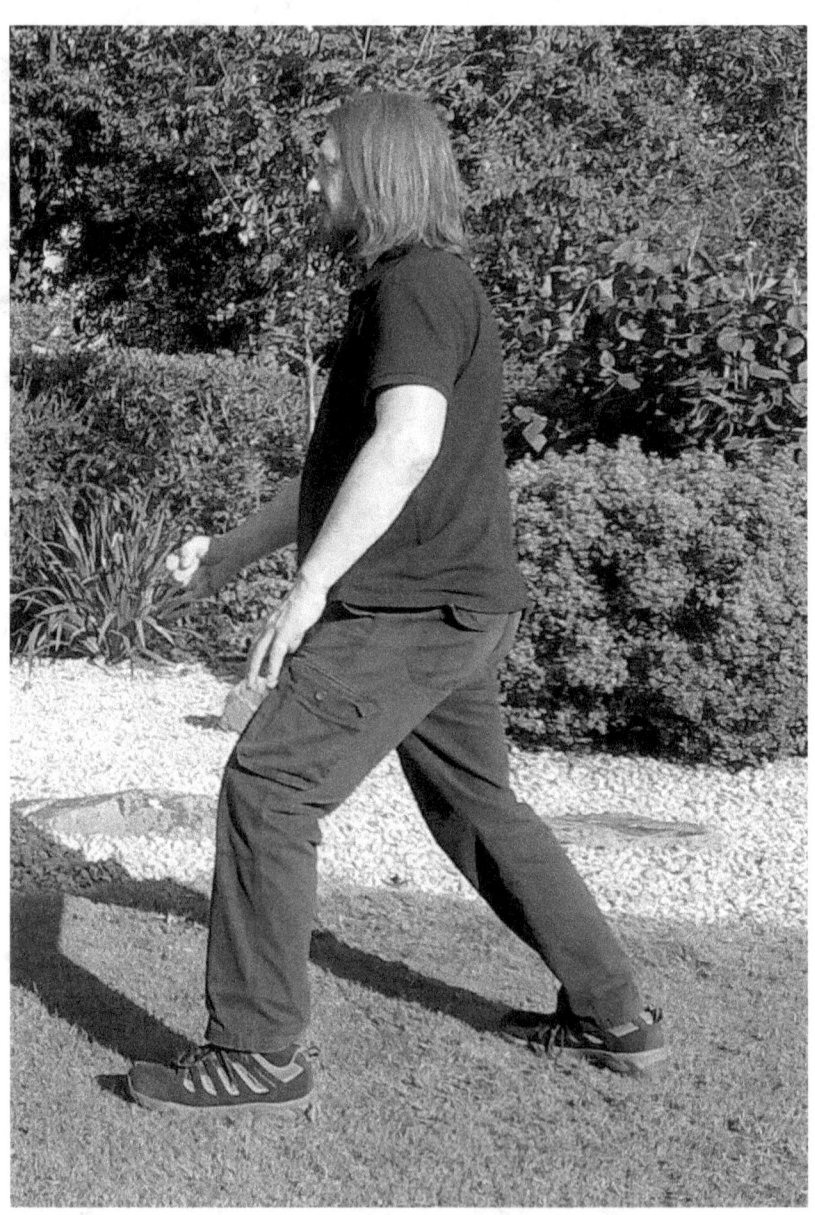

25) Grasp the Sparrows Tail

Hold a ball with the left hand on top, move back into your right foot and lift the toes of the left foot, turn your Dantien to turn your left foot forty-five degrees to your left. Roll your left foot down. Once you have completed this movement shift one hundred percent of your weight fully into the left foot.

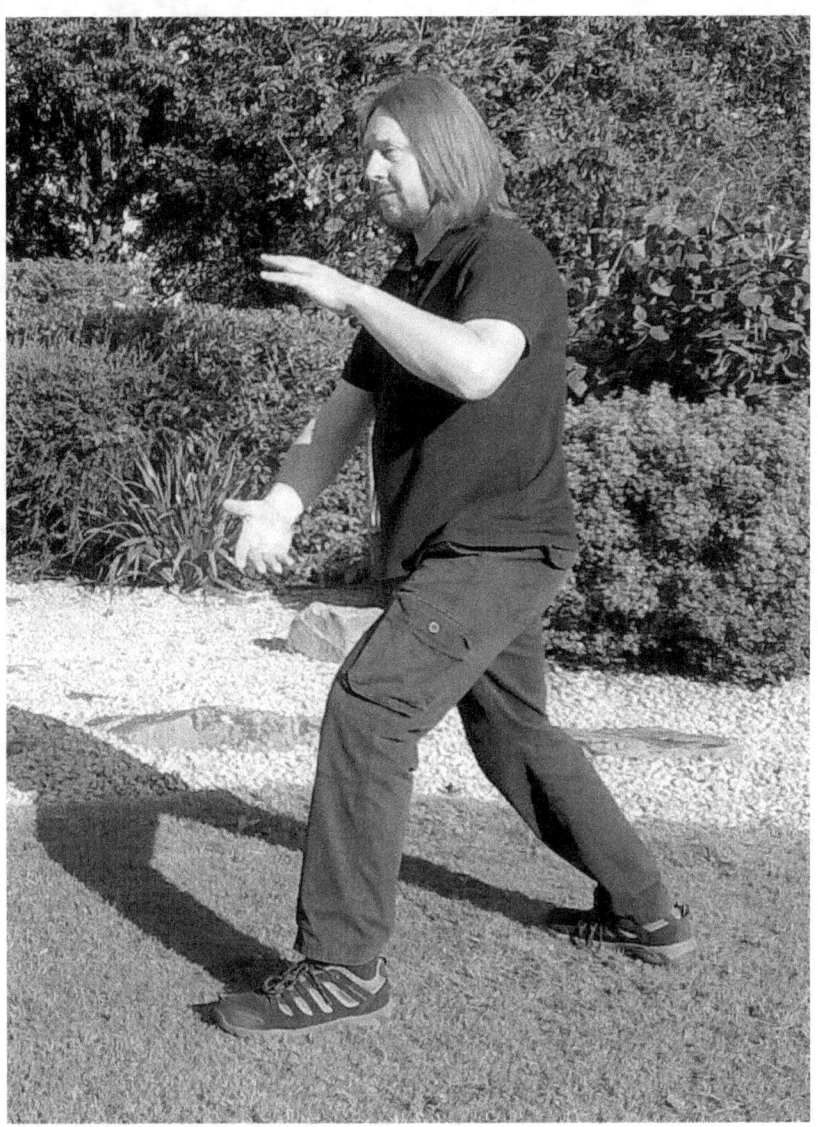

Ward Off Right

Step straight forward with the right foot into a Bow stance, keeping a shoulder width space between the feet.

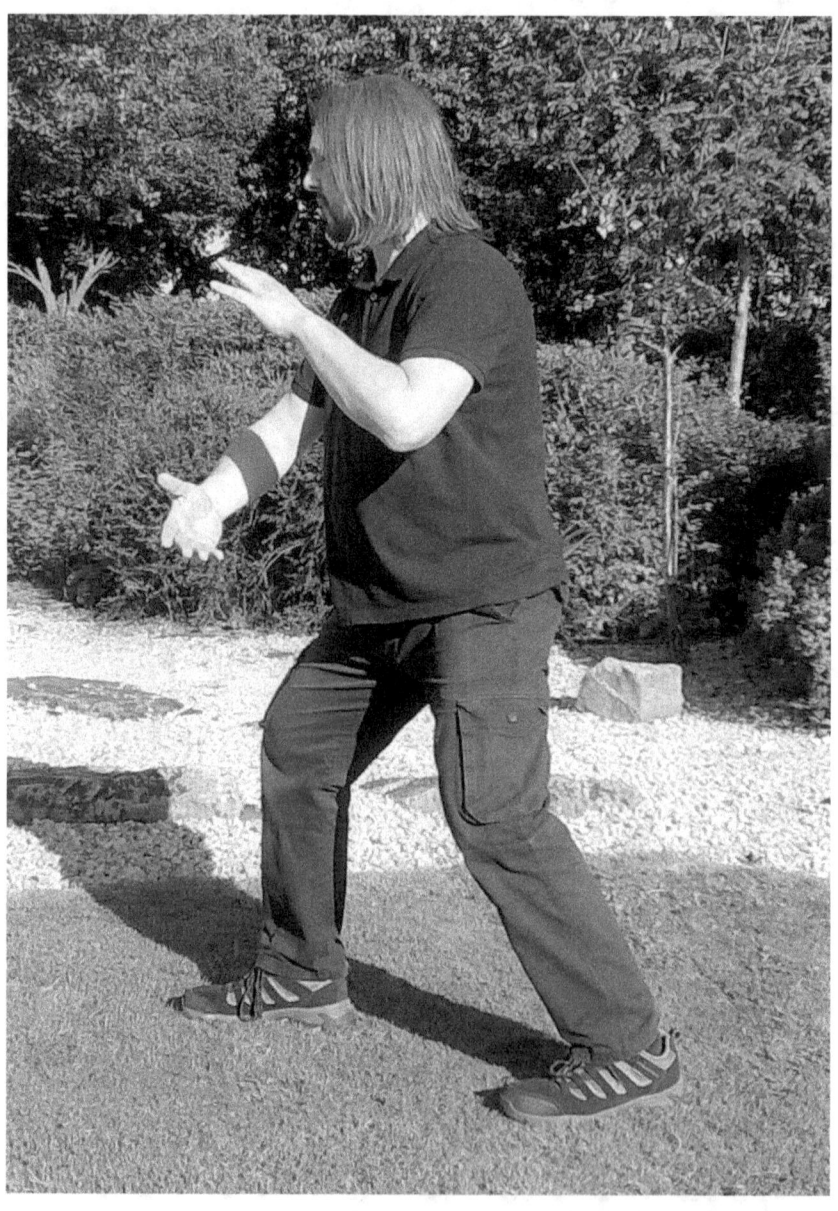

Leave the left hand in front of your chest and roll your right hand upwards in a curve to the 11 o'clock position in front of your right upper chest. The fingers of your left hand point to your right wrist and your elbows are heavy.

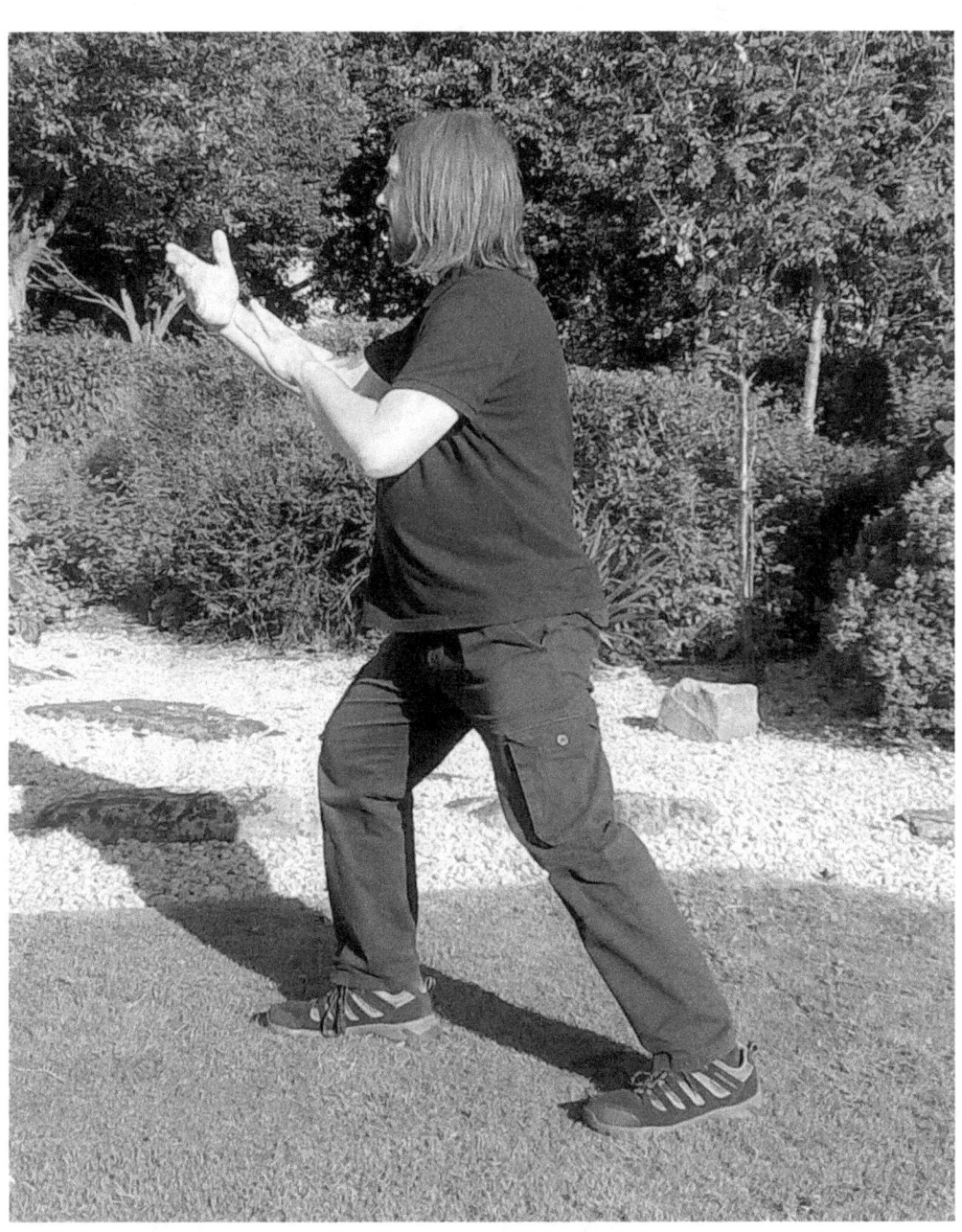

Rollback

Slowly lower your hands towards your Dantien. Maintain a space between the arms and your body and keep a distance roughly that of your own elbow and wrist between the hands.

At the same time, shift back slowly, until seventy percent of your body weight is in your left leg and turn your body to your left corner.

Keep your nose and belly button aligned.

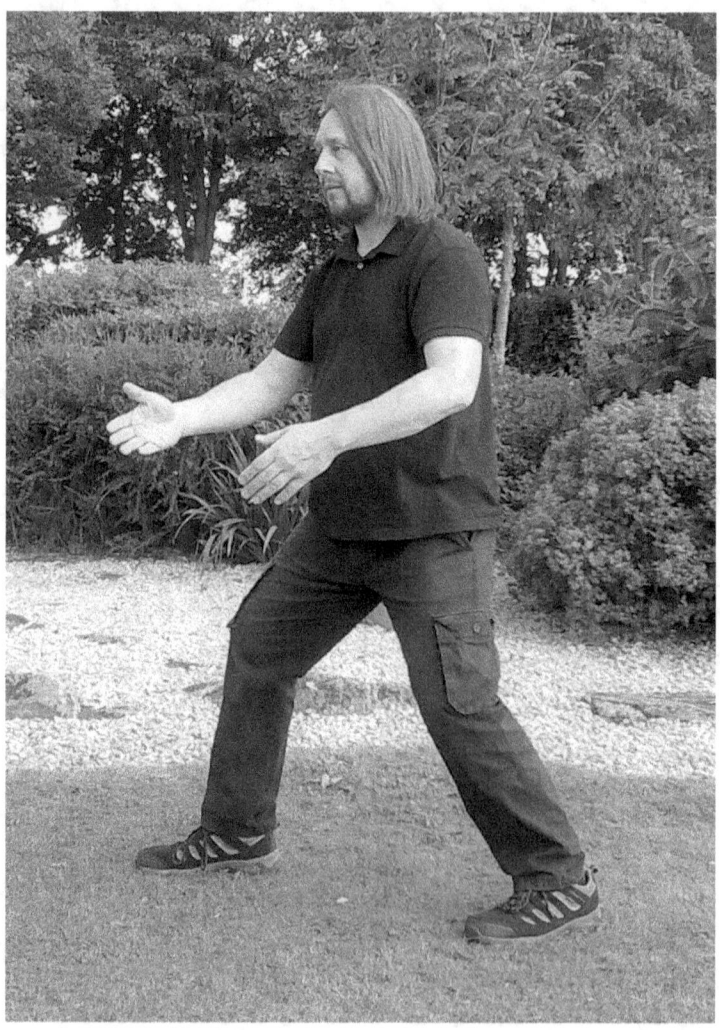

Press

Circle your left hand round and place your palm on your right inner wrist. Turn your body to square again and move your weight forward from the left leg into seventy percent front weighted, right Bow stance.

At the same time, bring your connected hands up in front of your chest, and expand them forward slightly. Your arms form a triangle shape.

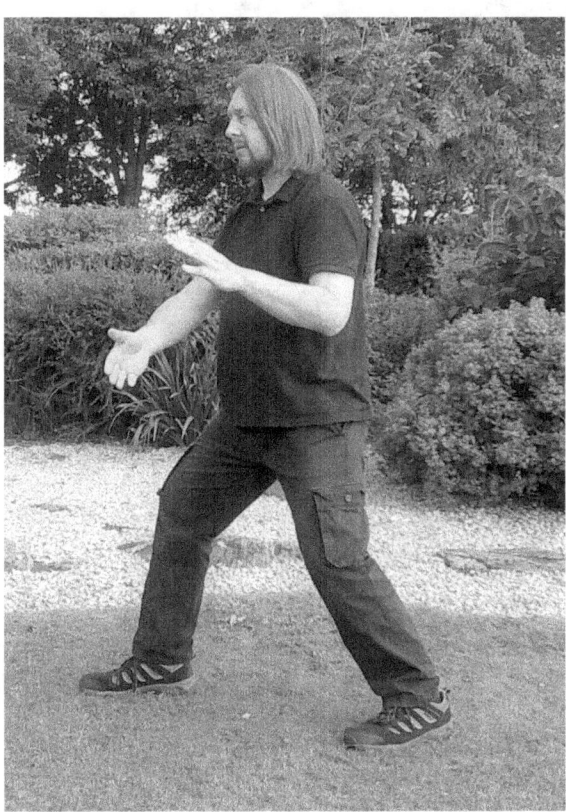 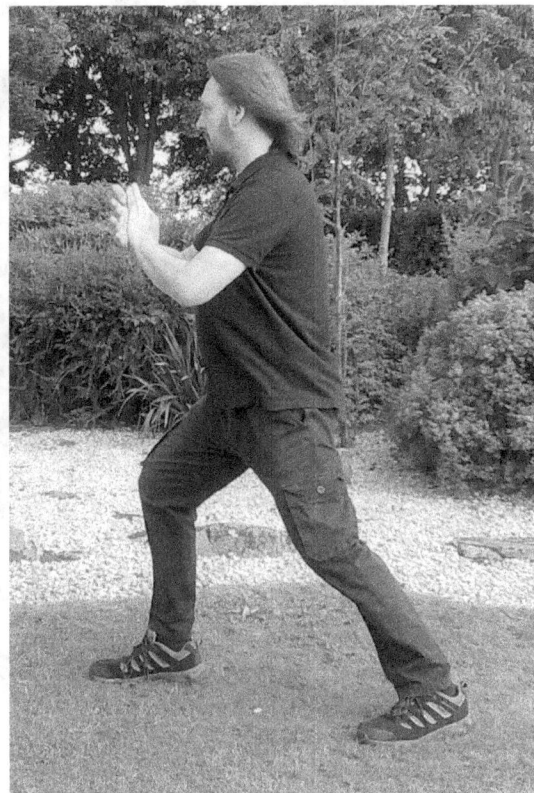

Separate hands

Rotate your hands to palms down and at the same time, cross your wrists with the left hand on top.

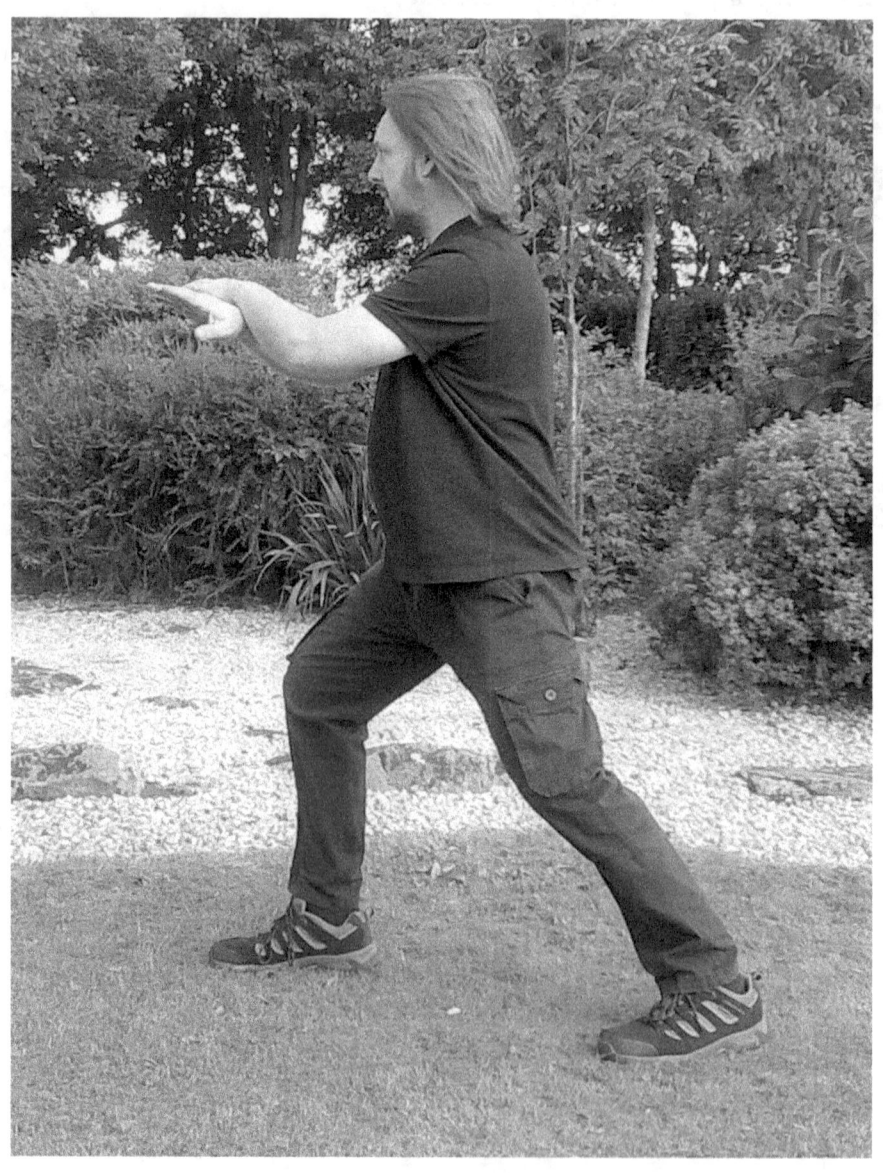

Immediately uncross your arms and separate your hands to shoulder width. At the same time, move backwards into your left leg.

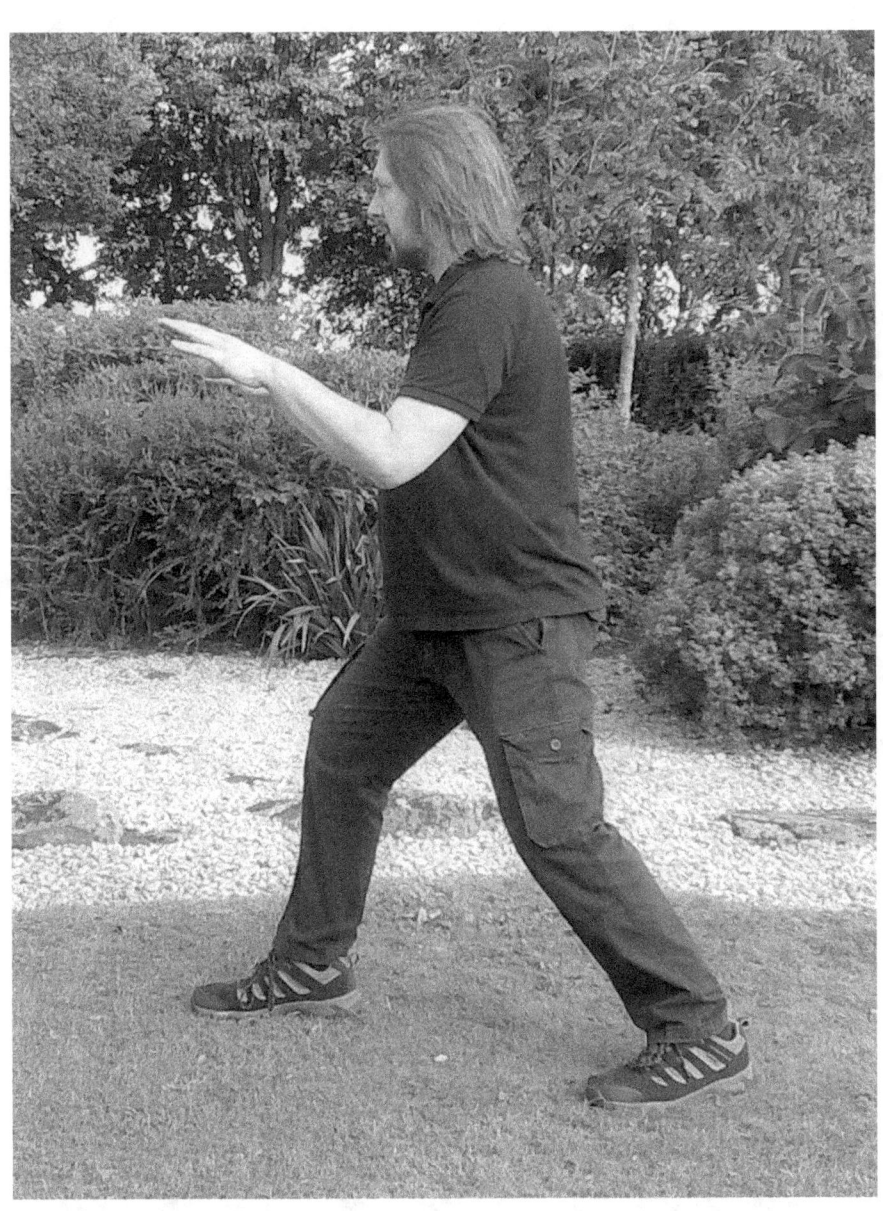

Push

Push forward, gradually shifting seventy per cent of your weight into your right leg, the hands follow the movement of your body and rise up a few inches.

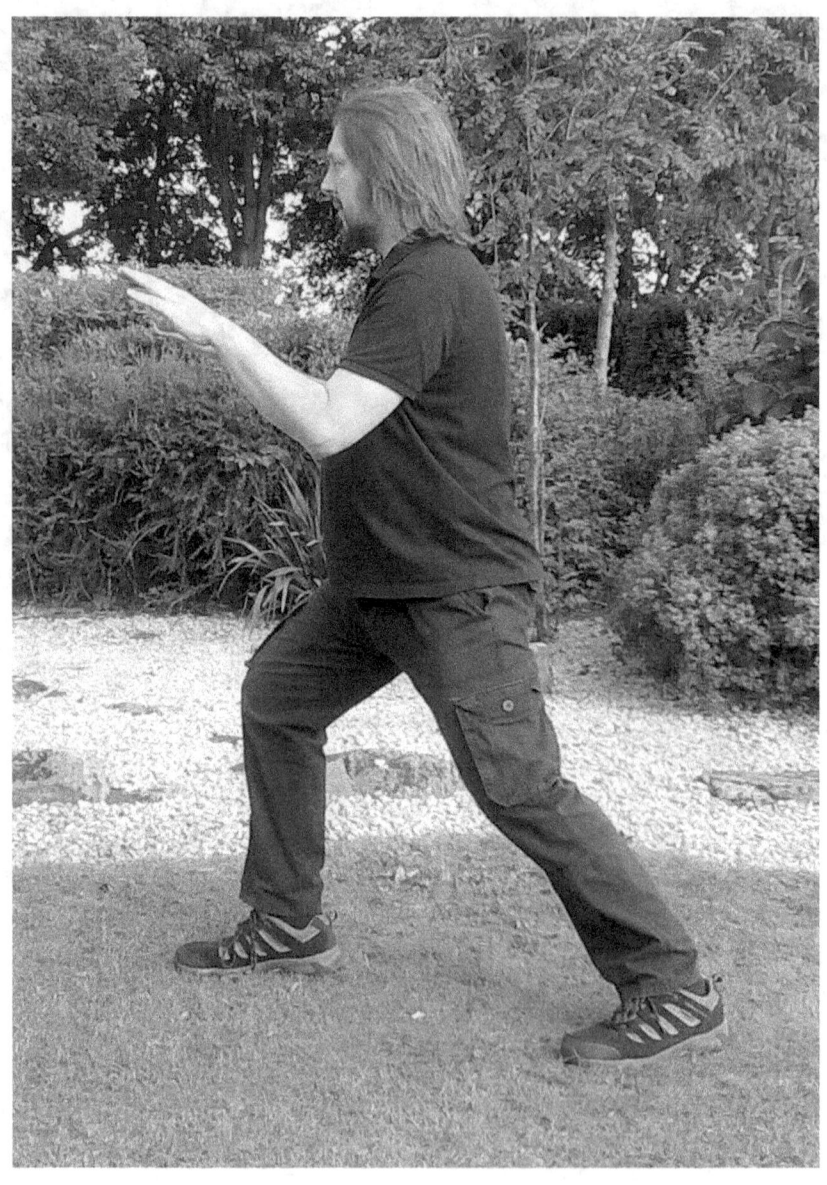

26) Single Whip

Shift your weight backwards seventy percent into your left foot.

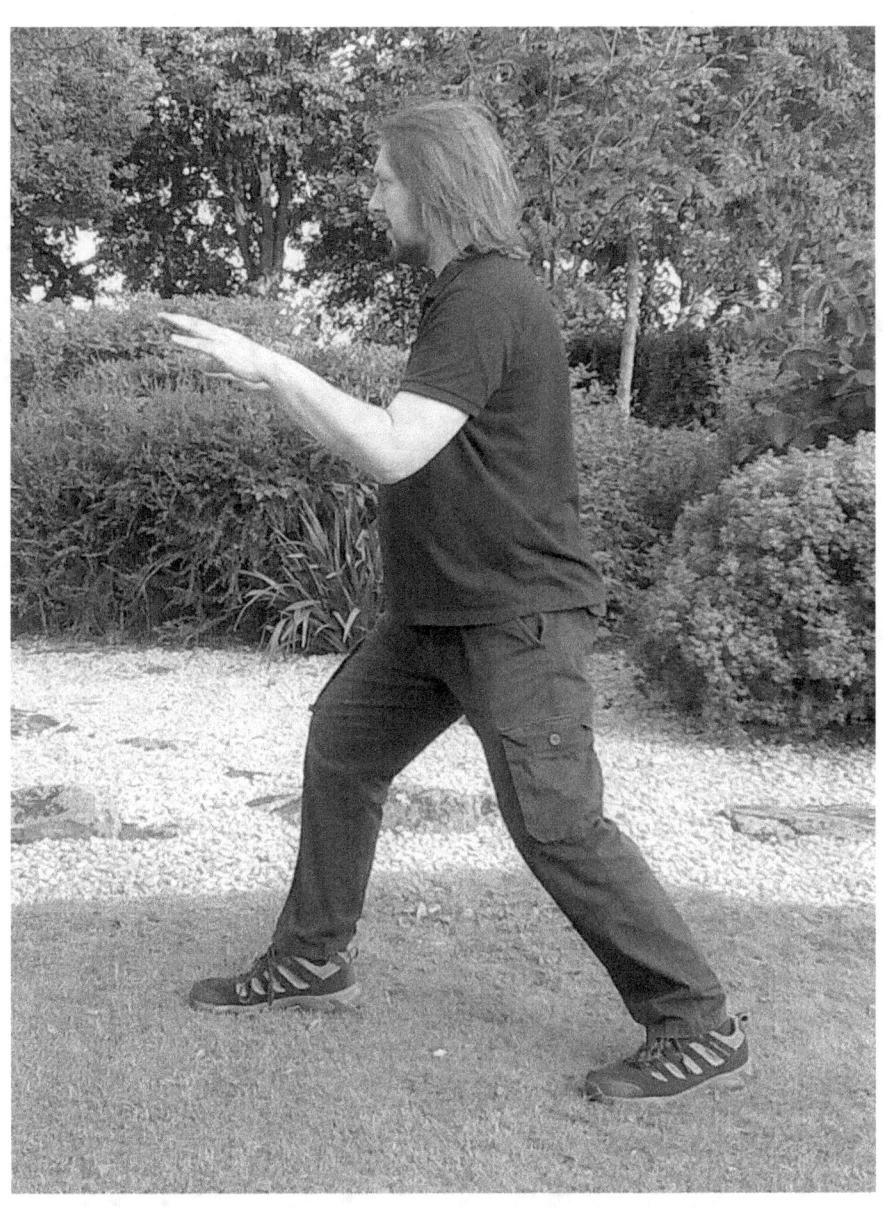

Lift the toes of your right foot. Turn to your back left corner; your hands remain in front of your shoulders.

Your right leg follows the bodies turning by pivoting on the right heel.

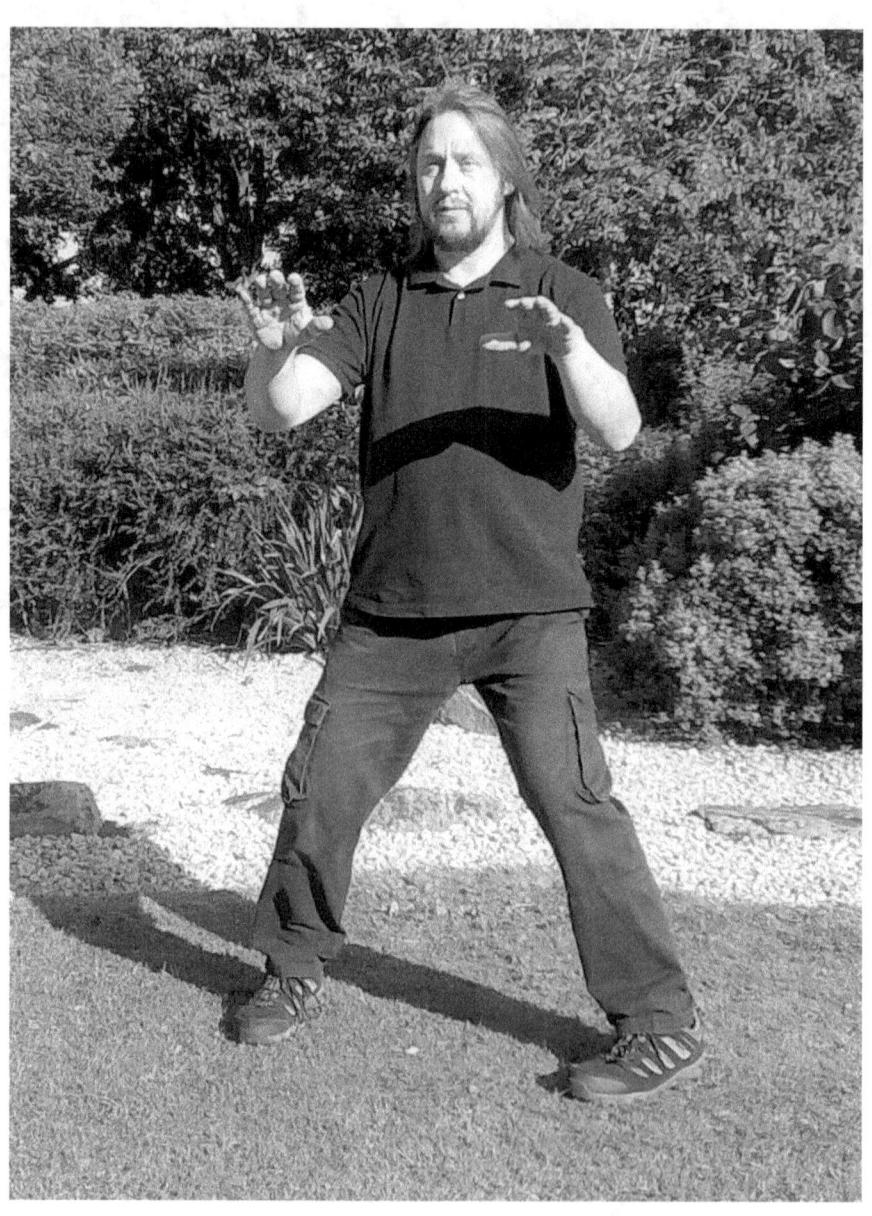

Hold a ball with the right hand on top and the left hand on the bottom.

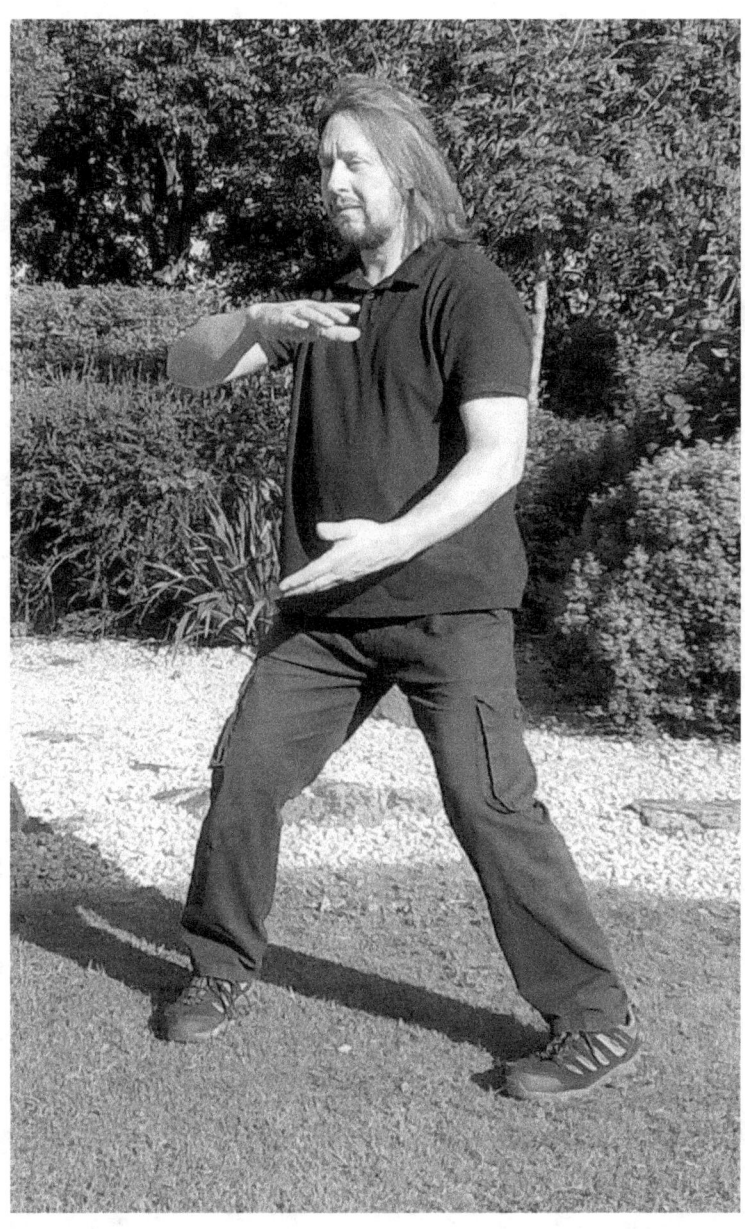

Push your right hand out until the arm is straight (but not locked out). At the same time bend your right wrist until the thumb points down and place your fingertips around the tip of the thumb to form a beak.

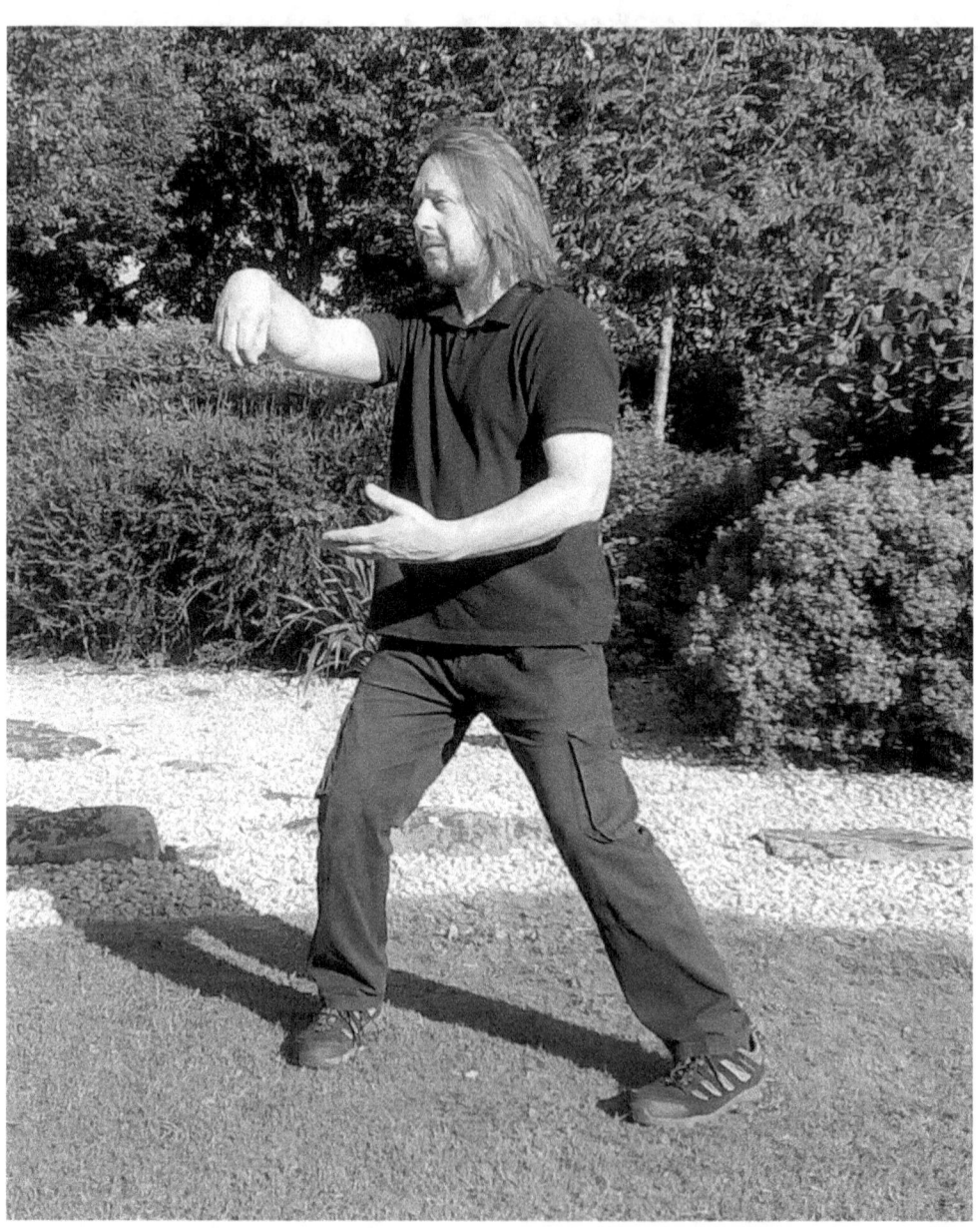

Turn back towards the left, your weight stays in the right leg. Lift up your left heel, pivot on the ball of the foot to the left and step forwards, place down your heel, and roll into a left footed seventy percent front weighted Bow stance.

As you step out your left hand rises in a Ward off shape, curving up and across your body to your left side, finally you should rotate your hand until the palm faces away from you in front of your left shoulder.

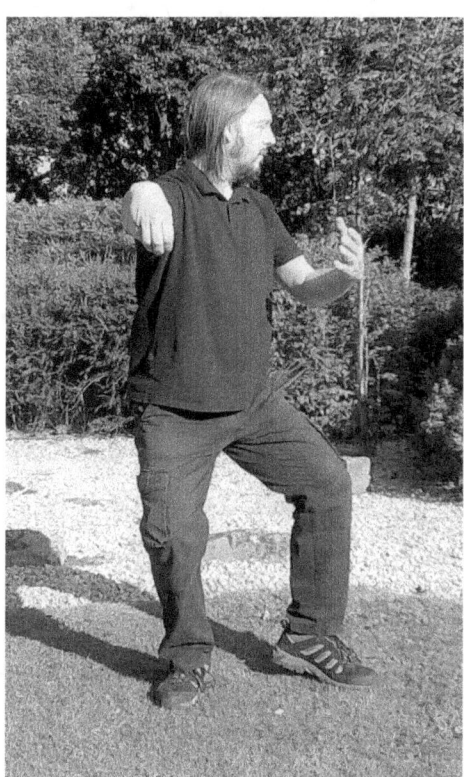 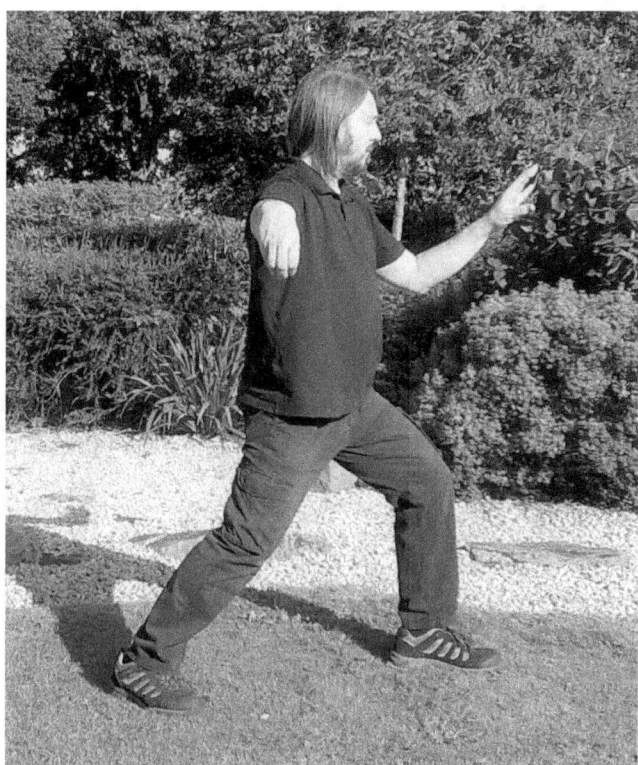

27) Fair Lady Works Shuttles x 4

One

Hold a ball with your right hand on top and the left hand underneath.

Shift backwards into your right leg, lift up your left toes, and turn on the heel towards your right side.

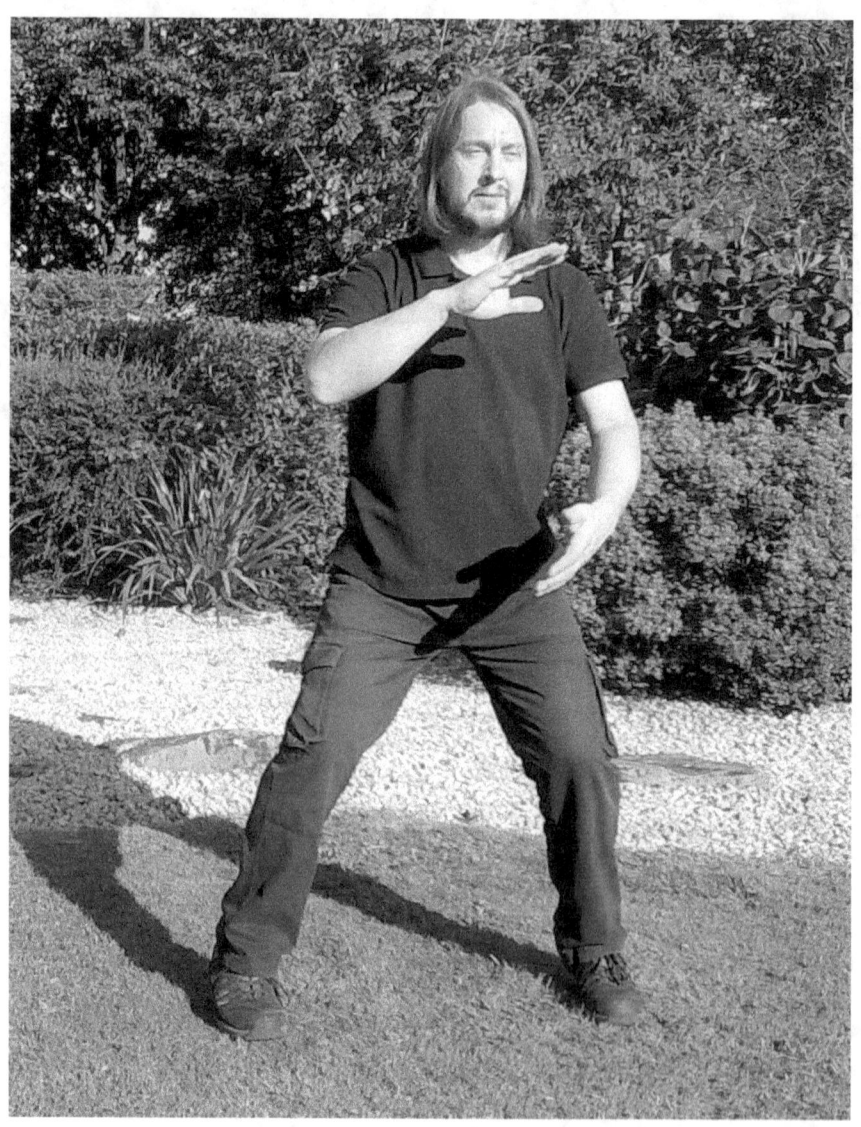

Roll your left foot down and shift your weight across onto it, turn the right foot outwards, roll your right foot down and move your weight into the right leg.

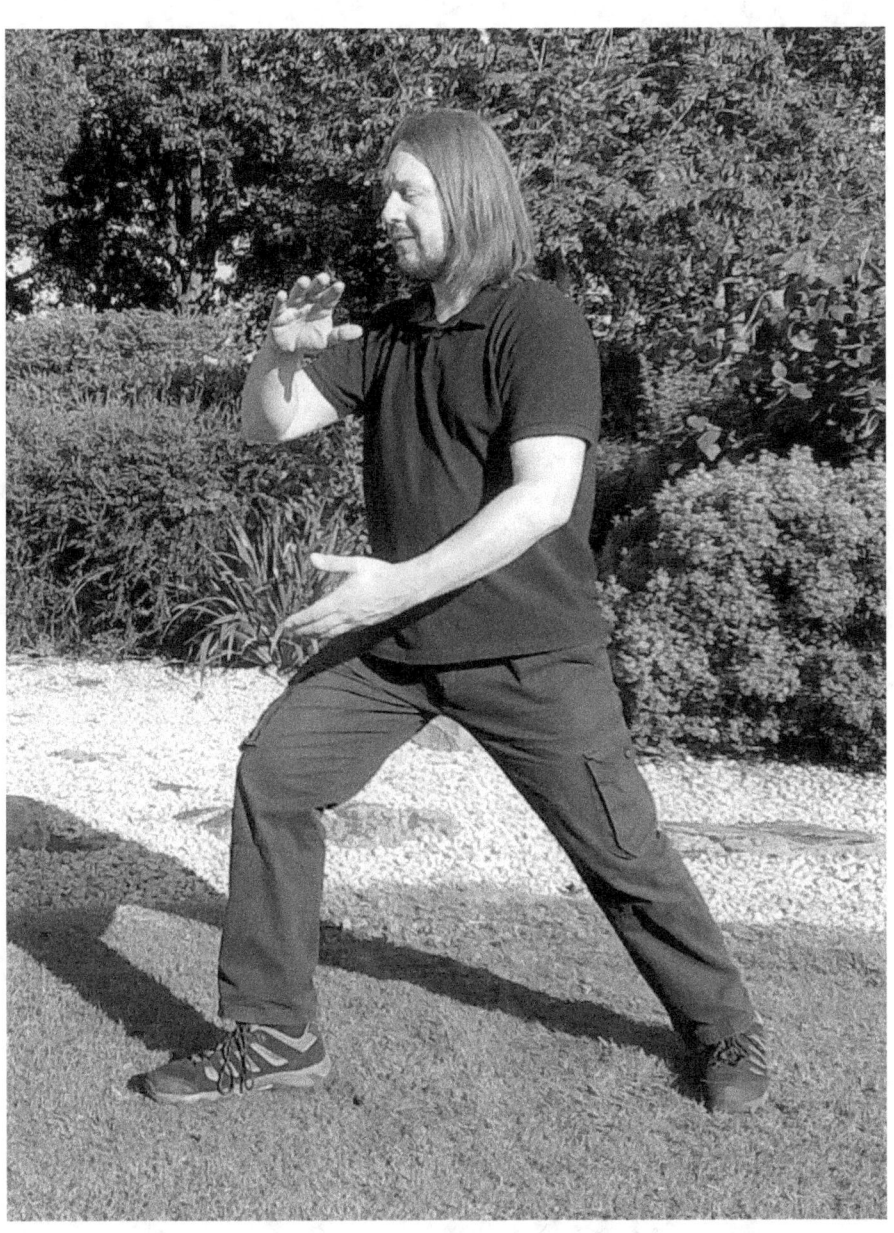

Step forward with the left foot into a left seventy percent front Bow stance. Bring your left hand up, across, and past the outside edge of your left forehead. As you lift the left hand, rotate it until the palm faces outward. At the same time, your right hand pushes forward in front of your upper chest, both hands are an equal distance from your body.

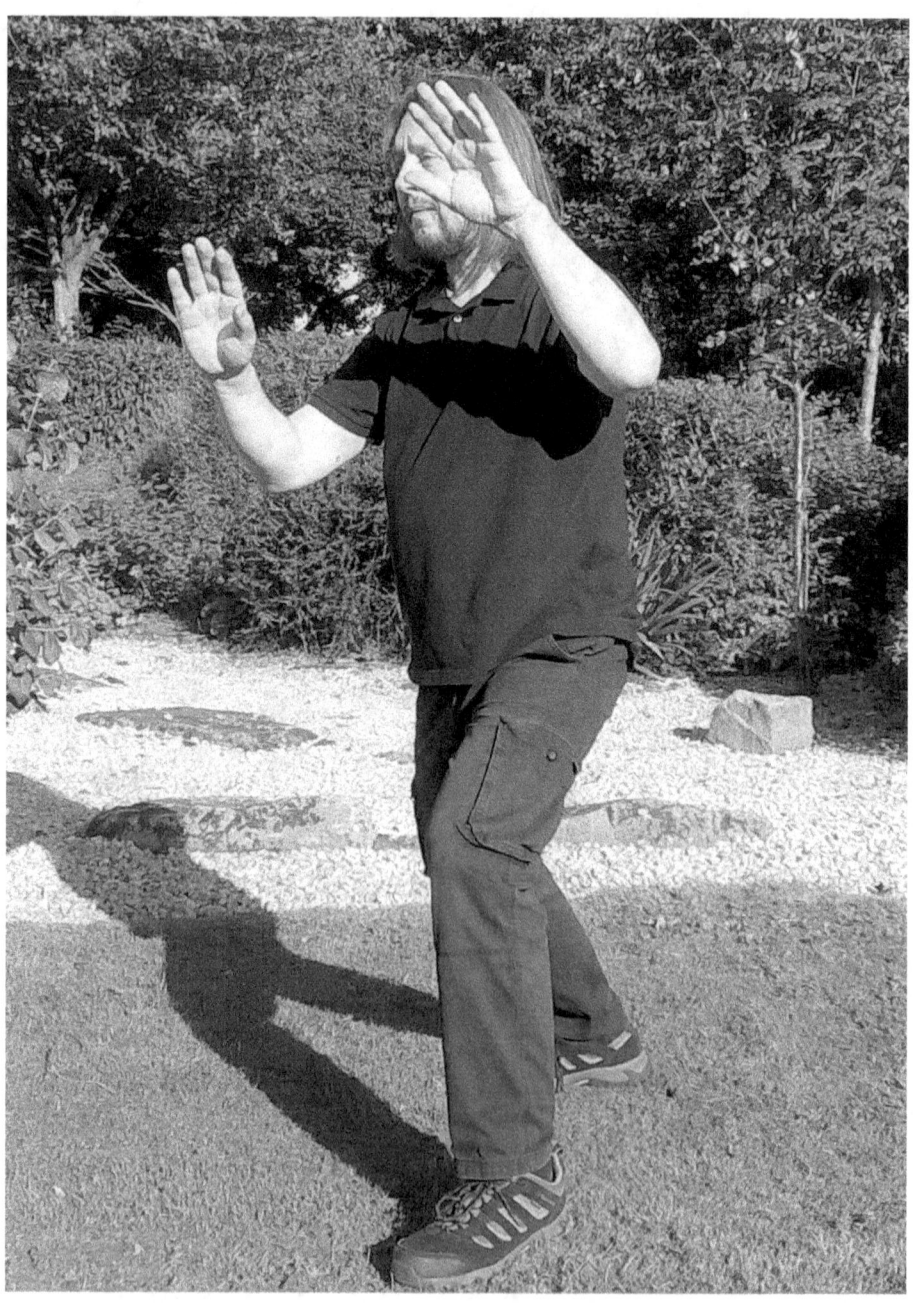

Two

Hold a ball with your left hand on top and your right hand on the bottom.

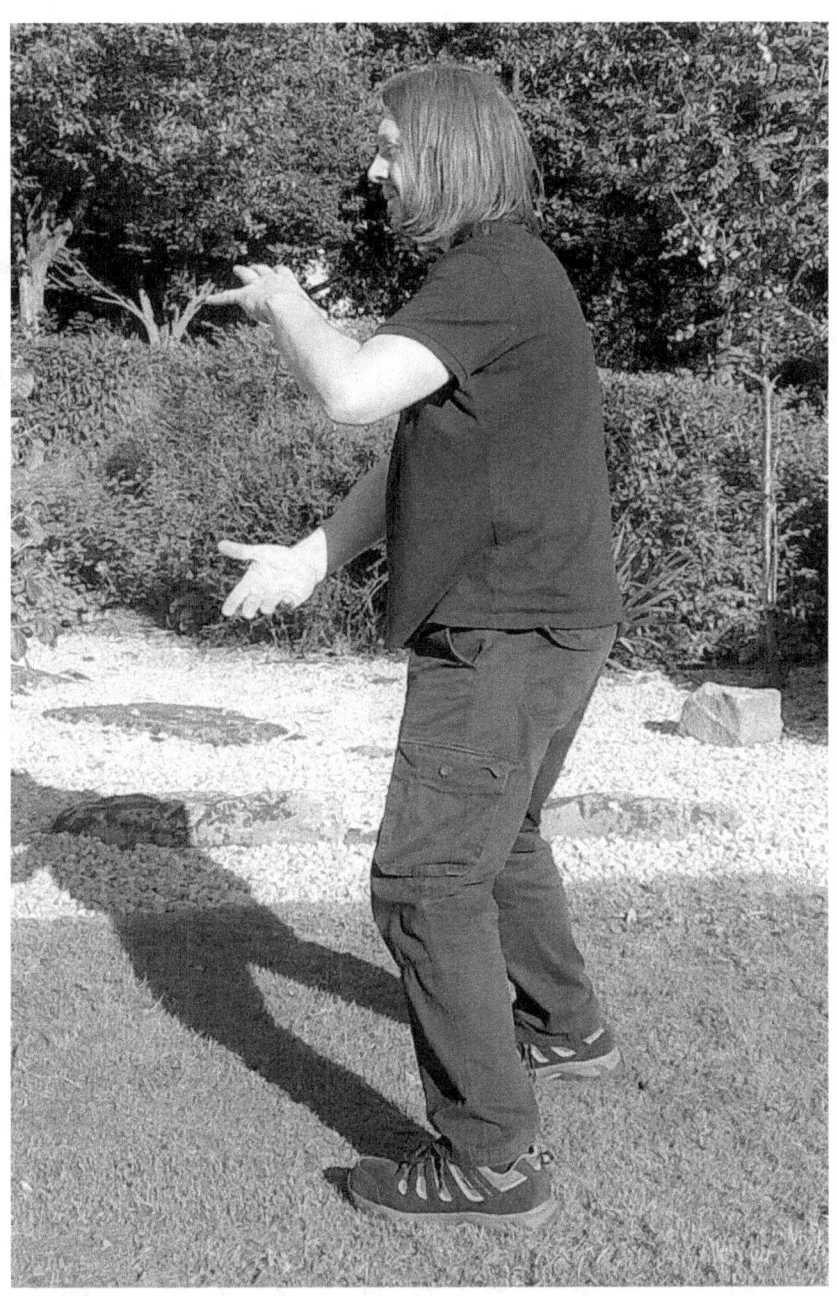

Shift all of your weight backwards into your right leg, step around to your right rear corner and move slowly into a right Bow stance.

Bring your right hand up, across, and past the outside edge of your right forehead. At the same time, your right hand pushes forward in front of your upper chest, both hands are an equal distance from your body.

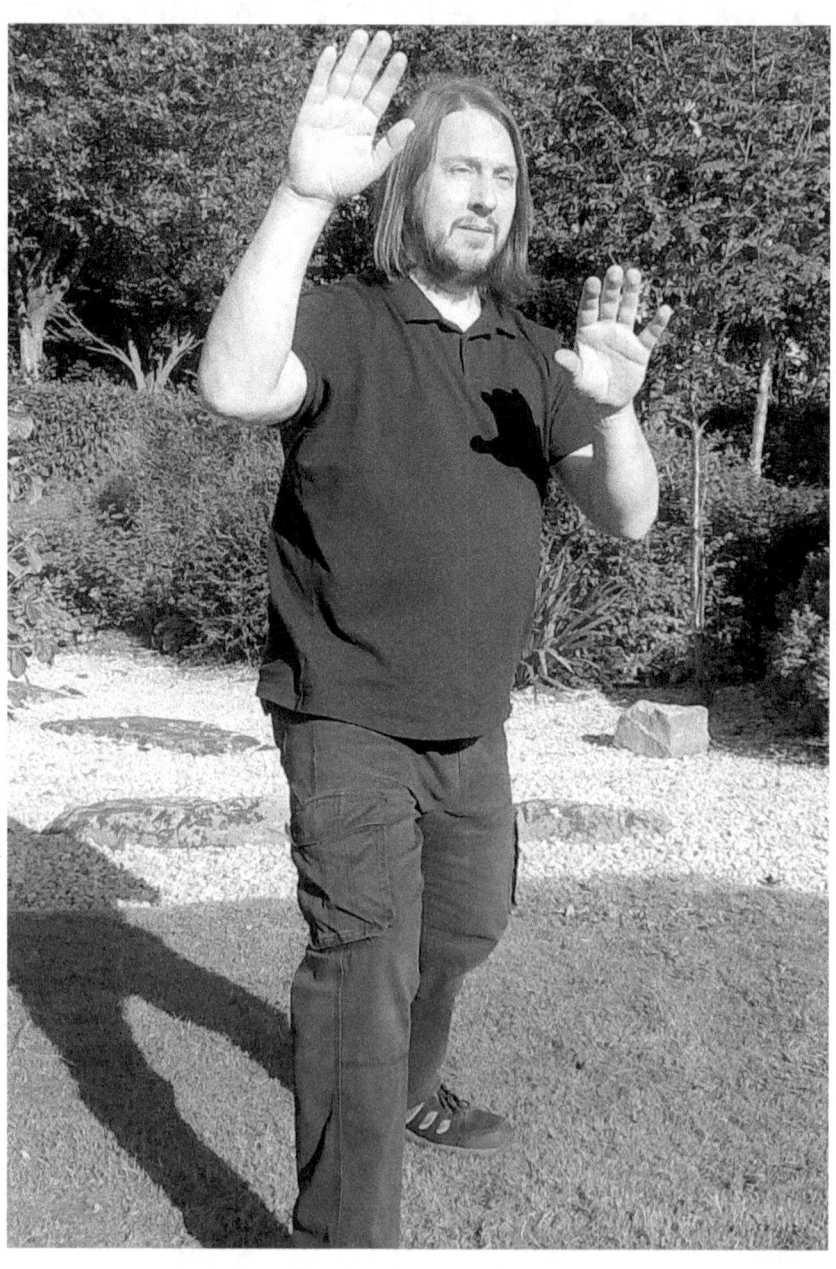

Three

Hold a ball with the right hand on top. Shift your weight to the left foot.

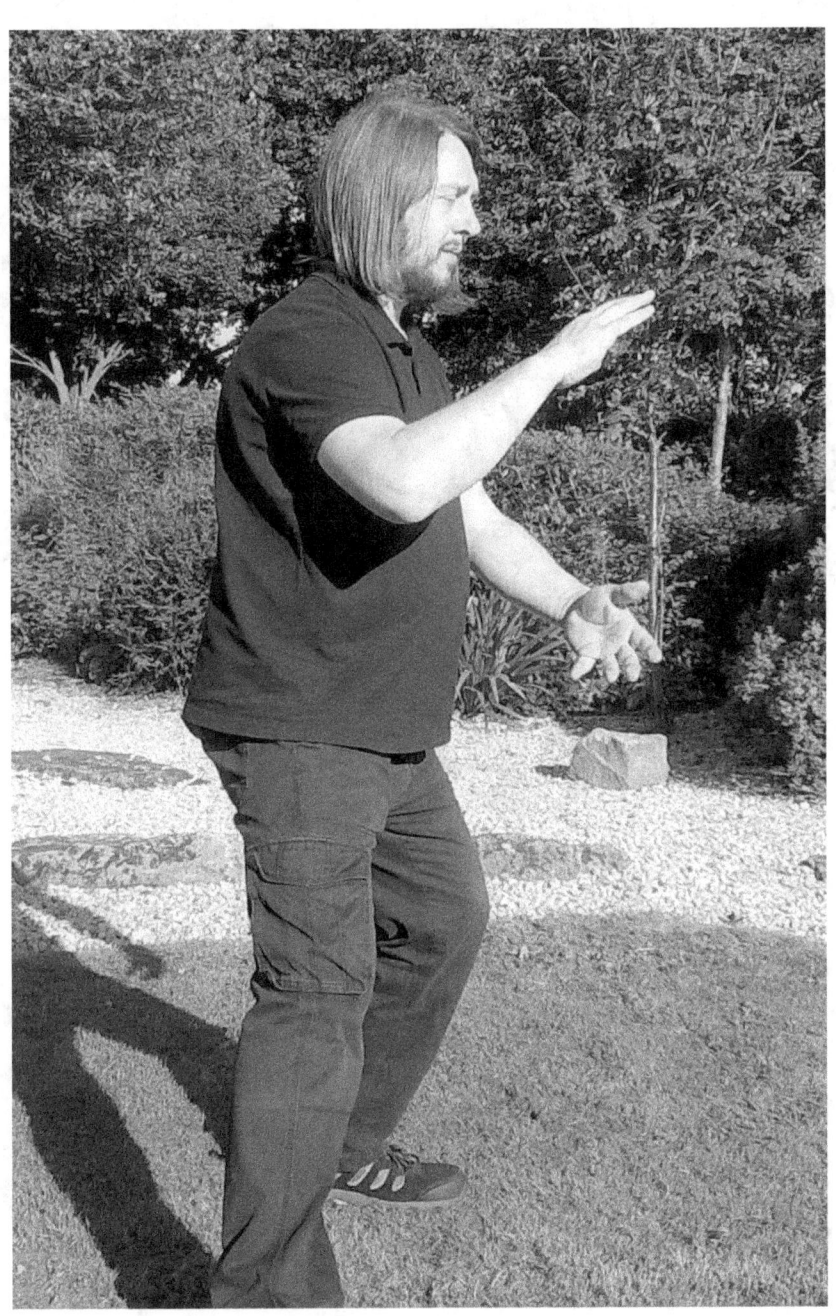

Keep a shoulder width stance and take half a step to the left corner with your right foot.

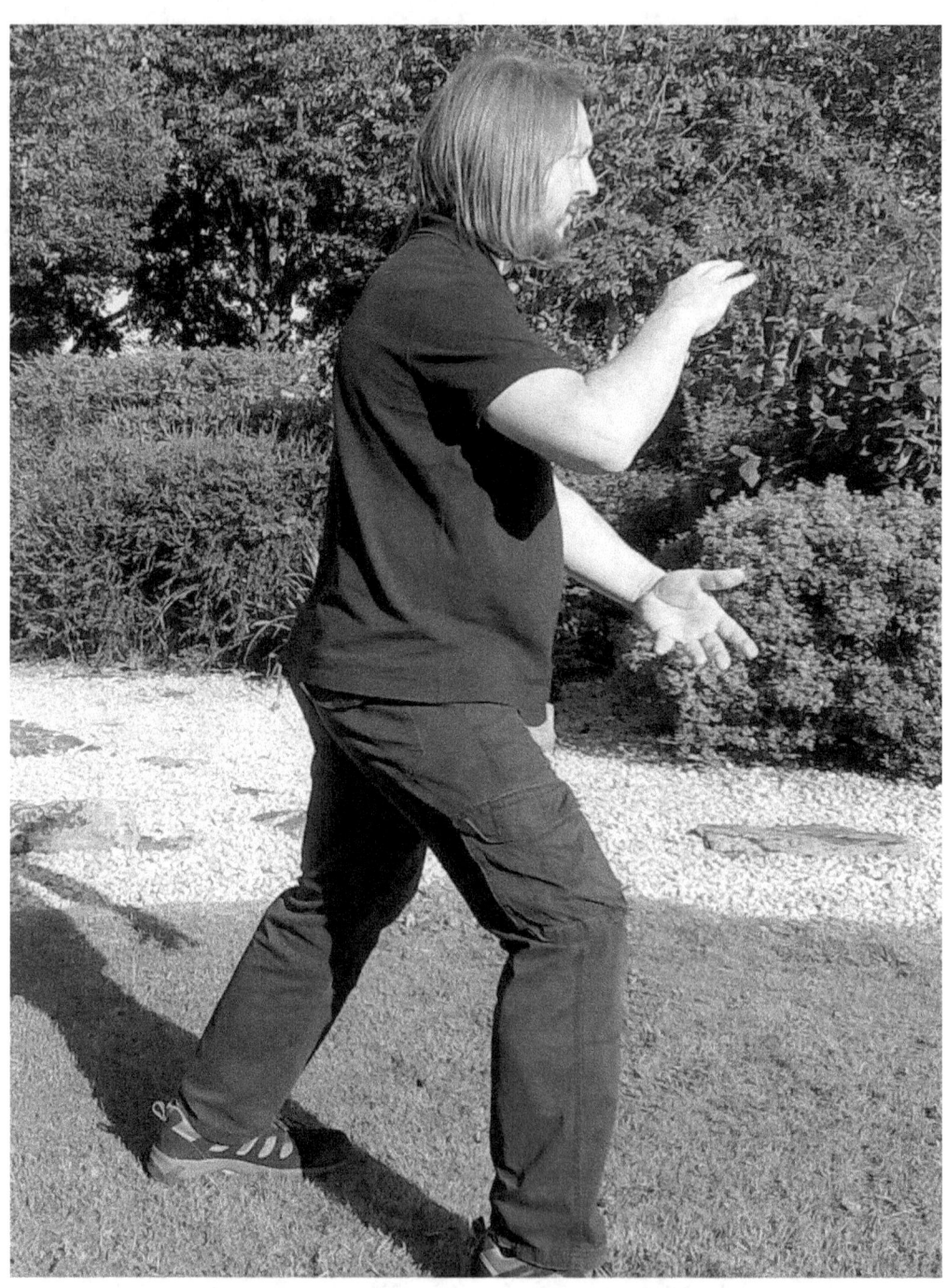

Place your heel down and roll the rest of your foot down. Move seventy percent of your bodyweight gradually into the right foot and step forward with the left foot into a Bow stance. Bring your left hand up, across, and past the outside edge of your left forehead. Your right hand pushes forward in front of the centreline, both hands are the same distance away from you.

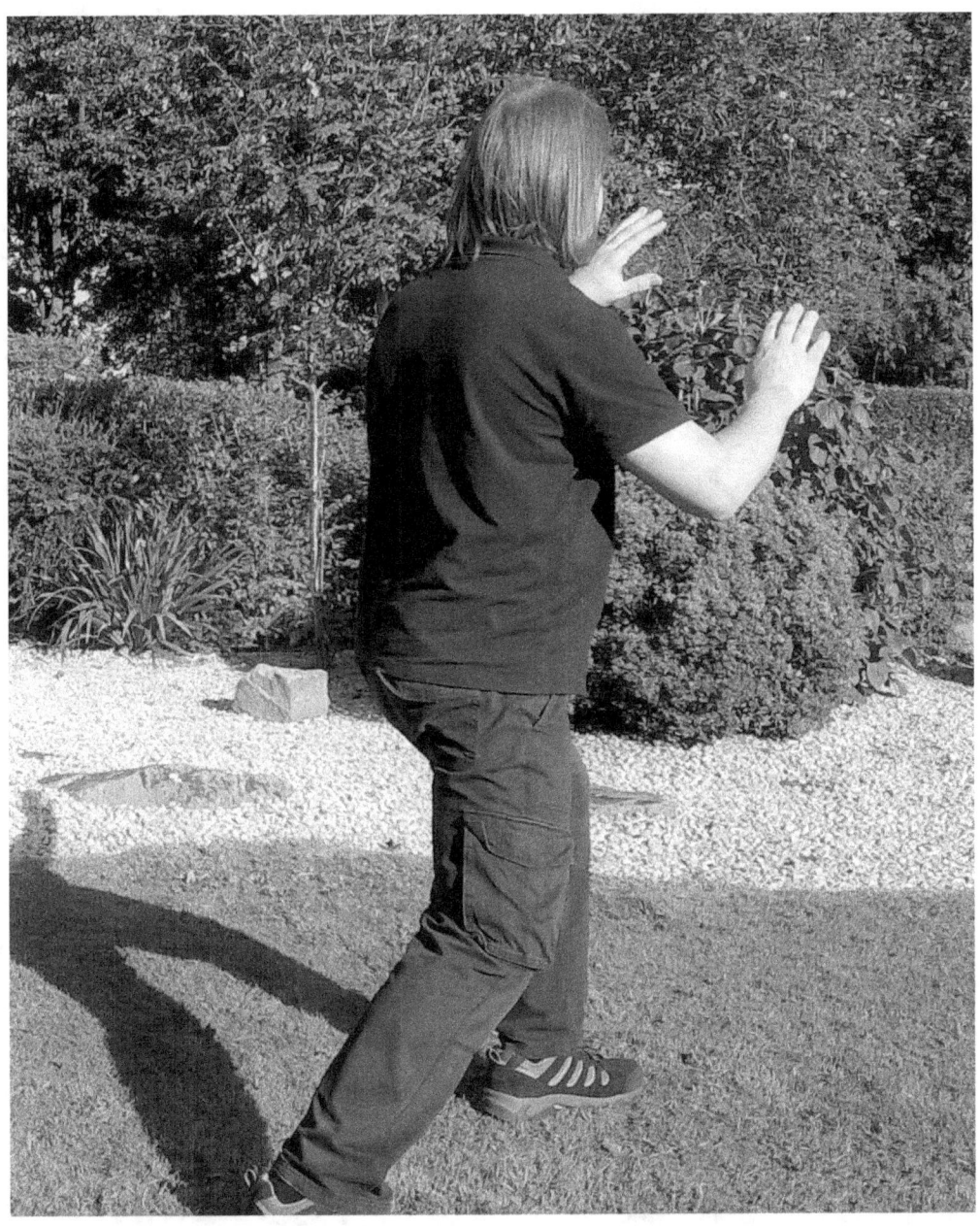

Four

Now hold the ball with the left hand on the top and your right hand underneath. Move your weight slowly back to your right leg and turn the toes of the left foot across to your right side.

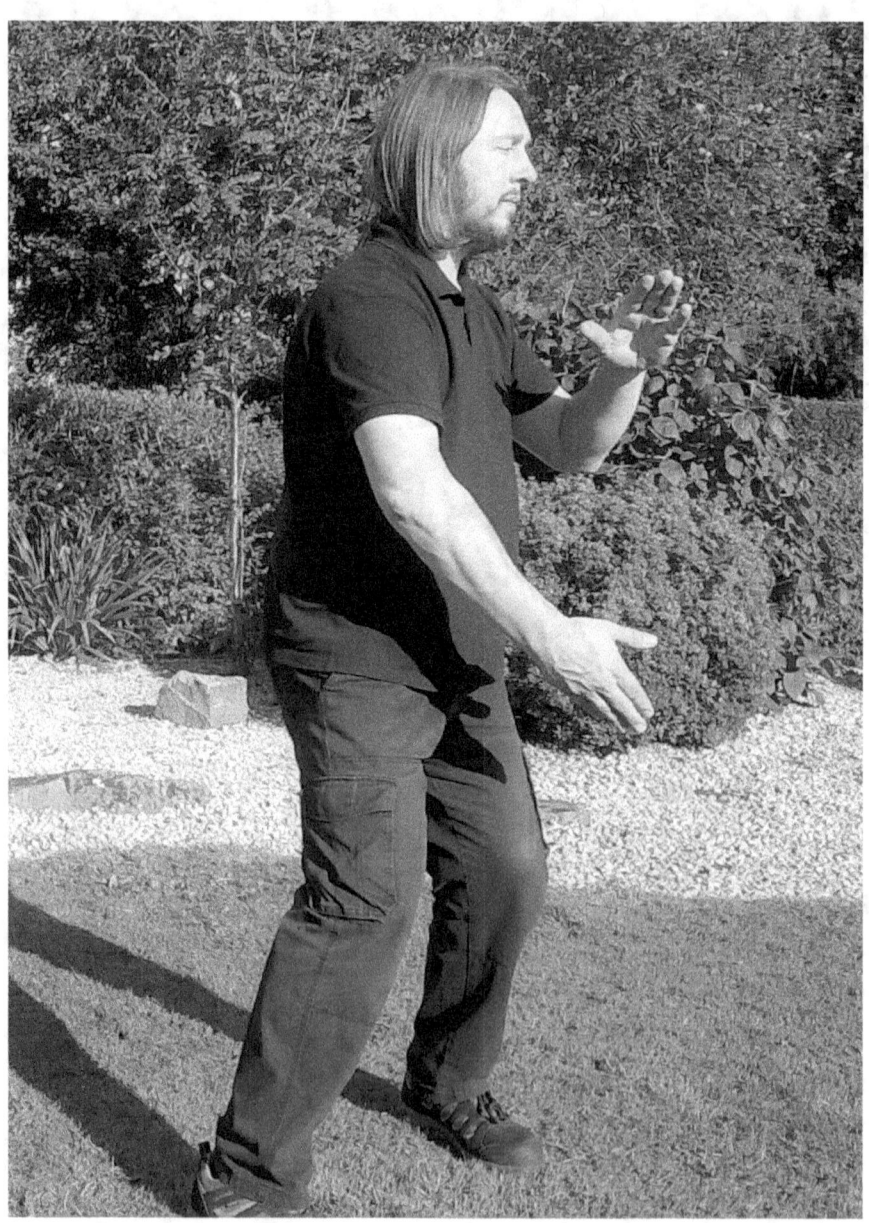

Shift your weight fully into the left foot and then take a big step around to your left rear corner with your right foot.

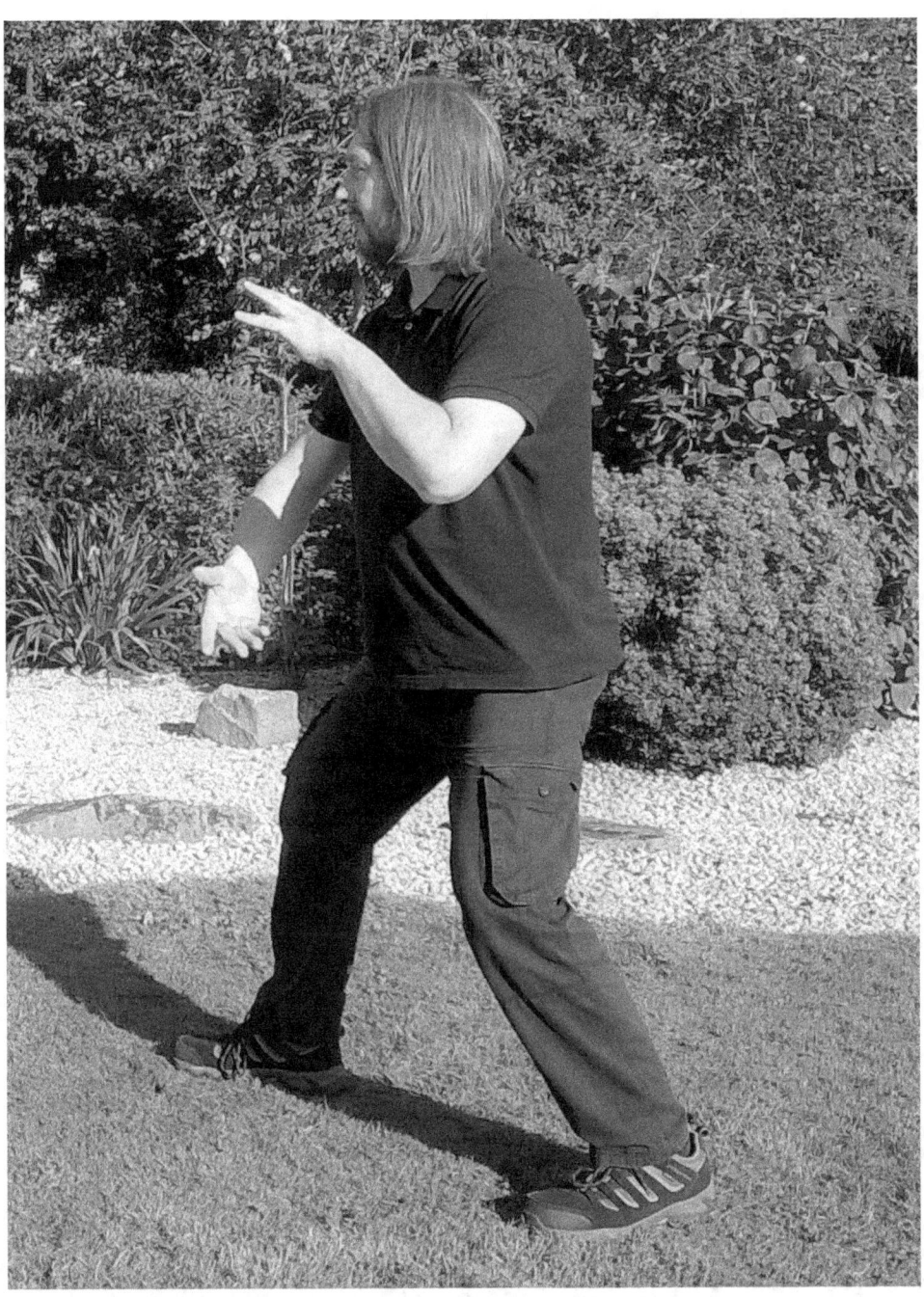

As you step into this seventy percent weighted forward Bow stance, bring your right hand up, across, and past the outside edge of your left forehead. Your left hand pushes forward in front of the upper chest, both hands end their movement at the same time.

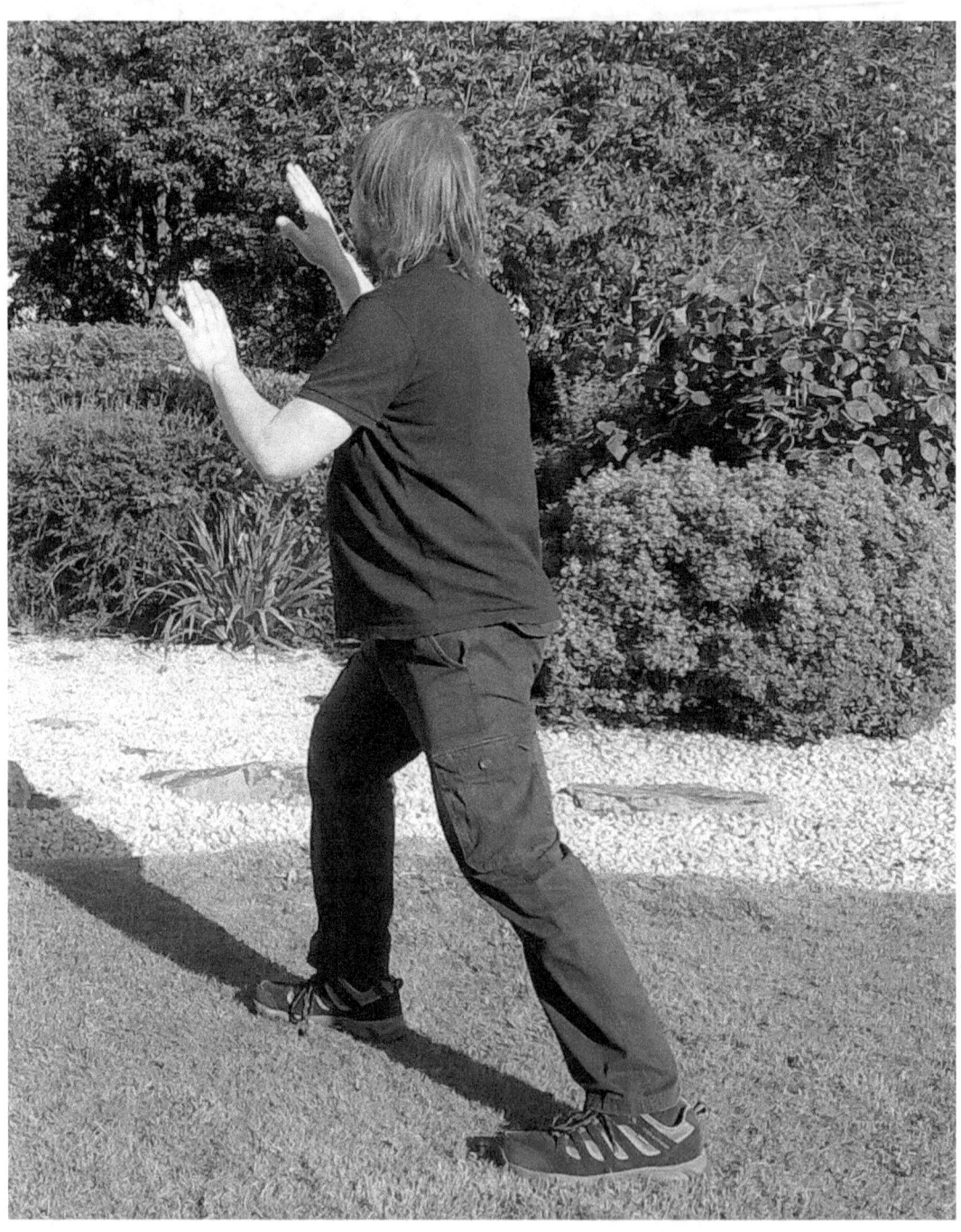

28) Ward Off Left

Hold a ball with your right hand on top and left hand underneath.

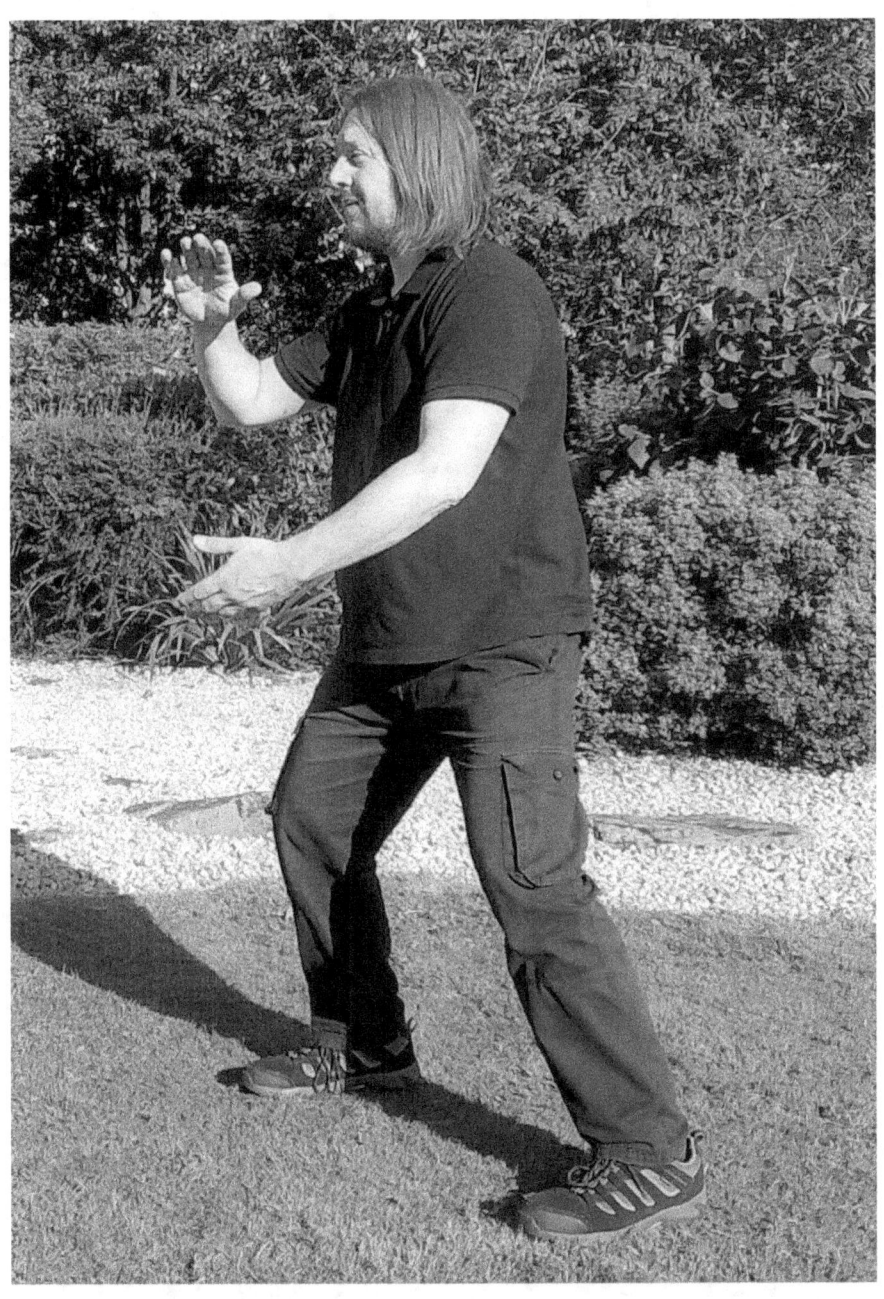

Shift slowly to your left leg, pivot on the right heel to your right side, and then shift your weight into your right leg. Keep a shoulder width space between your feet as you step.

Step forward with your left foot and roll the foot down, transferring seventy per cent of your weight into it, bring your left hand up in an arc to sit palm facing inwards, in front of your upper chest. The elbow should be lower than the hand.

At the same time, lower the right hand down by your right side.

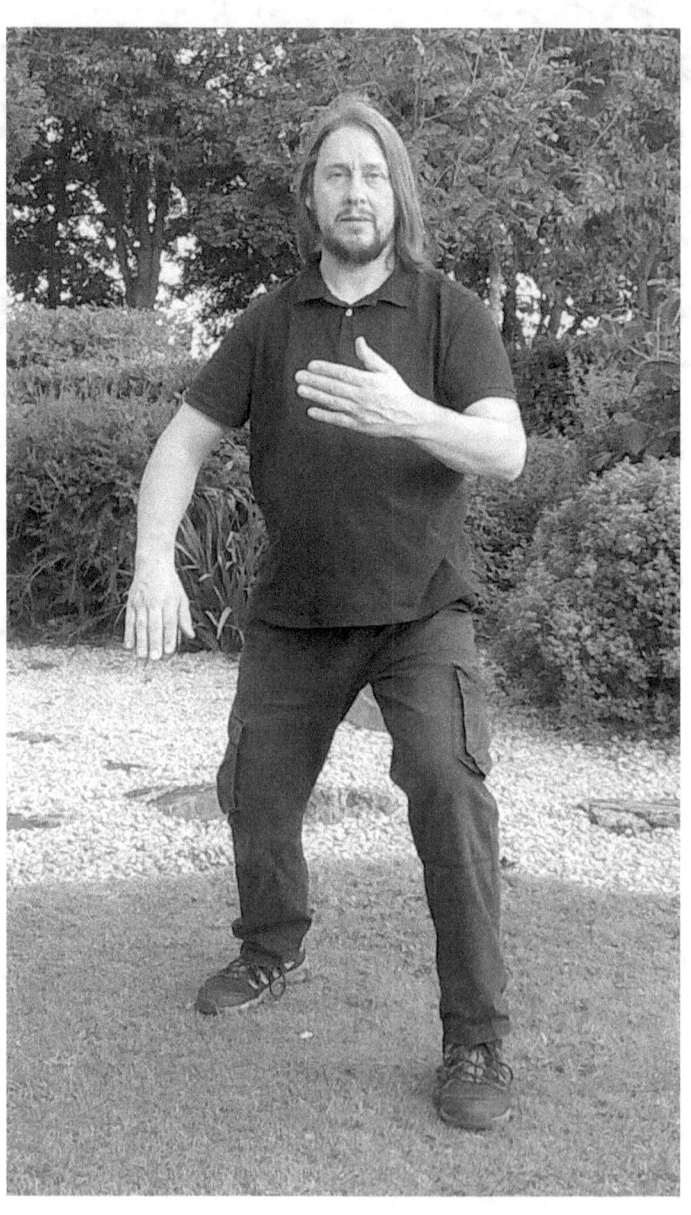

29) Grasp Sparrows Tail

Ward off Right

Hold the ball, with your left hand on top with the palm facing down, and your right hand palm upwards at the base of the ball.

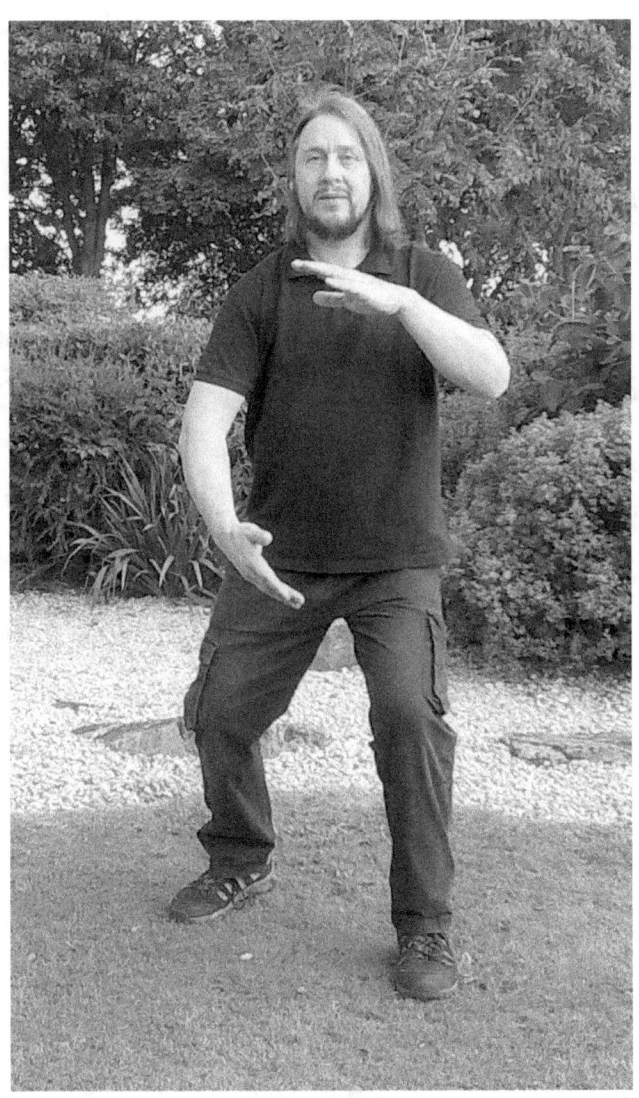

Move your weight backwards until it is fully in the right leg. Turn to your right side, lift your left toes, and pivot around on your heel, following your bodies turning.

Next, you should shift gradually into your left leg. Then lift up your right heel and turn around until you face square on again.

Step forward into a right Bow stance, keep a shoulder width space between the legs. Leave the left hand on top of the ball, and roll your right hand upwards in a curve, to the 11 o'clock position in front of your upper right chest. The fingers of your left hand point towards your right wrist.

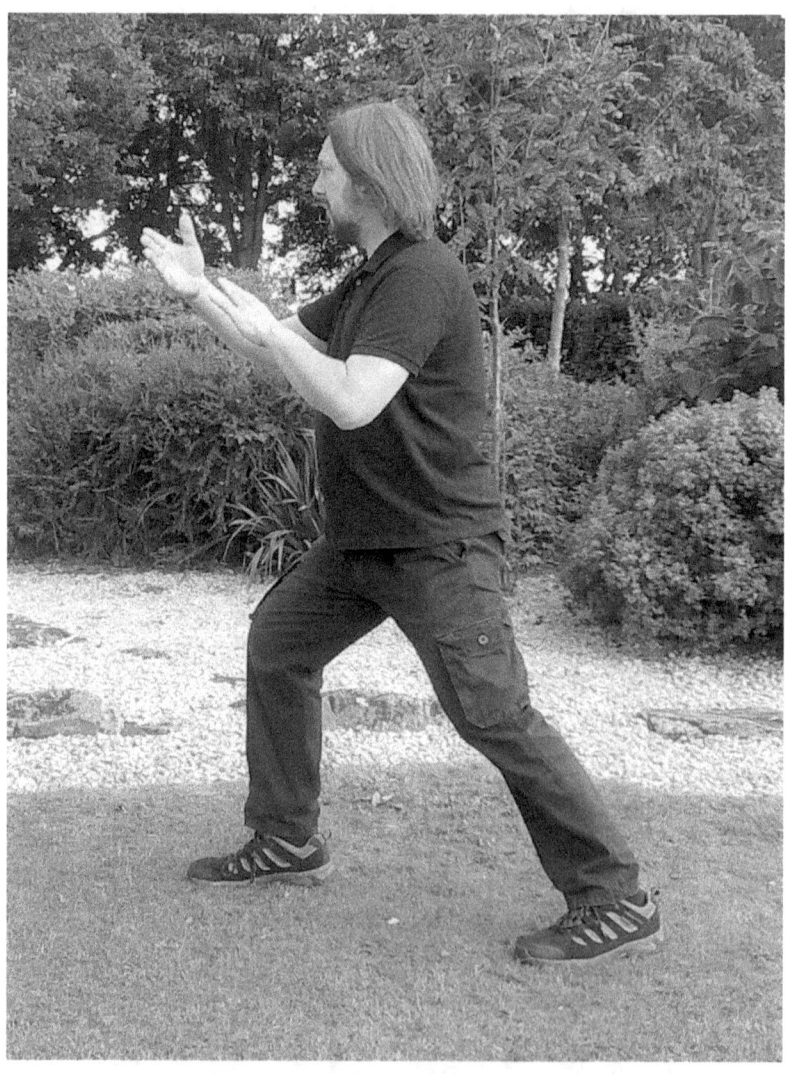

Rollback

Slowly lower your arms, keep a space between the hands, and do not let them move in towards your body.

Shift backwards onto your left leg into a seventy percent back weighted stance and turn your body towards your left corner. Keep your centreline aligned throughout this movement.

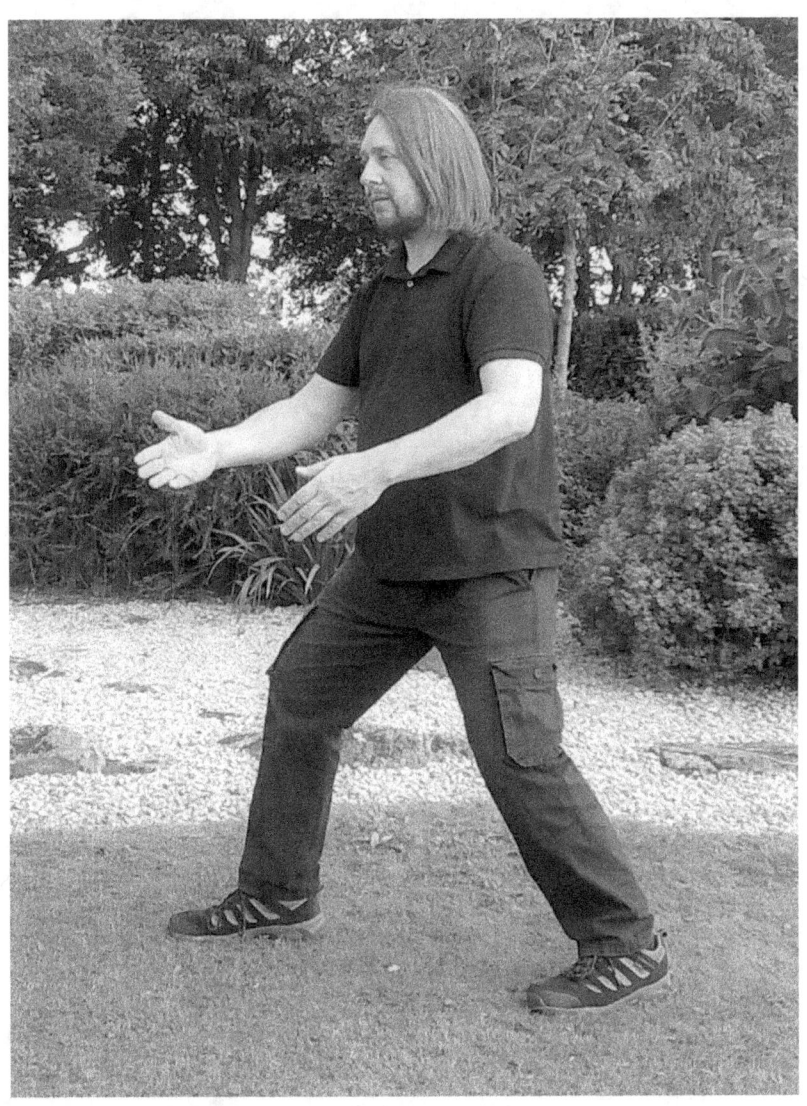

Press

Circle your left hand round and place the palm of the hand on the inside of your right wrist.

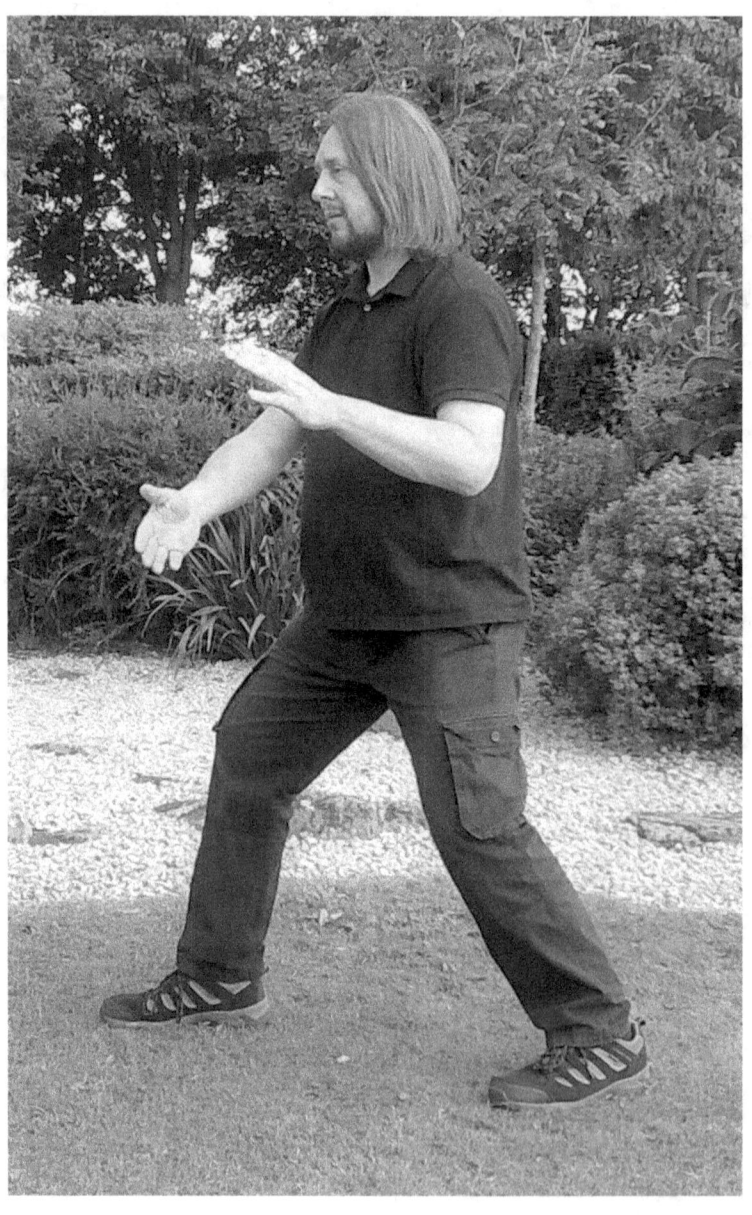

Turn your body back to square again and move forward from the left leg into a seventy percent weighted front right Bow stance.

At the same time, bring your connected hands up in front of your chest. Your arms form a triangle shape, as you press them forward slightly.

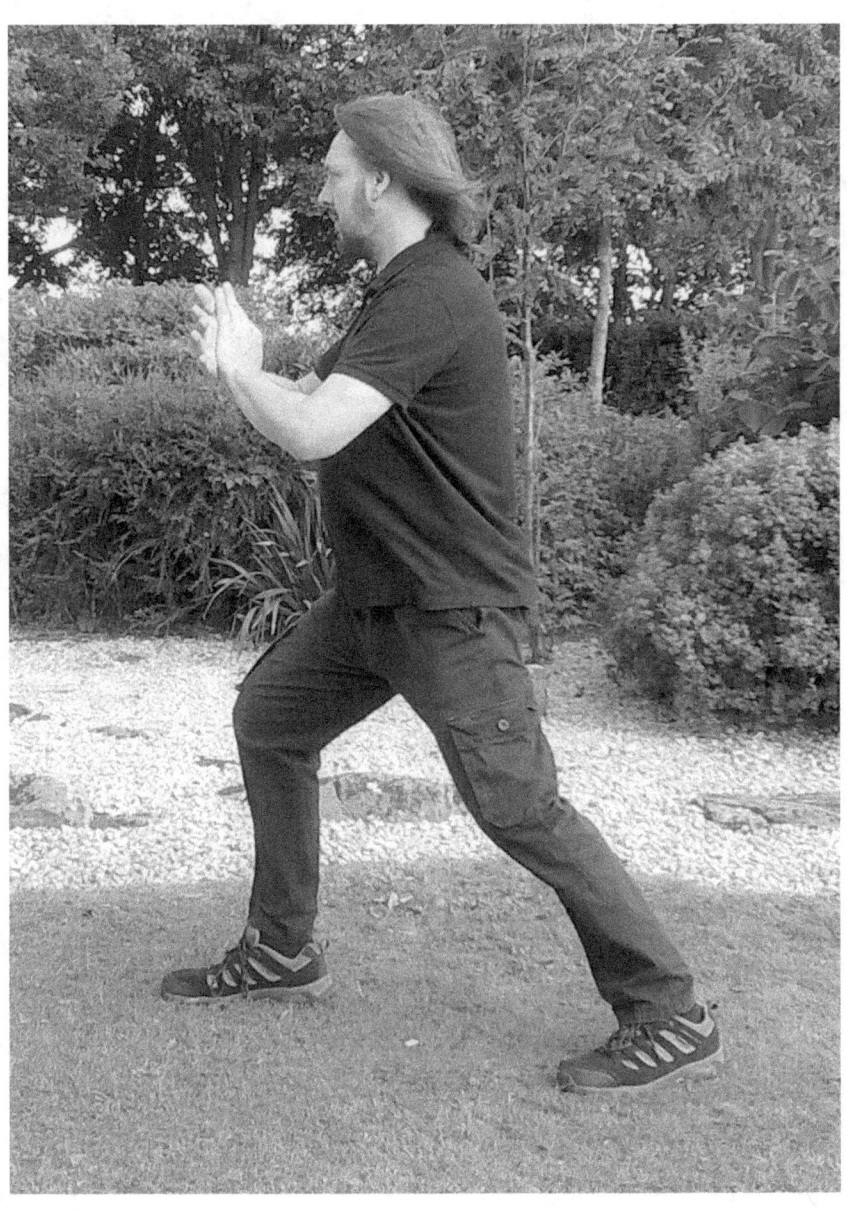

Separate Hands

Rotate both of your hands until your palms face downward, and cross them at the wrists with your left hand on top.

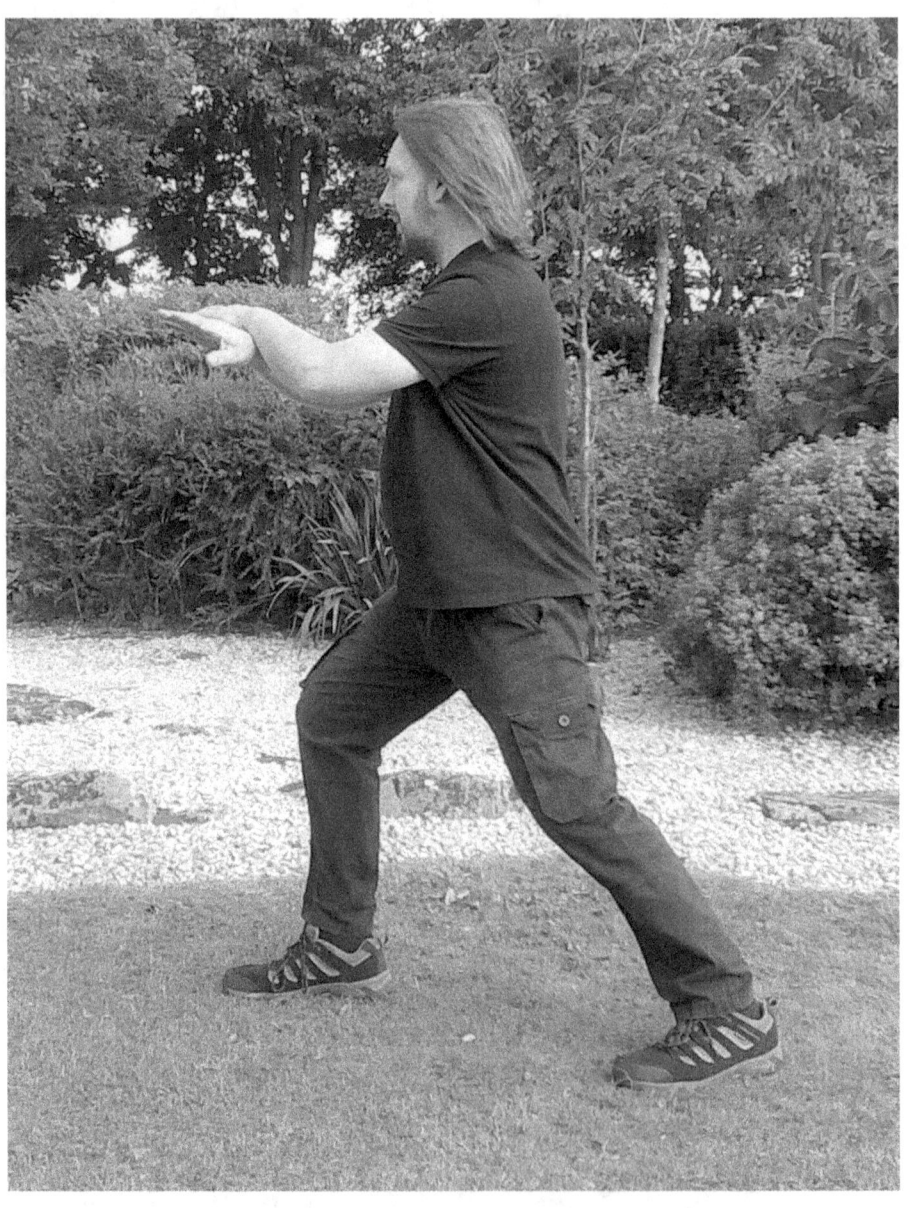

Separate both hands out to shoulder width, and at the same time move backwards, until you have seventy per cent of your weight in your left leg.

.

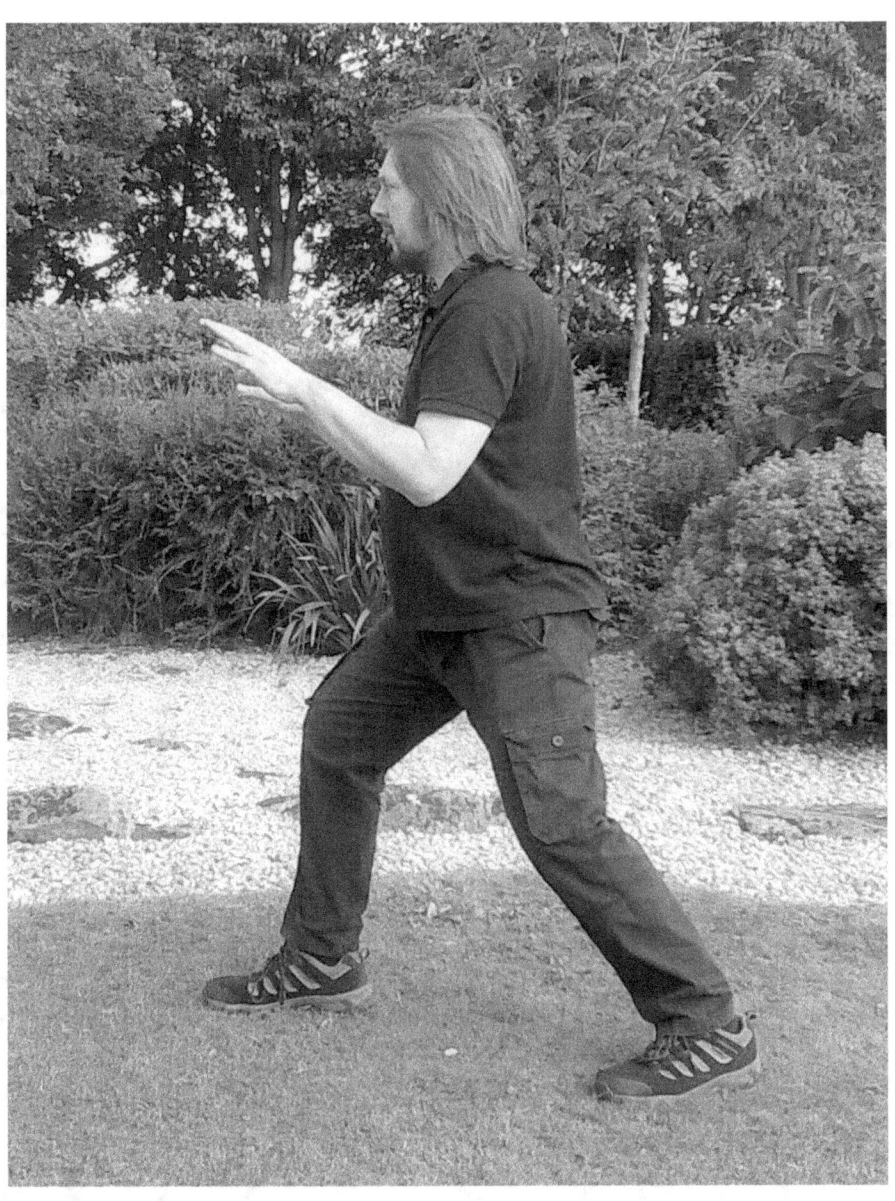

Push

Push forward, shifting into your right leg, the hands follow the movement of your body. As you push forwards, both hands rise up slightly in front of your shoulders.

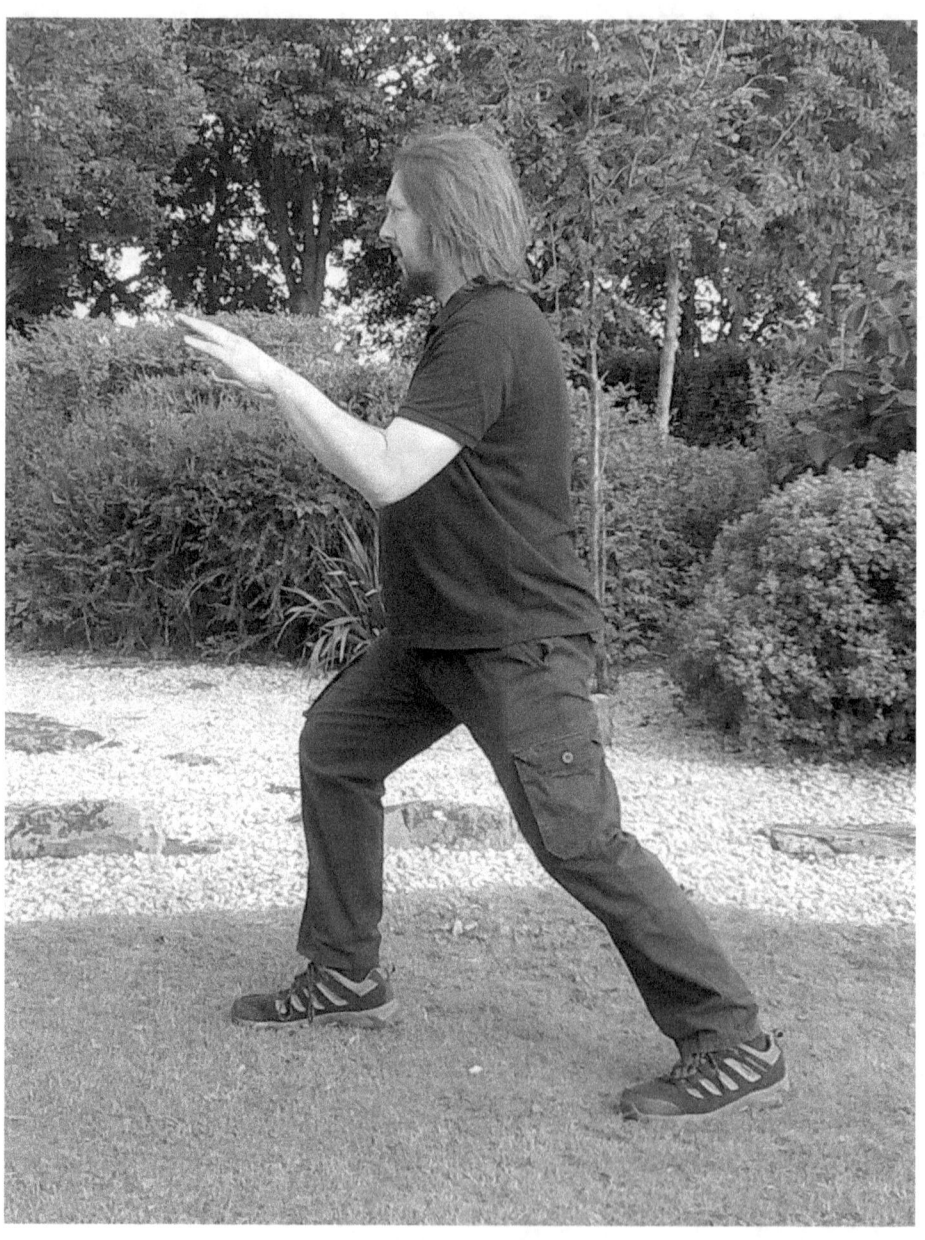

30) Single Whip

Shift your weight back into your left foot.

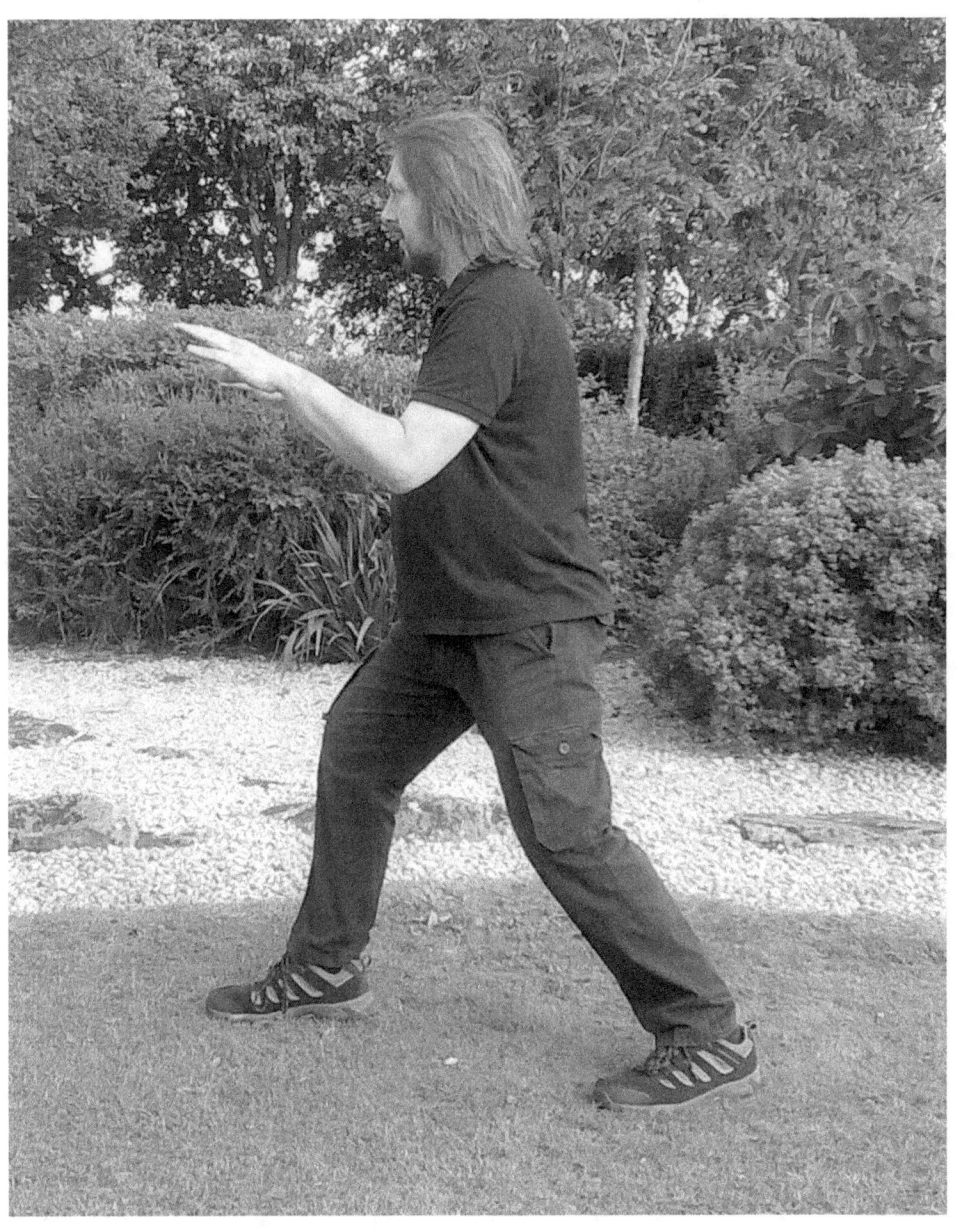

Lift the toes of your right foot and turn to your back left corner, your right leg follows the body's turning by pivoting on the heel. Your hands remain in front of your shoulders.

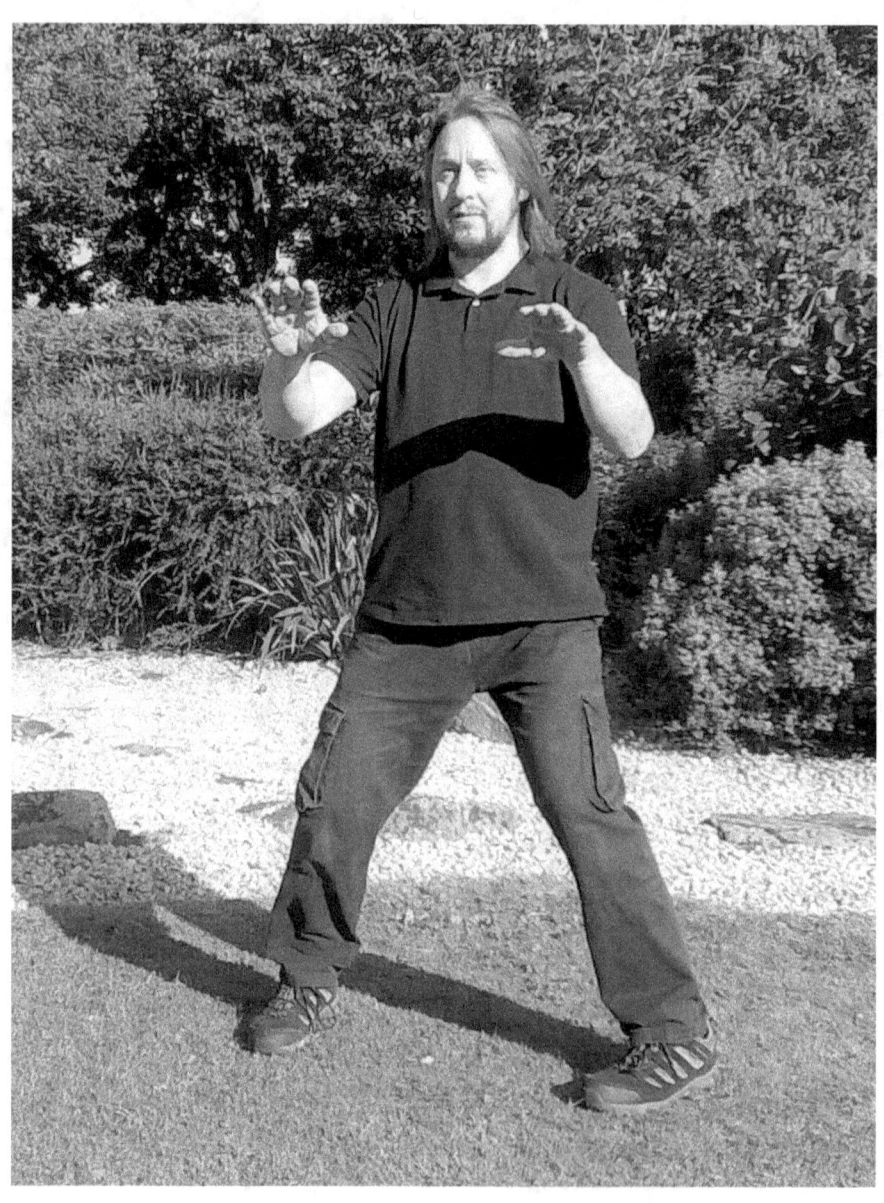

Hold a ball with the right hand on top and the left hand on the bottom.

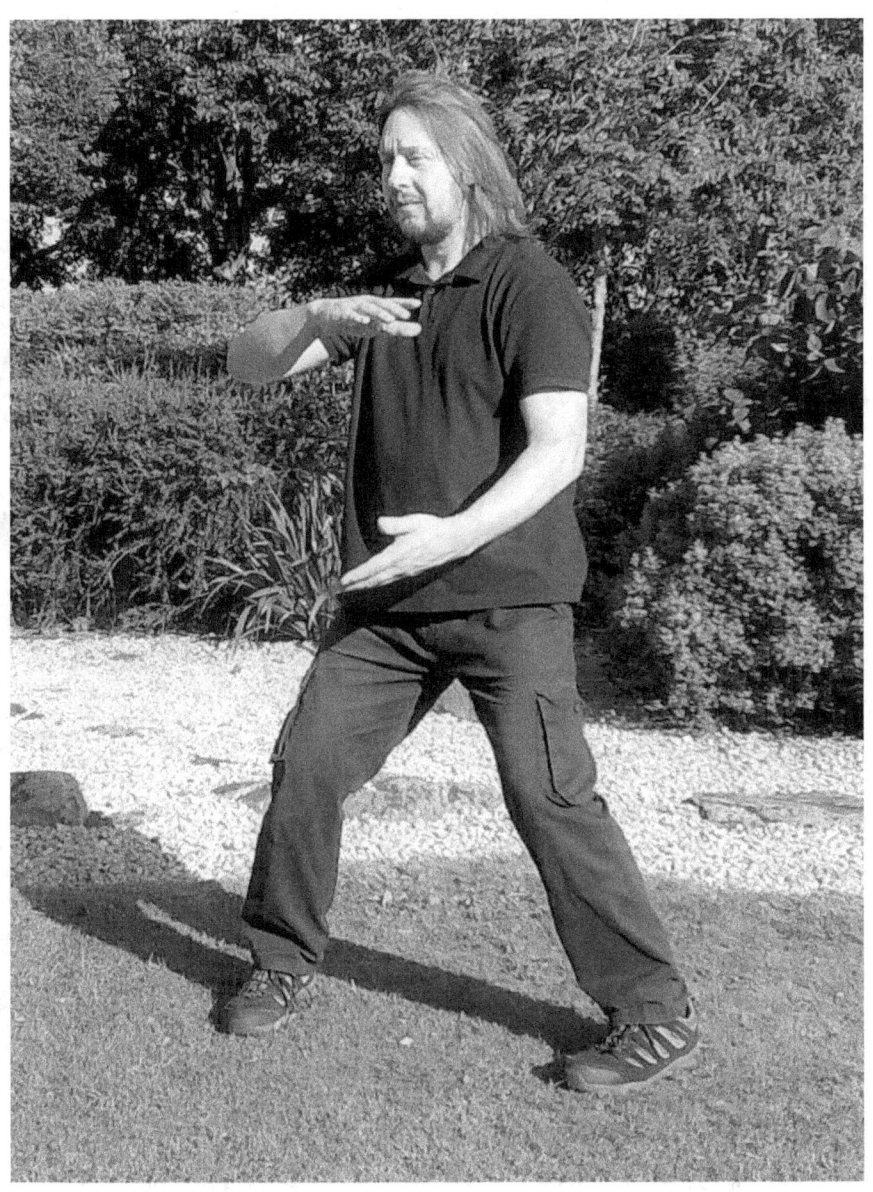

Push your right hand out until the arm is straight (but not locked out). At the same time bend your right wrist until the thumb points down, and place your fingertips around the tip of the thumb to form a beak.

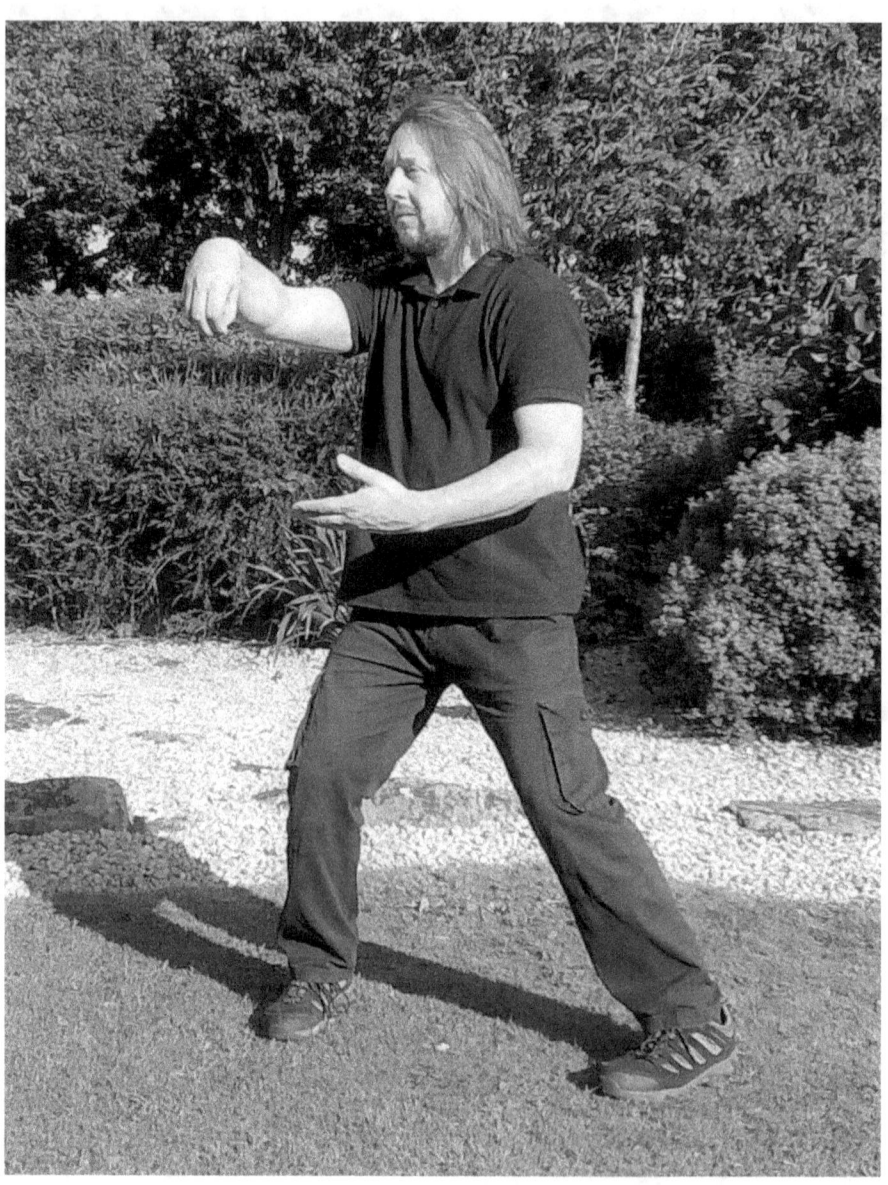

Turn back towards the left, your weight stays in the right leg. Lift up your left heel, pivot on the ball of the foot to the left and step forwards, place down your heel, and roll into a left footed Bow stance.

As you step your left hand rises in a Ward Off shape, curving up and across your body to your left side, finally rotate your palm until it faces away from you in front of your left shoulder.

Step forwards and diagonally to make a left footed Bow stance.

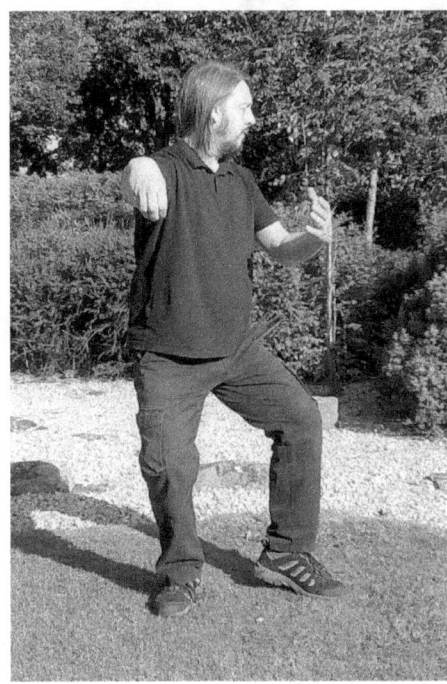 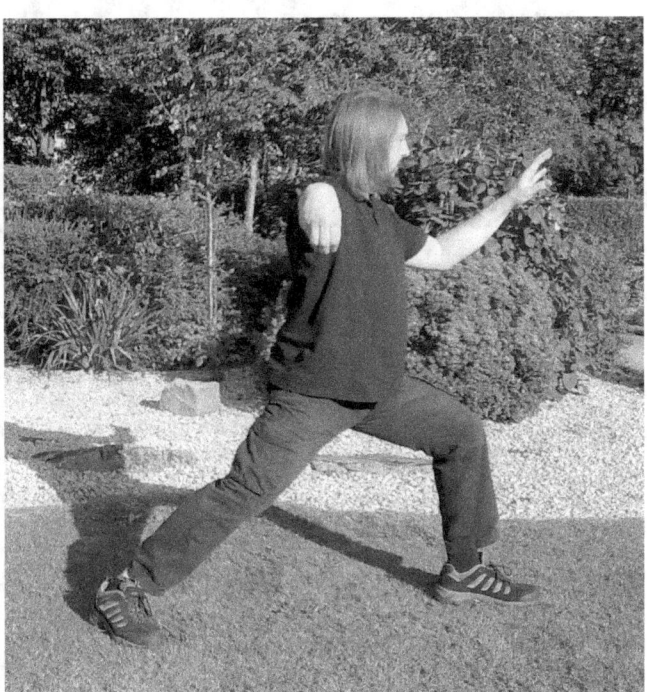

(To help you to get lower for Snake Creeps Down you can step back with your right foot to make a deeper stance)

31) Snake Creeps Down

Shift your weight back into your right foot, and turn your body to your right side. Pivot on your left heel and turn your toes to the right. Bring your left hand across to point the fingers at your right wrist.

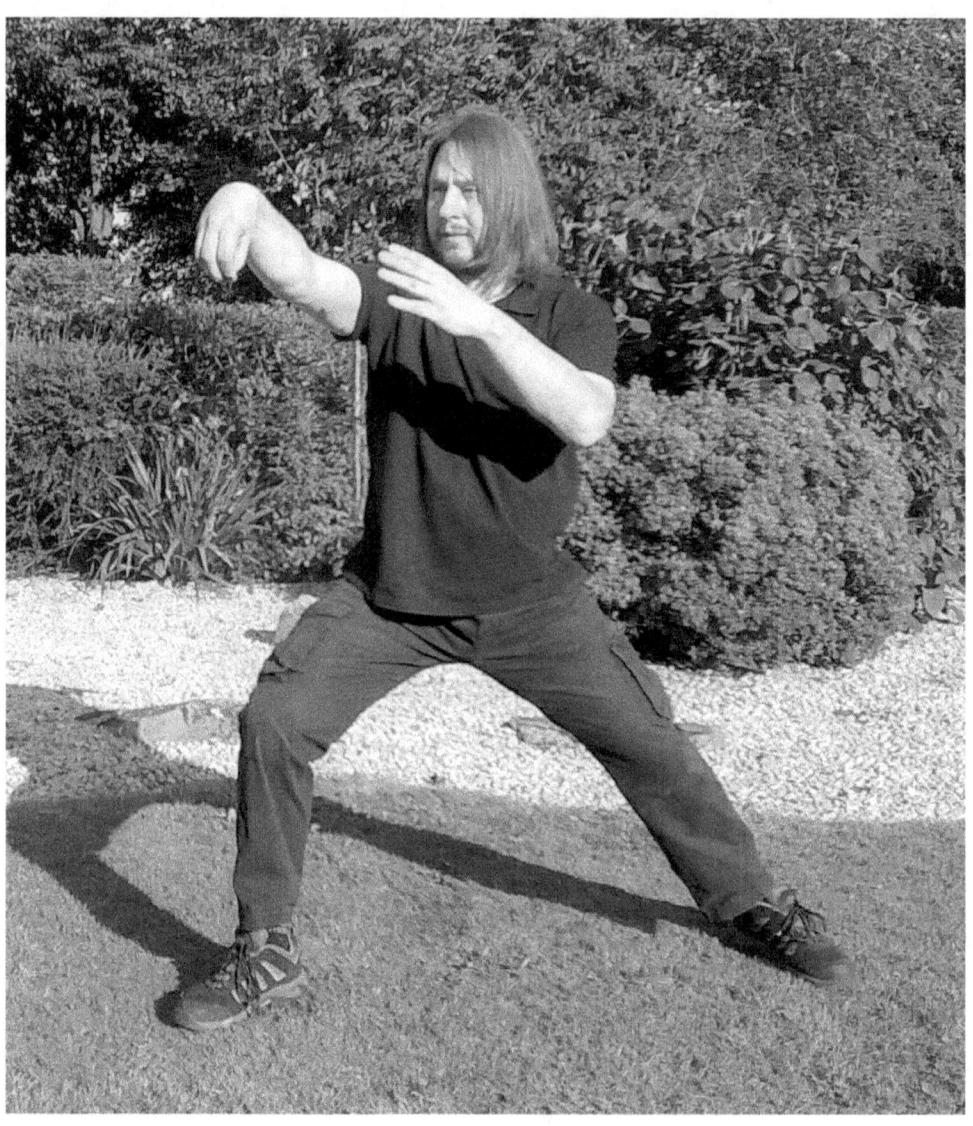

Sit down deeply on the right leg.

Turn the toes of your left foot back towards it's starting position and at the same time move your left hand down and forward to the inside of the left leg.

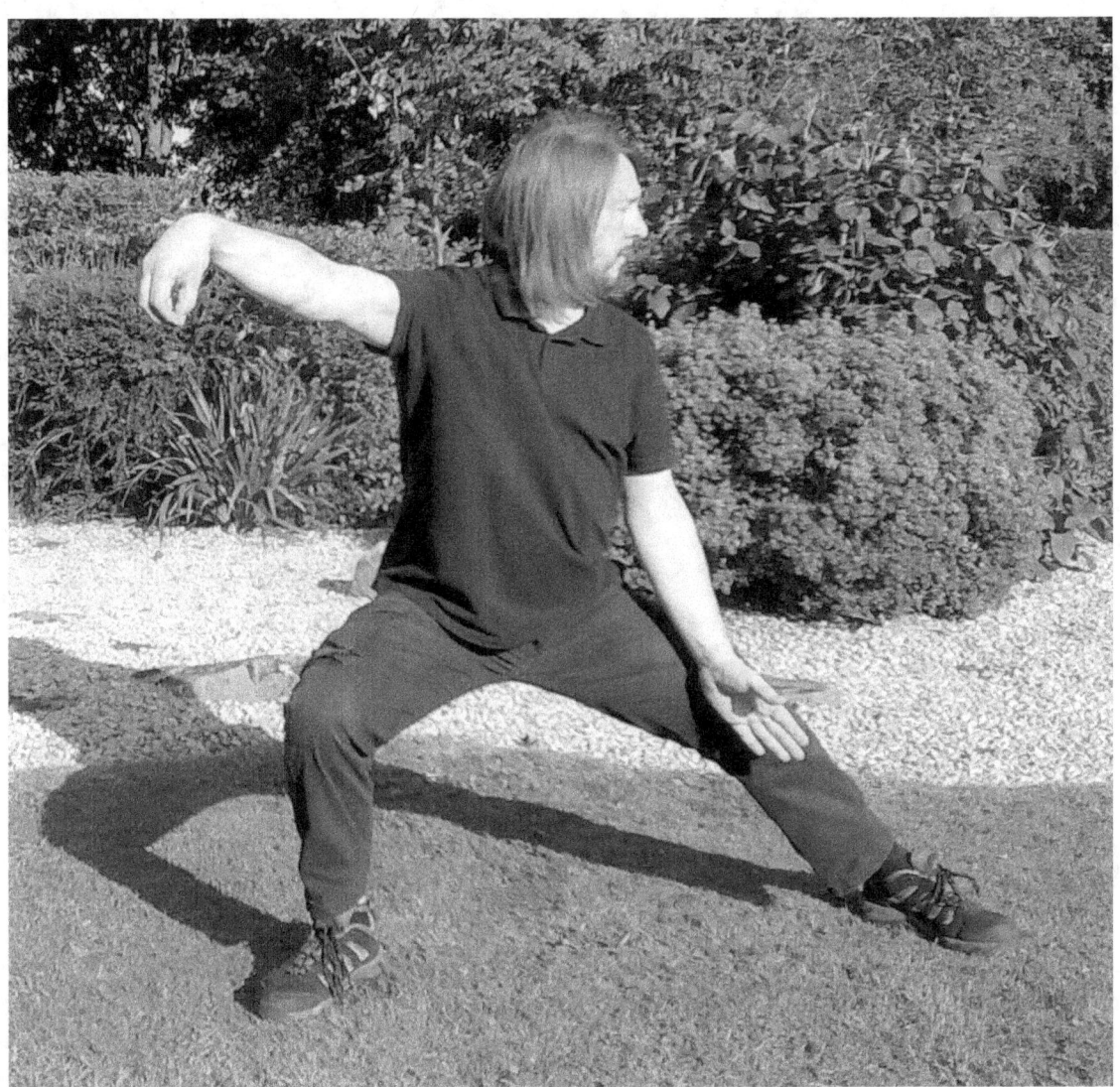

Start to move your bodyweight back into the left leg, as you do this the fingers of the left hand should point forward. Return your right toes back to their starting position, and make a fist with your left hand. At the same time, turn your right hand over, until the beaked fingers face backwards.

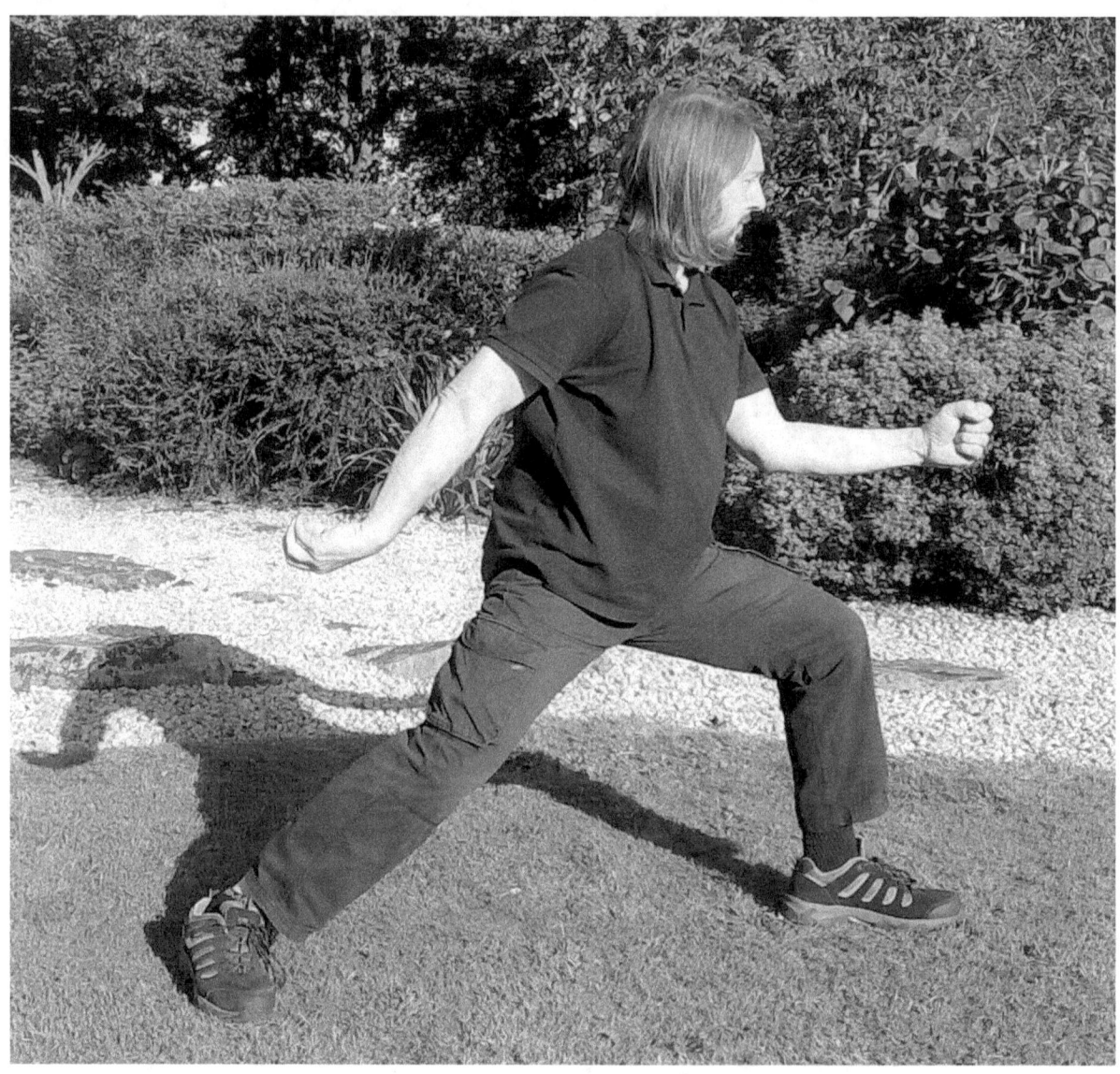

32) Step Up to Seven Stars

Lift your left fist up in front of your centreline and turn the left foot out to forty-five degrees.

As you bring the right hand forwards past your right hip, let go of the beak and make a relaxed fist.

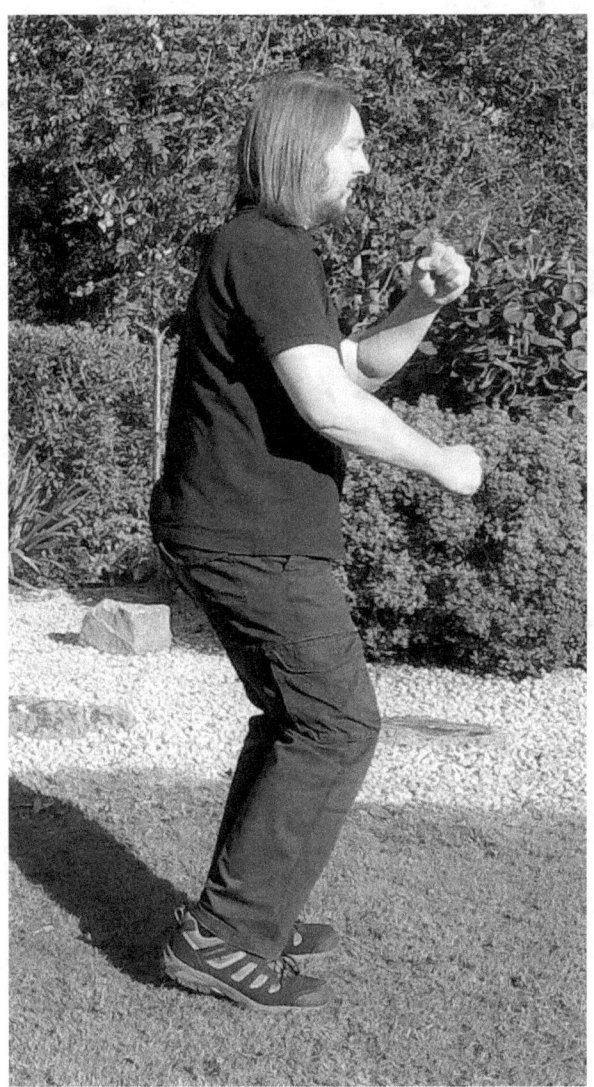

Rise up and put your full weight into the left leg, and then step through into a right heel up Cat stance.

At the same time as you step forwards with the right foot, bring your right hand up and across to the middle of your upper chest, and cross your wrists with the right hand on the outside. The backs of the hands face upwards, and your arms form a triangle shape.

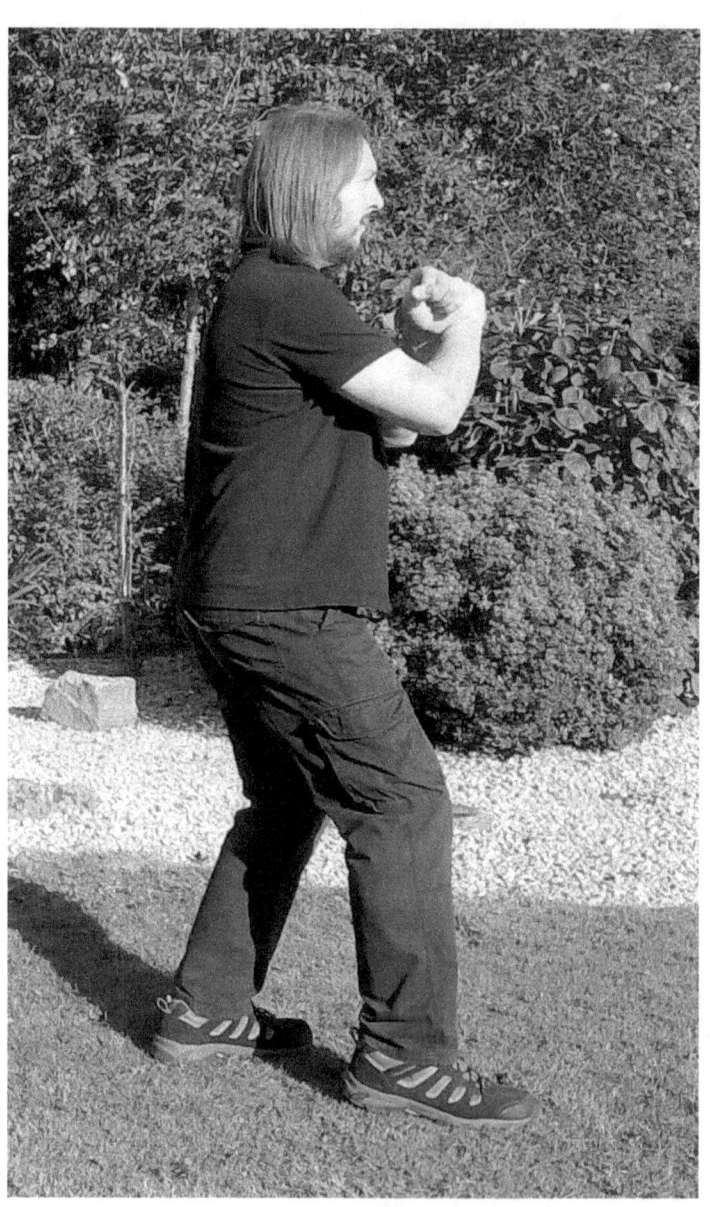

33) Retreat to Ride a Tiger

Step backwards with your right foot, shift it behind your left foot and place it down at a forty-five degree angle. Straighten your left foot and lift the heel to make a Cat stance.

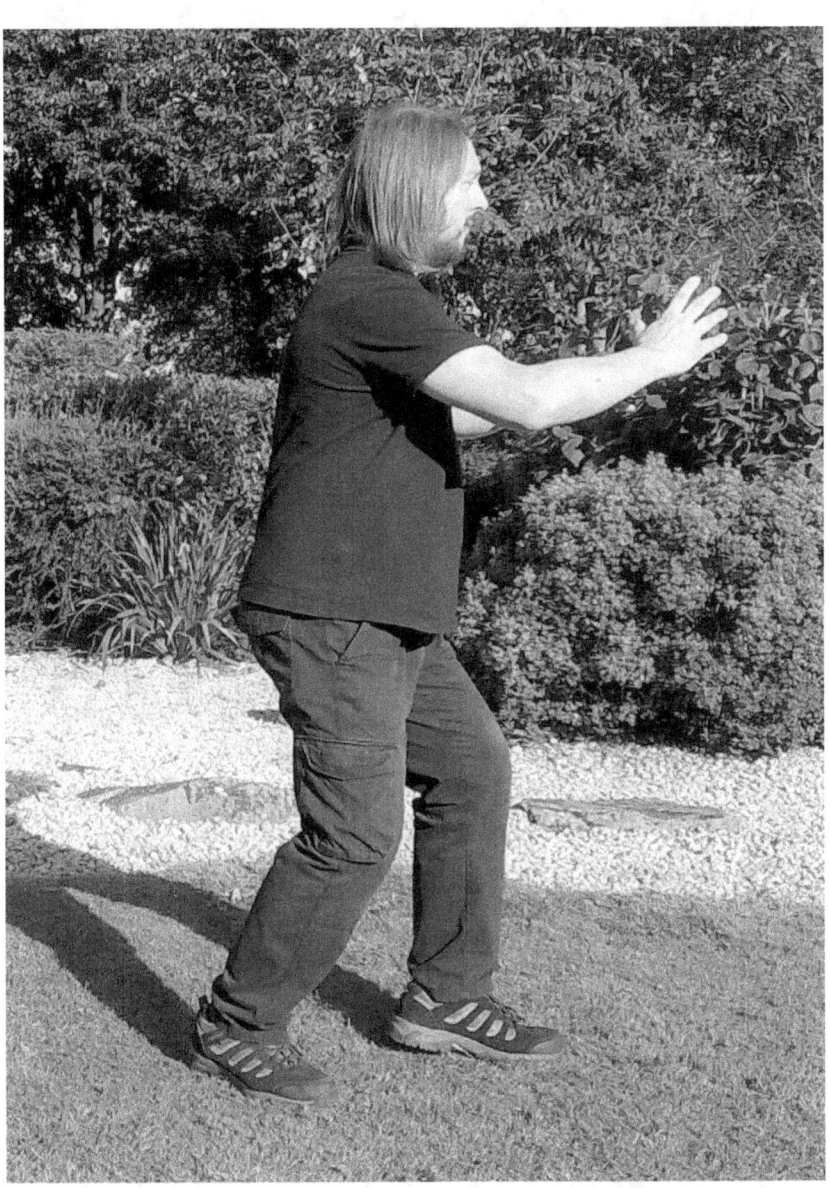

At the same time open up your hands and separate them, your right hand moves out to your right side, and the left arm sweeps down and out, past the front left side of your body.

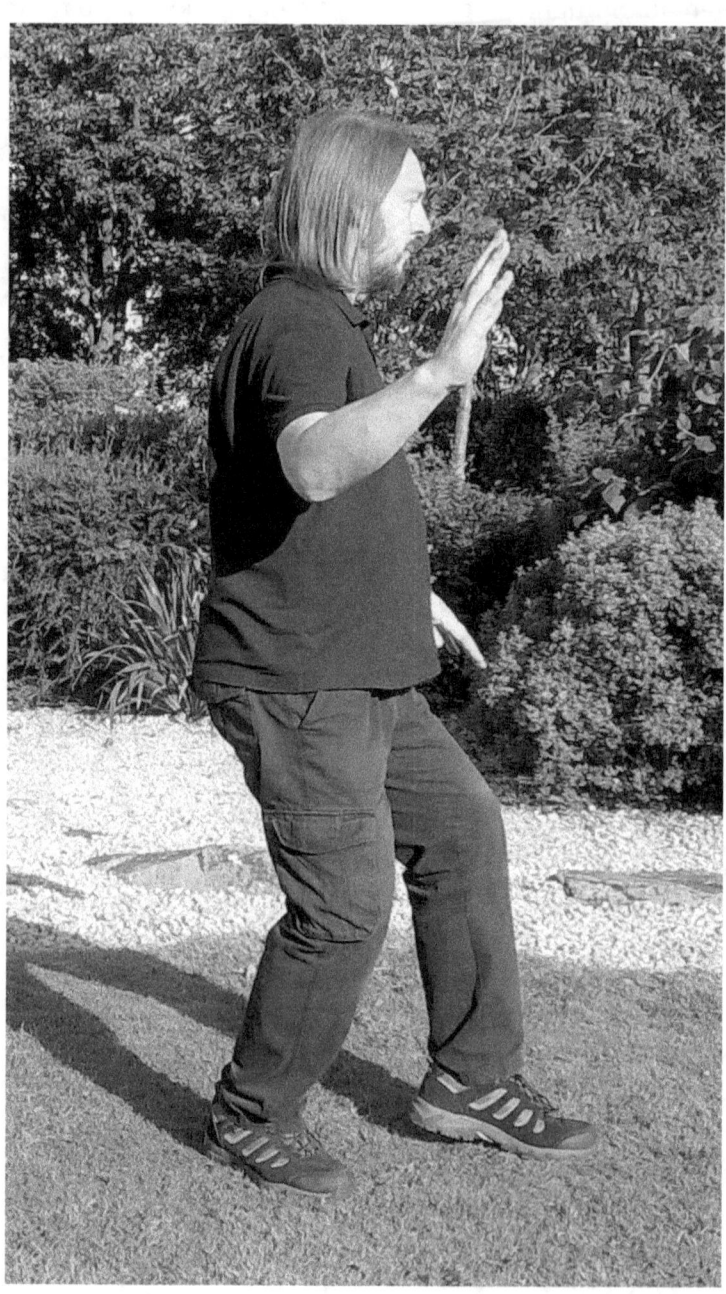

34) Turn and Sweep Lotus with Leg

Bring both arms in and lift them up in front of your shoulders.

Turn your body to the left, this helps you to wind up, unwind your body to your right side, and spin around on your right heel three hundred and sixty degrees.

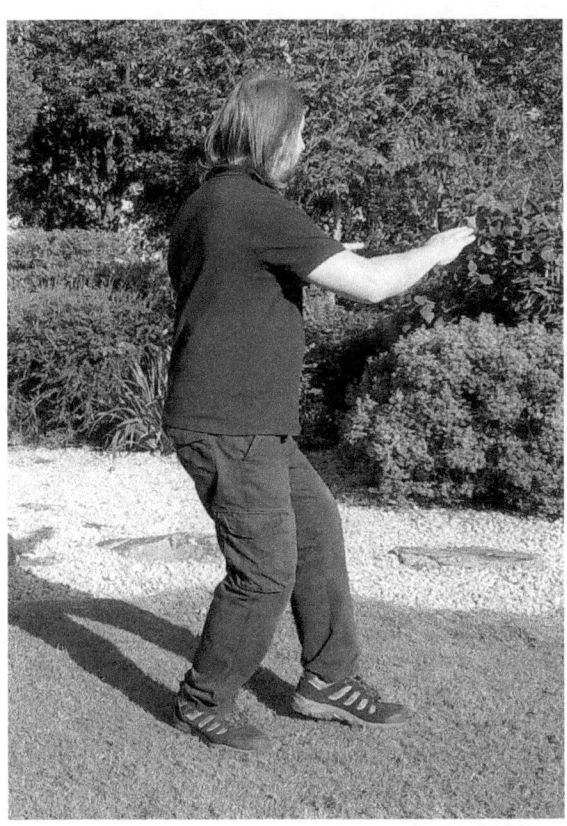 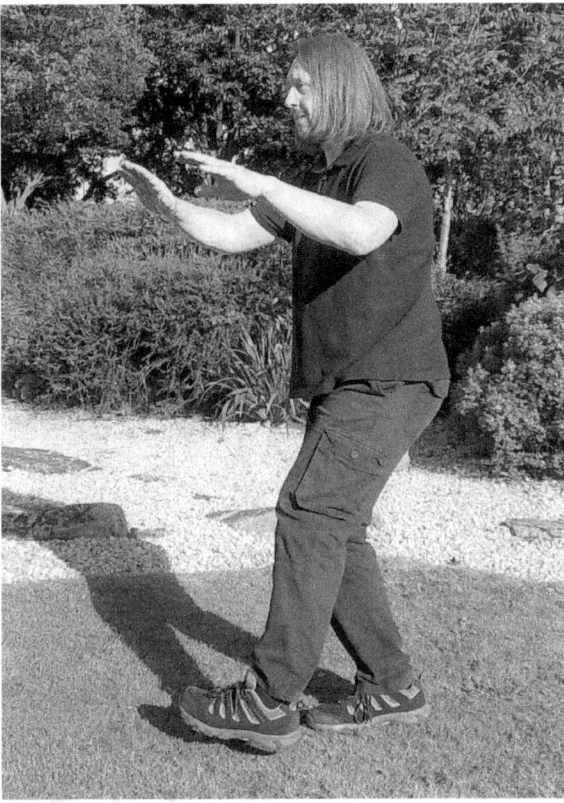

When you are three quarters of the way through the spin, put your left foot on the floor, heel down first. Move your weight into it, and lift up your right heel.

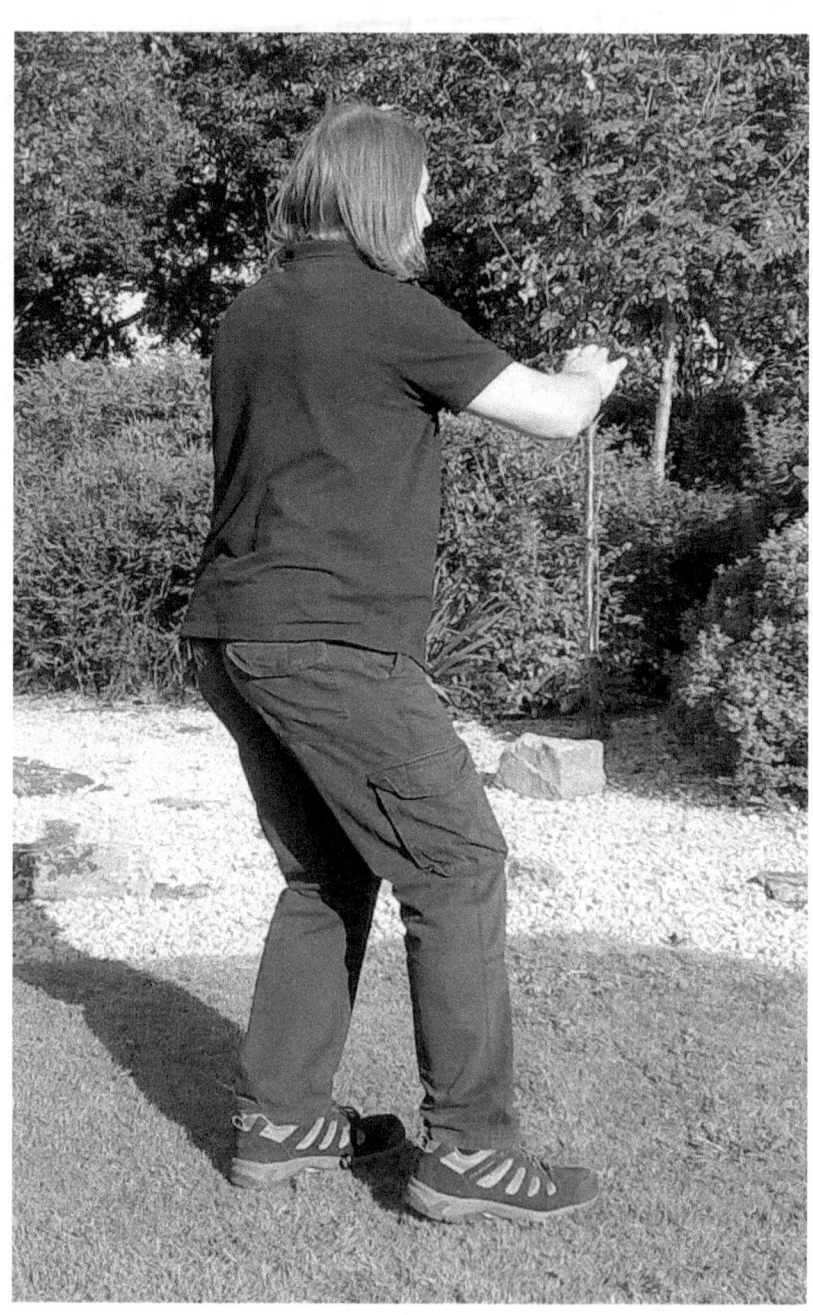

You are now in a left footed one hundred percent back weighted Cat stance, with the right toes on the floor.

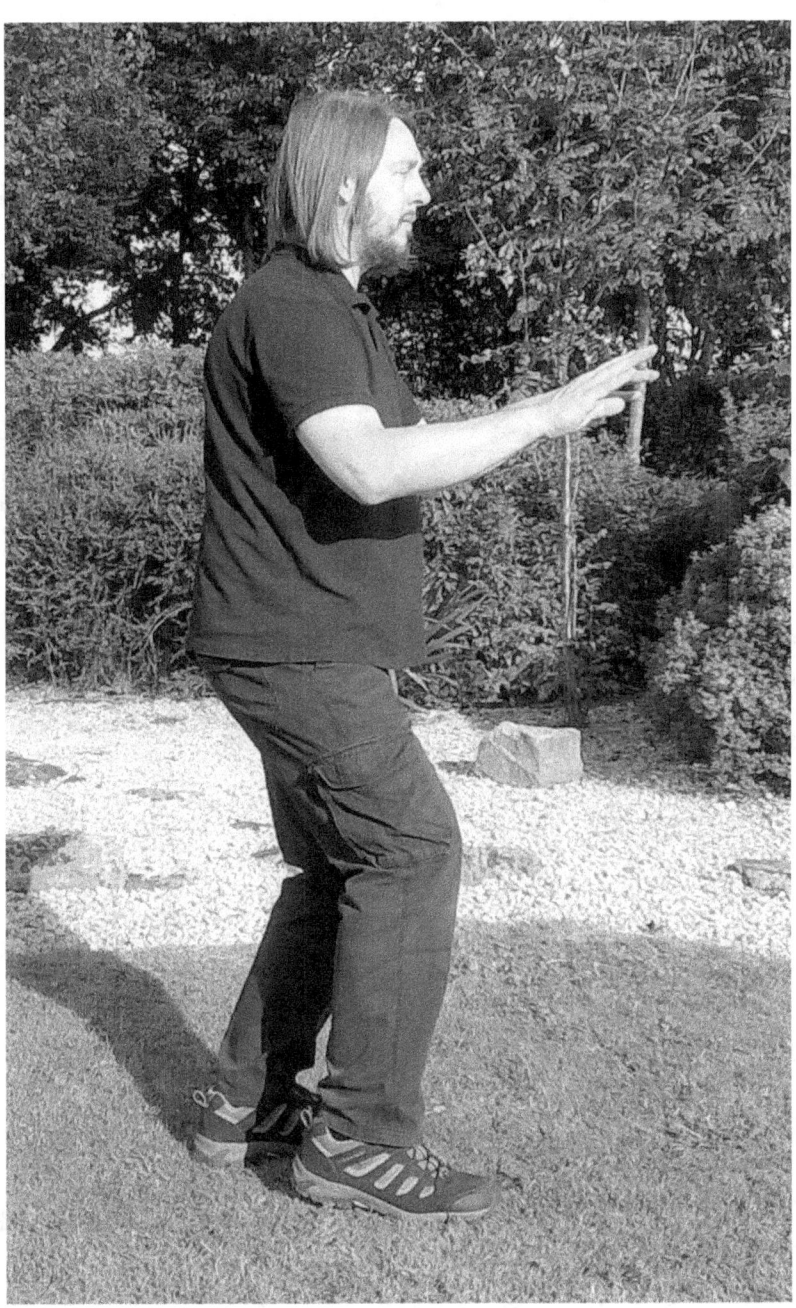

Your hands remain in front of your upper chest. Sit down on your left leg and make a circular left to right kick with your right foot, the toes of the right foot point upward.

As you kick, touch the fingertips of both hands lightly, with the upright toes of your right foot.

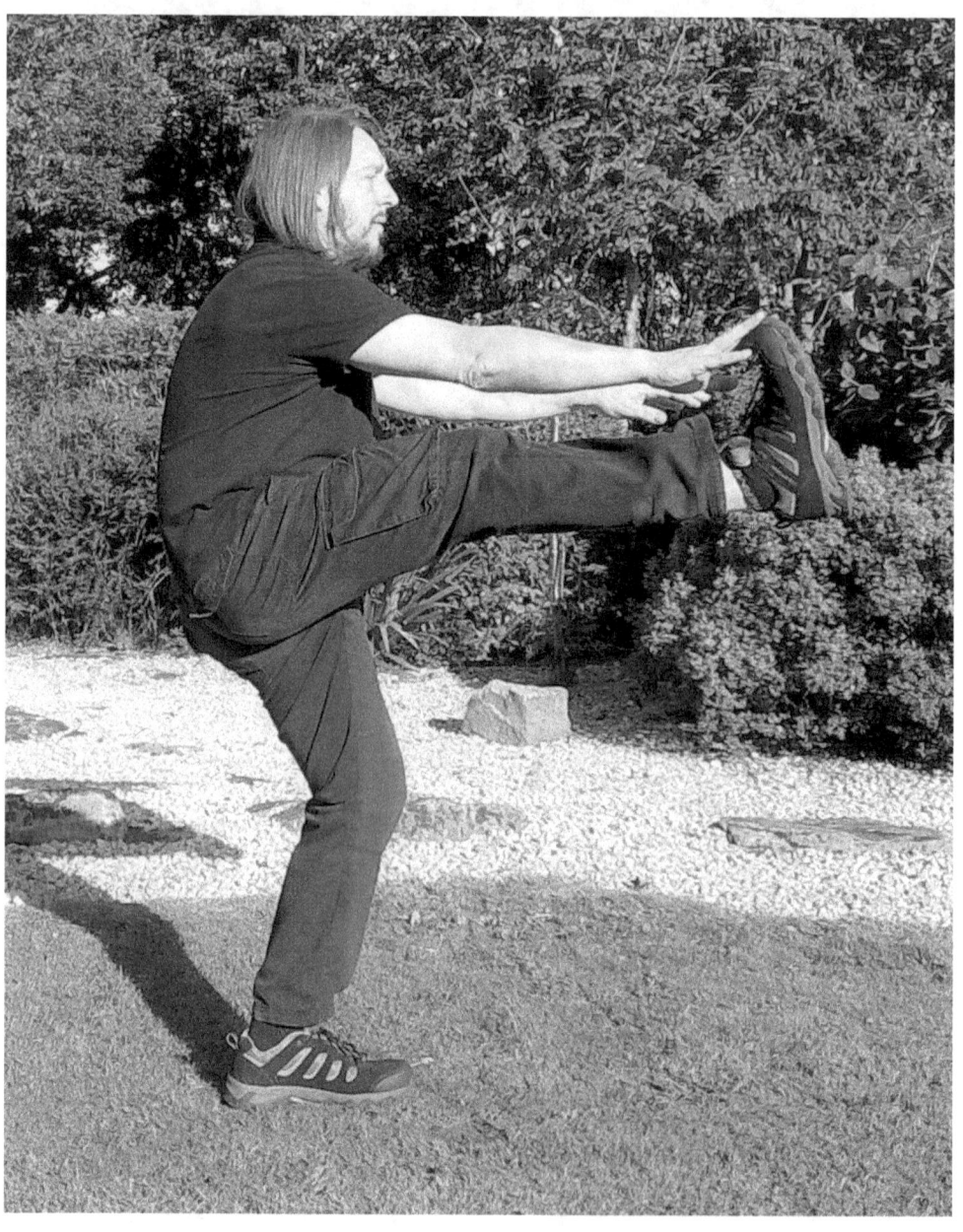

35) Bend Bow to Shoot the Tiger

Turn your body to face your left corner, make loose fists, and place them in front of your lower Dantien palms facing upwards.

Step into a right forward Bow stance.

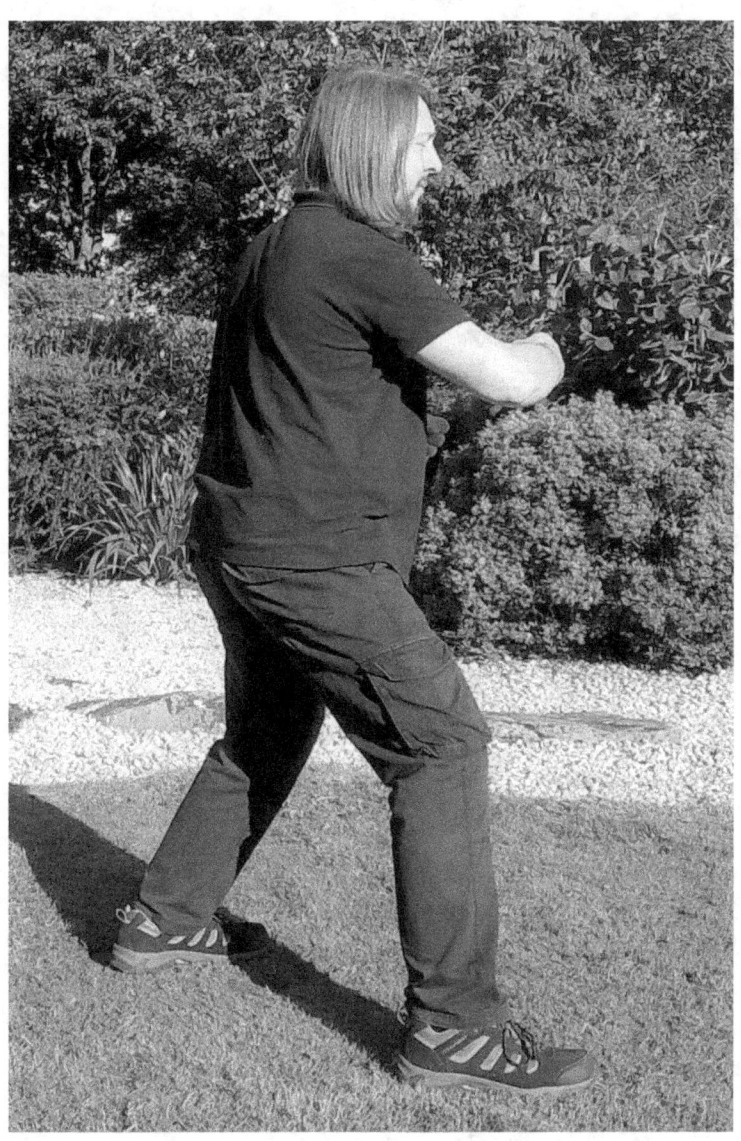

Your right hand rises up and across, past the right outside edge of your forehead. As the hand rises, it rotates until the fingers turn outward.

At the same time, the left hand punches forward and up, the movement ends at the height of your upper chest. As you punch, your hand rotates so that the thumb side of the hand faces upward.

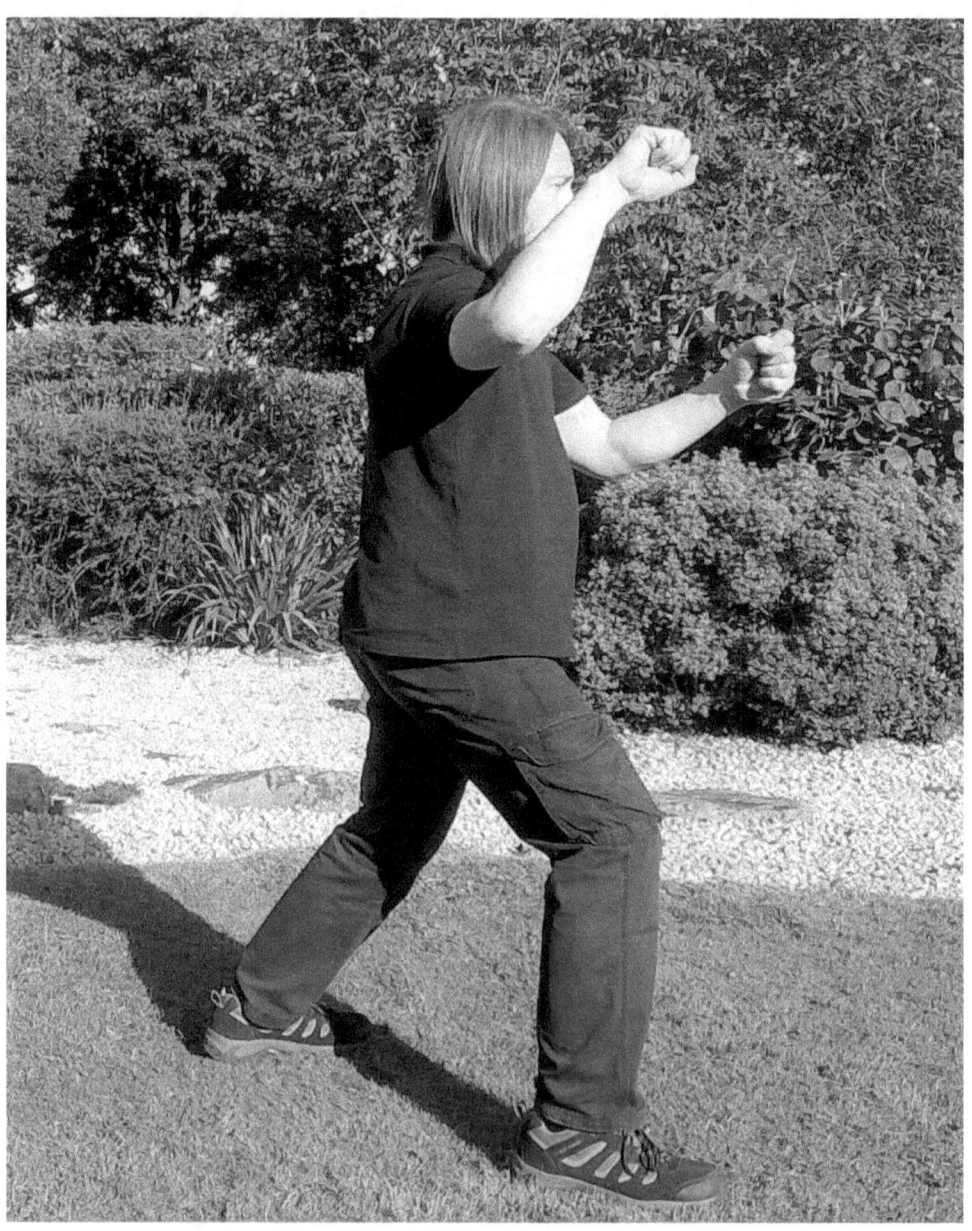

36) Deflect Parry and Punch

Turn your body slightly to your left side and then turn to your right corner, your hands follow the movement of the body in a deflecting and parrying movement. The left hand follows your right hand, as if an invisible chord connects them.

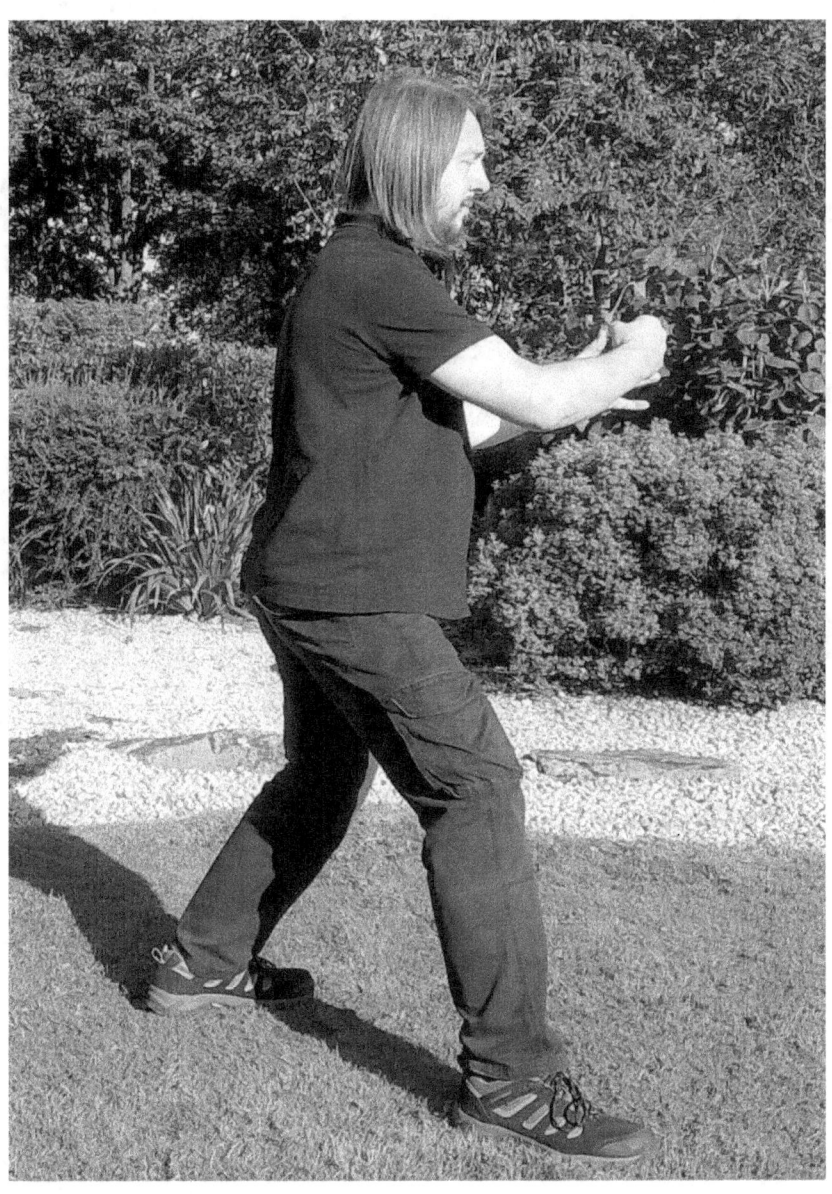

Move your right fist to the side of the right hip, with the thumb facing upwards. Your left hand follows the right fist to stop halfway across the body, palm down in front of the centreline.

Roll your right foot down, shift your weight fully into the right leg, and then step forward into a left Bow stance. At the same time, punch the right hand forwards and upwards, underneath the palm of your left hand.

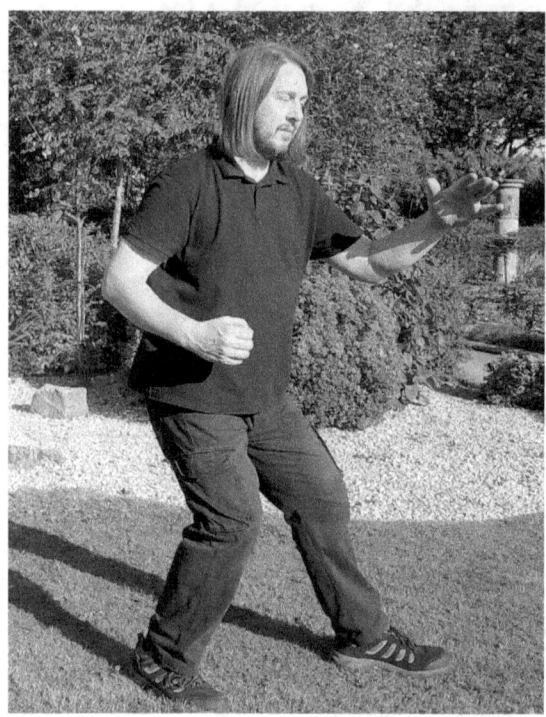
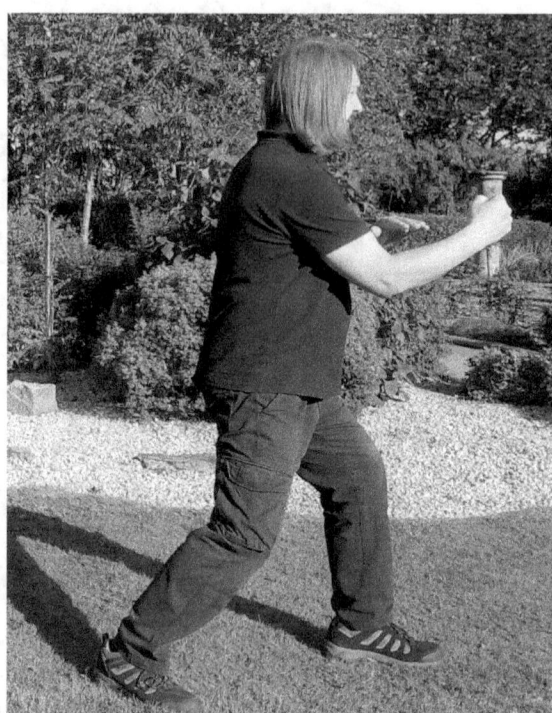

When the punch is completed, rotate your left hand until your palm faces upwards, and move it underneath your right elbow,

Shift smoothly backwards into the right foot, making a seventy percent back weighted Bow stance. Bring the left hand forward so that both arms cross at the wrists in front of your chest, with the left hand on the outside of the right hand.

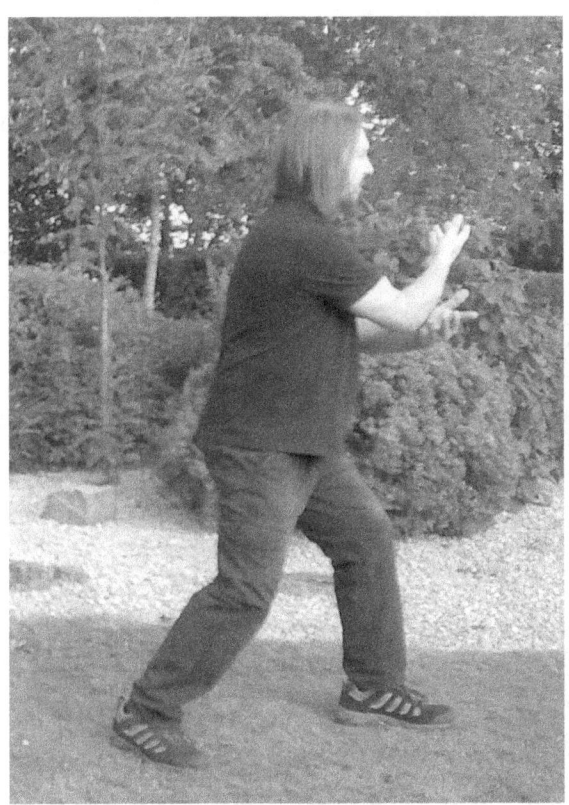 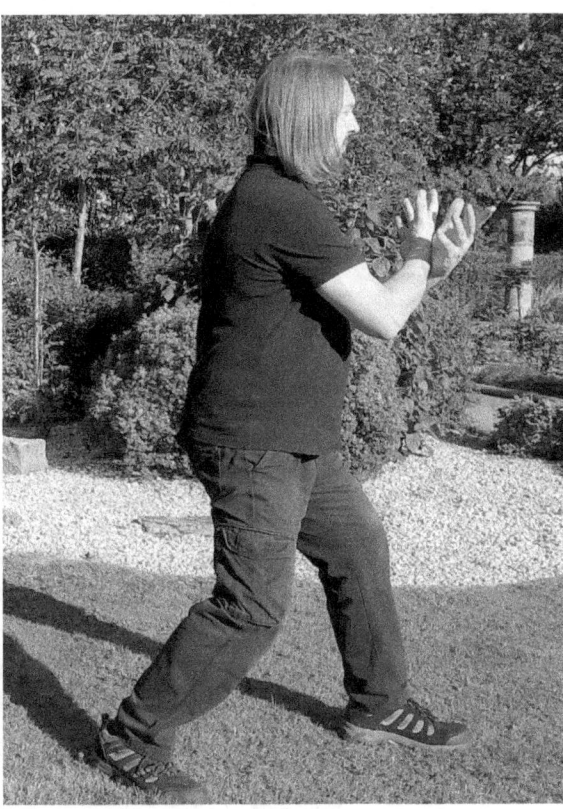

Push

Separate both hands to shoulder width, with your fingertips pointing forward, and shift backwards into your right leg.

Move forward again from your right leg into a left leg forward, seventy percent weighted Bow stance, at the same time your hands follow the movement of your body, rising up two inches as they push forward.

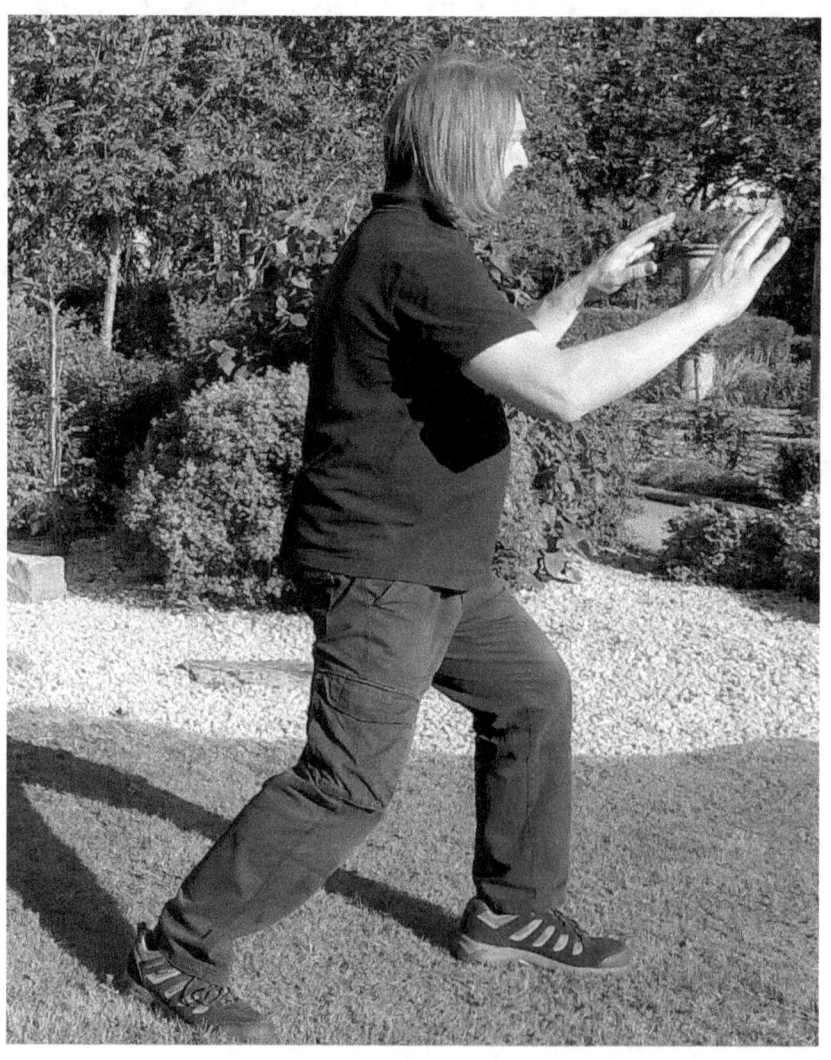

37) Seal the Knot

Shift your weight into the right foot, and lift up the toes of your left foot. Turn your body to your right side, your left leg follows by pivoting on the heel.

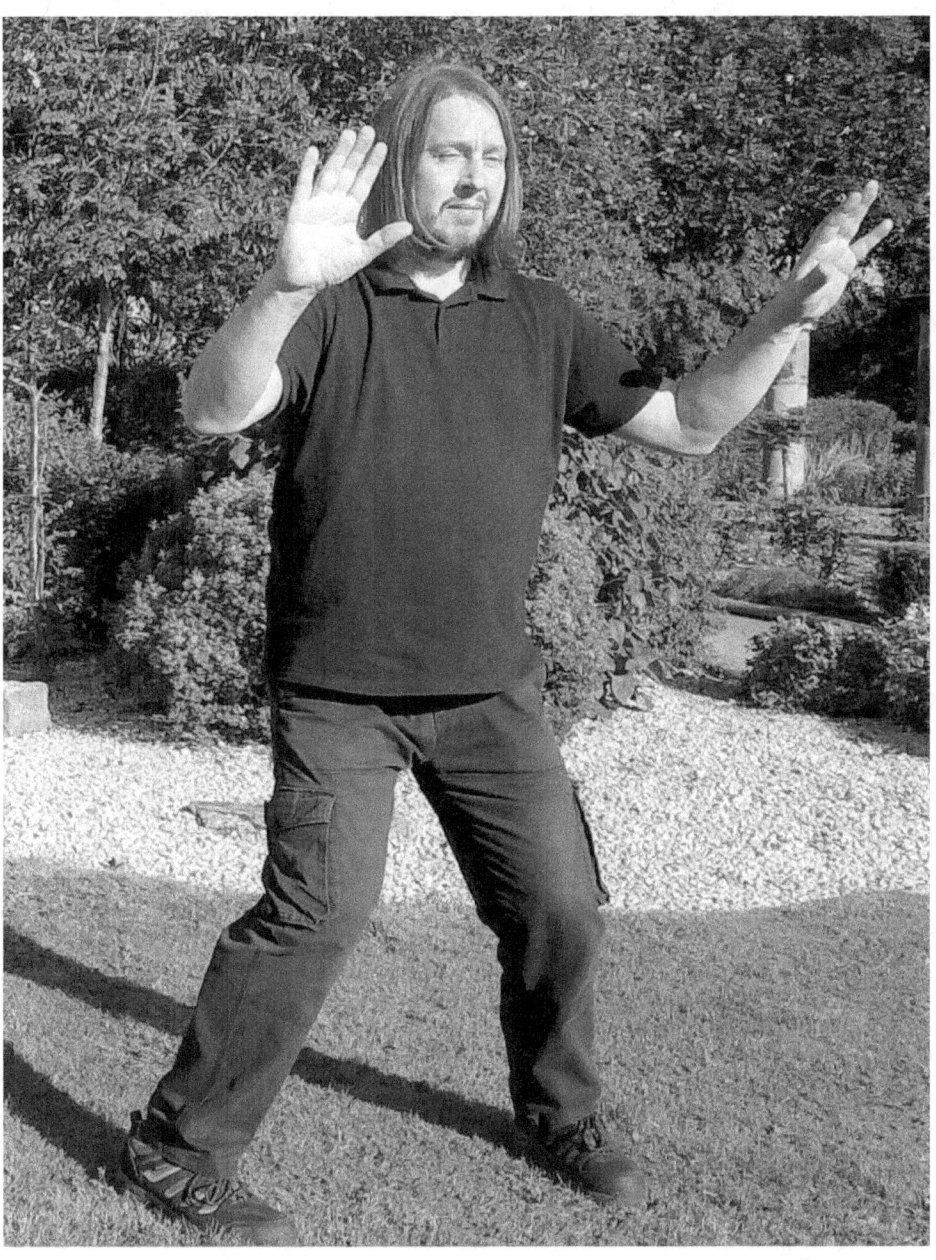

Shift the weight fully into the left foot.

Step with your right foot into a parallel shoulder width stance, with equal weight in each foot.

Circle both arms down and then bring them both back up in front of your centreline.

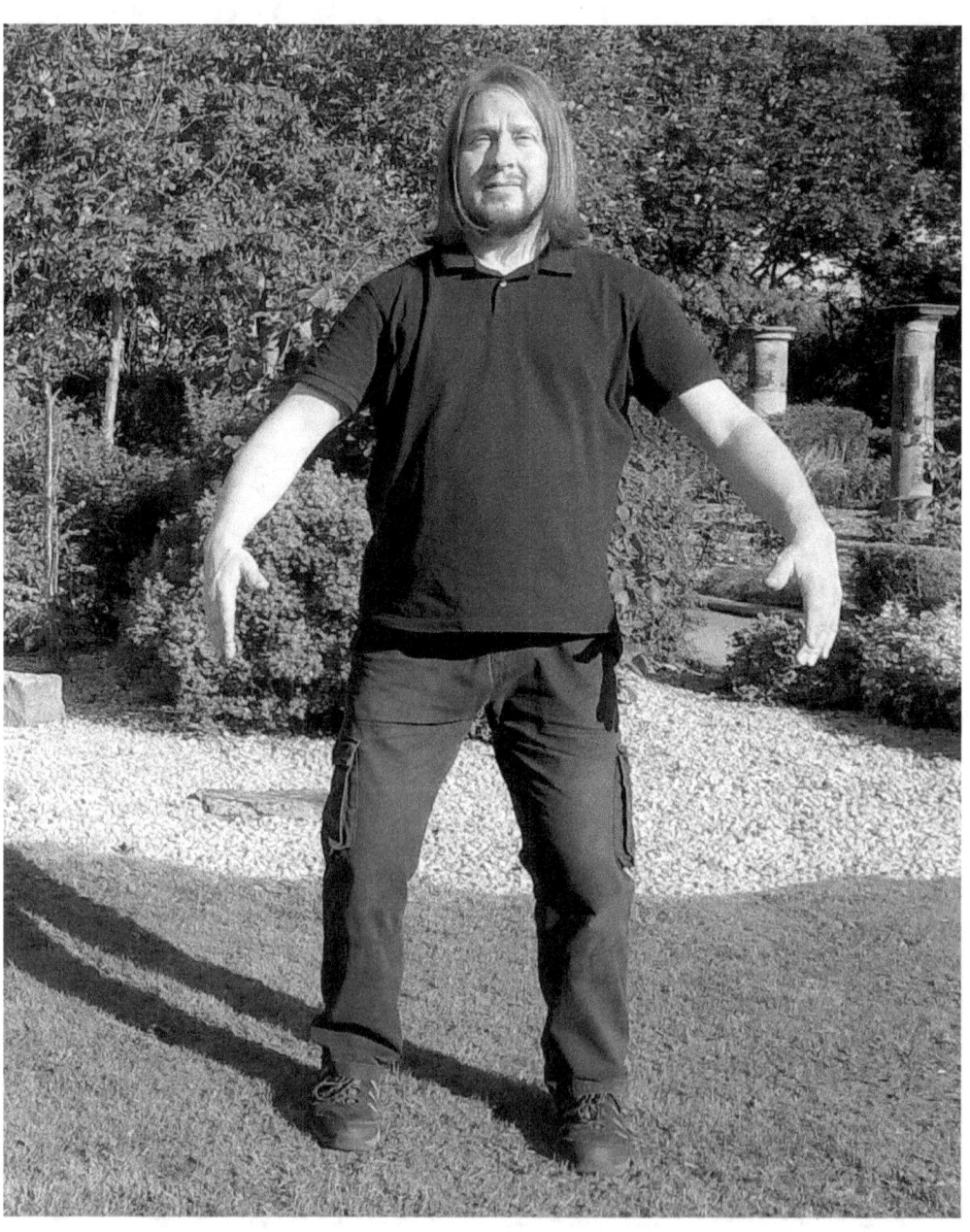

Cross your arms at the wrists, forming a triangle in front of the upper chest. The right wrist should be on the outside of the left wrist.

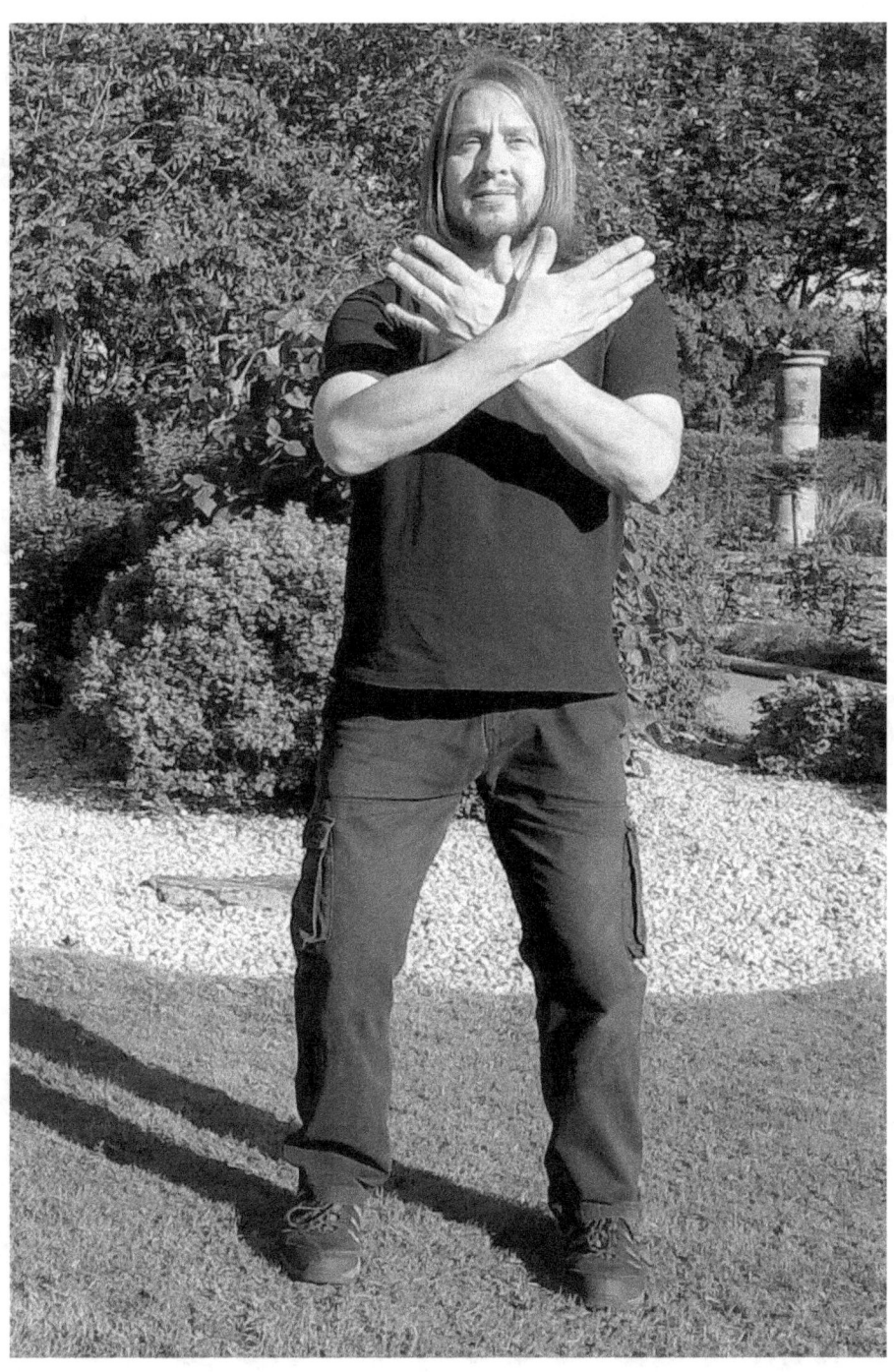

Turn your palms to face the ground, separate your hands, and slowly lower them down to your sides.

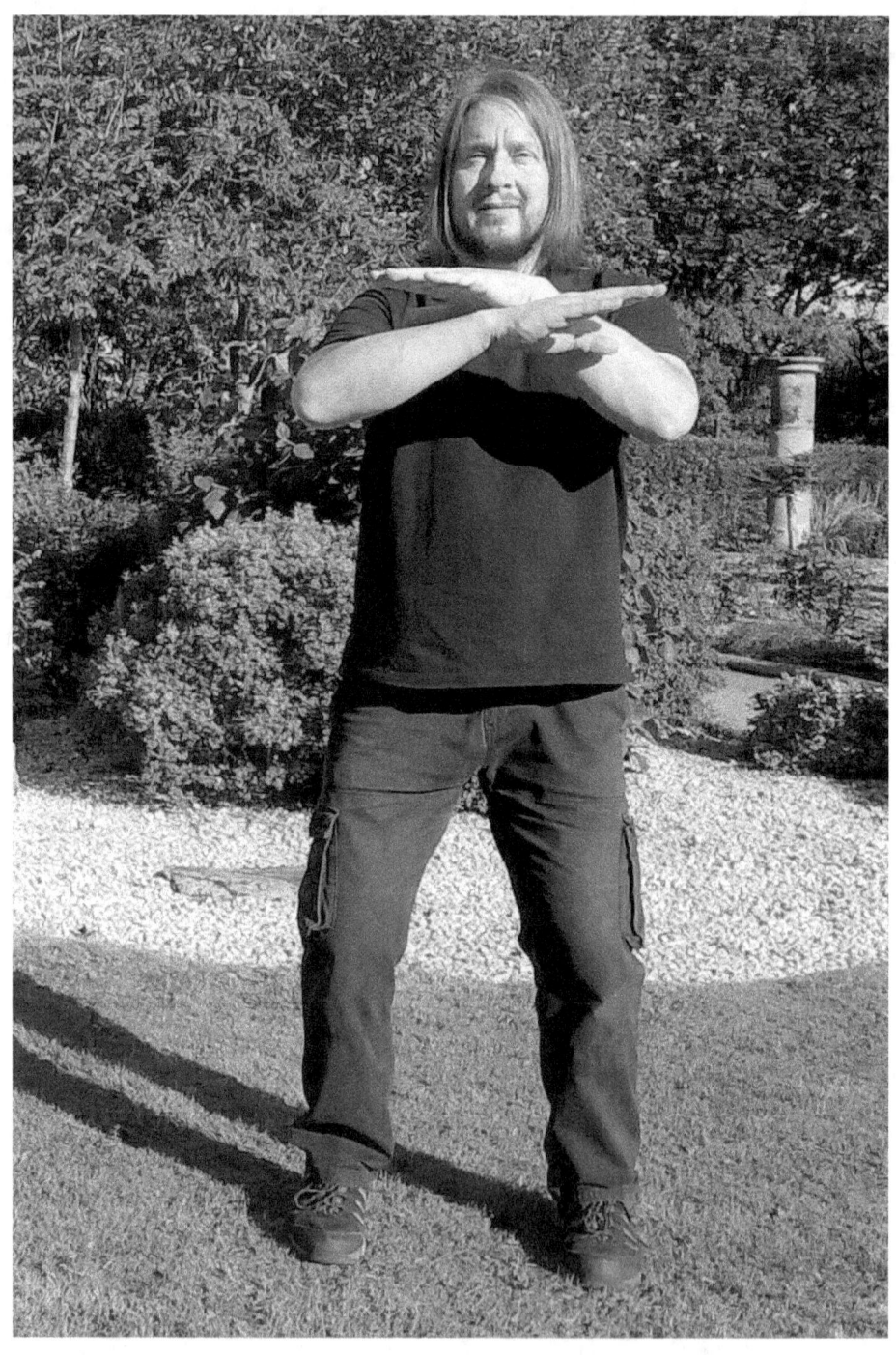

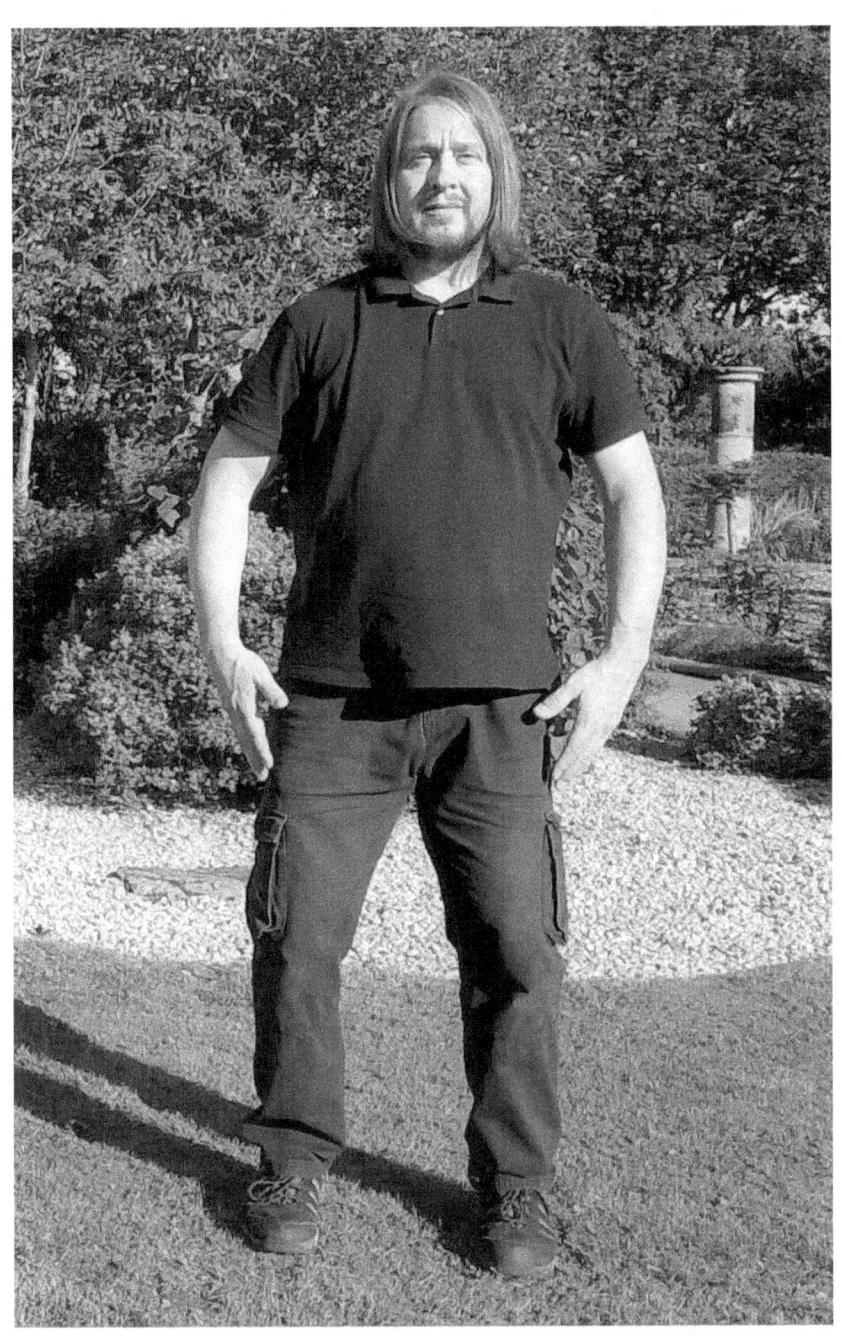

Step back in with your left foot and place your feet together, with your arms by your sides and your hands touching the corners of your thighs.

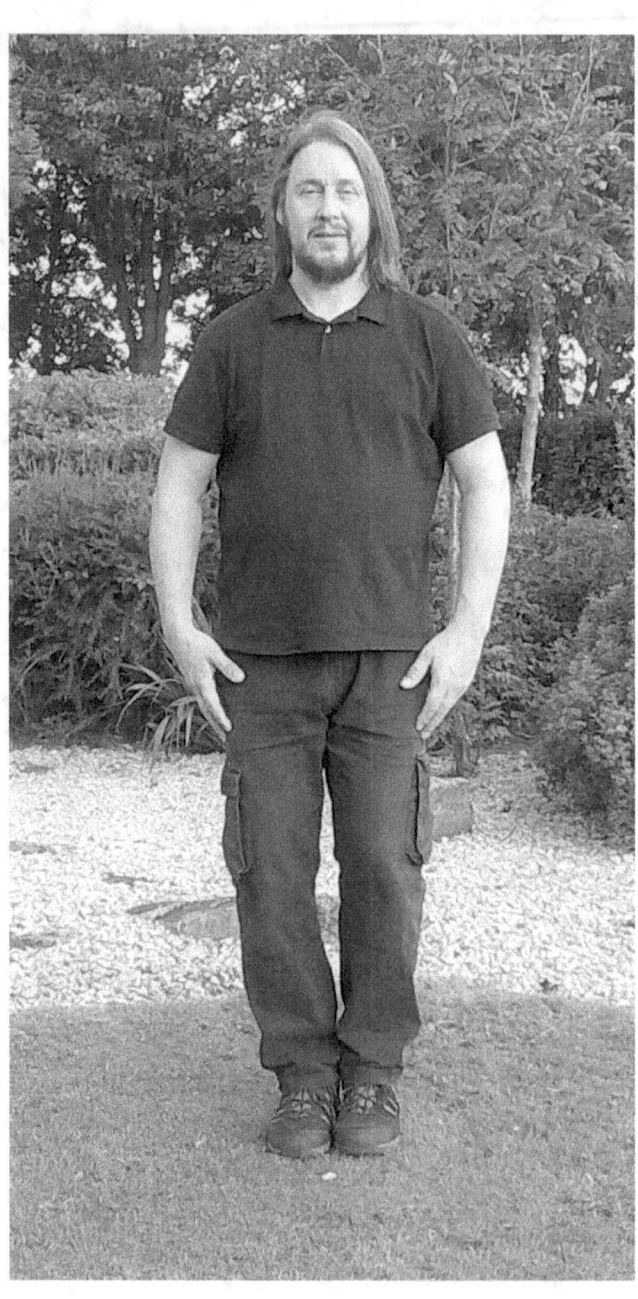

For more information, visit...

WWW.RichMorleyTaiChi.Com

Edited by Pancho B Gubbins Esq

Photography by Raffles

©Richard Morley 2016

www.ingramcontent.com/pod-product-compliance
Lightning Source LLC
Chambersburg PA
CBHW051944280526
45789CB00009B/3162